DATE DUE		
JUN 1 4 1994			
FEB 2 2 1999			
NOV 0 2 1999			
0 4 OCT 2002			
JUN 2 2 2003			
1 0 JUL 2003			

1987
YEAR BOOK OF
UROLOGY®

The 1987 Year Book Series

Anesthesia: Drs. Miller, Kirby, Ostheimer, Roizen, and Stoelting

Cancer: Drs. Hickey, Saunders, Clark, and Cumley

Cardiology: Drs. Schlant, Collins, Engle, Frye, Gifford, and O'Rourke

Critical Care Medicine: Drs. Rogers, Allo, Dean, Gioia, McPherson, Michael, Miller, and Traystman

Dentistry: Drs. Cohen, Hendler, Johnson, Jordan, Moyers, Robinson, and Silverman

Dermatology: Drs. Sober and Fitzpatrick

Diagnostic Radiology: Drs. Bragg, Keats, Kieffer, Kirkpatrick, Koehler, Miller, and Sorenson

Digestive Diseases: Drs. Greenberger and Moody

Drug Therapy: Drs. Hollister and Lasagna

Emergency Medicine: Dr. Wagner

Endocrinology: Drs. Bagdade, Ryan, Molitch, Braverman, Robertson, Halter, Kornel, Horton, Korenman, Morley, Rogol, Burger, and Metz

Family Practice: Drs. Rakel, Couchman, Driscoll, Avant, and Prichard

Hand Surgery: Drs. Dobyns, Chase, and Amadio

Hematology: Drs. Spivak, Bell, Ness, Quesenberry, and Wiernik

Infectious Diseases: Drs. Wolff, Tally, Keusch, Klempner, and Snydman

Medicine: Drs. Rogers, Des Prez, Cline, Braunwald, Greenberger, Wilson, Epstein, and Malawista

Neurology and Neurosurgery: Drs. DeJong, Currier, and Crowell

Nuclear Medicine: Drs. Hoffer, Gore, Gottschalk, Sostman, and Zaret

Obstetrics and Gynecology: Drs. Mishell, Kirschbaum, and Morrow

Ophthalmology: Drs. Ernest and Deutsch

Orthopedics: Dr. Coventry

Otolaryngology–Head and Neck Surgery: Drs. Paparella and Bailey

Pathology and Clinical Pathology: Drs. Brinkhous, Dalldorf, Grisham, Langdell, and McLendon

Pediatrics: Drs. Oski and Stockman

Perinatal/Neonatal Medicine: Drs. Klaus and Fanaroff

Plastic and Reconstructive Surgery: Drs. McCoy, Brauer, Haynes, Hoehn, Miller, and Whitaker

Podiatric Medicine and Surgery: Dr. Jay

Psychiatry and Applied Mental Health: Drs. Freedman, Lourie, Meltzer, Nemiah, Talbott, and Weiner

Pulmonary Disease: Drs. Green, Ball, Menkes, Michael, Peters, Terry, Tockman, and Wise

Rehabilitation: Drs. Kaplan and Szumski

Sports Medicine: Drs. Krakauer, Shephard, and Torg, Col. Anderson, and Mr. George

Surgery: Drs. Schwartz, Jonasson, Peacock, Shires, Spencer, and Thompson

Urology: Drs. Gillenwater and Howards

Vascular Surgery: Drs. Bergan and Yao

1987
The Year Book of
UROLOGY®

Editors
Jay Y. Gillenwater, M.D.
*Professor and Chairman, Department of Urology, University of Virginia
School of Medicine*
Stuart S. Howards, M.D.
Professor, Department of Urology, University of Virginia School of Medicine

Year Book Medical Publishers, Inc.
Chicago • London • Boca Raton

Printed in U.S.A.

International Standard Book Number: 0-8151-3465-7

International Standard Serial Number: 0084-4071

Editorial Director, Year Book Publishing: Nancy Gorham
Sponsoring Editor: Judy L. Plazyk
Literature Surveillance Supervisor: Laura J. Shedore
Assistant Director, Manuscript Services: Frances M. Perveiler
Associate Managing Editor, Year Book Editing Services: Linda H. Conheady
Assistant Managing Editor, Year Book Editing Services: Elizabeth Griffith
Production Manager: H.E. Nielsen
Proofroom Supervisor: Shirley E. Taylor

Table of Contents

The material covered in this volume represents literature reviewed through January 1987.

ADULT

PEDIATRIC

Journals Represented

Acta Pathologica et Microbiologica Scandinavica b. Microbiology
Acta Physiologica Scandinavica
Acta Radiologica
American Journal of Clinical Pathology
American Journal of Kidney Diseases
American Journal of Medicine
American Journal of Obstetrics and Gynecology
American Journal of Roentgenology
Annales Chirurgiae et Gynaecologiae
Annales de Radiologie
Annals of Internal Medicine
Annals of Plastic Surgery
Annals of Surgery
Archives of Disease in Childhood
Archives of Internal Medicine
Archives of Pathology and Laboratory Medicine
Archives of Surgery
British Journal of Surgery
British Journal of Urology
British Medical Journal
Cancer
Clinical Chemistry
Clinical Nephrology
European Urology
Experimental and Molecular Pathology
Fertility and Sterility
Hospital Practice
Human Pathology
Journal of the American Medical Association
Journal of Clinical Endocrinology and Metabolism
Journal of Pediatric Surgery
Journal of Thoracic and Cardiovascular Surgery
Journal of Trauma
Journal of Urology
Kidney International
Lancet
Mayo Clinic Proceedings
Medical Journal of Australia
Mount Sinai Journal of Medicine (New York)
National Kidney Foundation Newsletter
Nephron
New England Journal of Medicinee
Pediatrics
Plastic and Reconstructive Surgery
Prostate
Quarterly Journal of Medicine
Radiology
S.A.M.J./S.A.M.T.-South African Medical Journal
Scandinavian Journal of Infectious Diseases
Scandinavian Journal of Urology and Nephrology
Science

Surgery, Gynecology and Obstetrics
Transplantation
Transplantation Proceedings
Urologia Internationalis
Urologic Radiology
Urological Research
Urology
Western Journal of Medicine
World Journal of Surgery

Introduction

The 247 abstracts in the 1987 YEAR BOOK OF UROLOGY were selected from more than 2,600 articles reviewed to provide a quick reference source for the latest literature. All abstracts were selected for their clinical relevance. This is the first year that the textbook *Adult and Pediatric Urology* is updated by the YEAR BOOK OF UROLOGY. The order of presentation follows that of the new textbook.

A number of significant contributions were made this year. One of the most significant was the identification of a human prostatic growth factor by Story and associates of Milwaukee (Abstract 28–1). These investigators isolated a basic fibroblast growth factor having a molecular weight of 17,400 from human benign prostatic hyperplastic tissue.

Van der Maase and associates of Copenhagen (Abstract 34–5) diagnosed carcinoma in situ in the contralateral testis in 27 of 500 patients (5.4%) with unilateral testicular germ cell cancer. Whereas testicular cancer did not develop in 8 patients with carcinoma in situ, contralateral testicular cancer did occur in 7 of the remaining 19 patients. Lewi and associates from Glaasgow (Abstract 14–1) report that metastases developed in 4 of 22 patients (18%) with renal oncocytoma. Dahnert and associates from Baltimore (Abstract 28–3), using a correlation of ultrasound, x-ray studies, and histopathologic findings, concluded that the echogenic foci in prostatic sonograms represent prostatic calcifications, not prostatic cancer.

There were a number of exceptional papers on prostate cancer this year. De Voogt and associates (Abstract 29–15) reported on European cooperative studies on the cardiovascular side effects of diethylstilbestrol, cyproterone acetate, medroxyprogesterone, and estramustine phosphate. In the first study, lethal cardiovascular disease developed within 3 years in 20% of those taking diethylstilbestrol and in 11% of those taking estramustine phosphate. In the second study, by Hendriksson and associates of Hudding, Sweden, patients taking low-dose estrogen had a 25% major cardiovascular toxicity rate versus none for the orchiectomy group. Epstein and associates of Baltimore (Abstract 29–19) reported a 27.5% false negative rate with frozen sections in 310 prostatic cancer patients having pelvic node dissections.

Haapiainen from Helsinki (Abstract 29–3) studied 34 patients with stage A carcinoma of the prostate; 53% were focal and 47% were diffuse. The progression rate for the diffuse involvement was 38%, compared with 11% for the focal. Three of the 34 patients died of metastatic disease. Of the eight patients with progression of disease, six had diffuse cancer (more than three chips). Epstein and associates of Baltimore (Abstract 29–4) followed 94 patients with stage A1 prostatic cancer for more than 8 years. Sixteen percent had progression of the disease. Neither tumor volume nor tumor grade predicted progression. McNeal and Bostwick from Palo Alto (Abstract 29–6) identified cytologic atypia in the prostatic ductal and acinar lining epithelium that they believe is the antecedent lesion of most prostatic cancers.

As reported in Abstract 29–7, Skiddall and associates of Leeds, England, monitored prostate cancer patients with two specific antigens: prostate specific antigen and γ-seminoprotein. Prostate specific antigen is confined to the cytoplasm of the acinar and ductal epithelium of the prostate gland. Of patients with metastases, 90% had elevated concentrations of prostate specific antigen and 97% had elevated levels of γ-seminoprotein.

Scardino and associates of Houston (Abstract 29–11) studied the prognostic significance of a positive postirradiation biopsy specimen in 45 patients with prostatic cancer. Positive specimens were found in 35% of patients. Within 10 years, local recurrences developed in 82% of those with a positive biopsy result and in 32% of those with a negative biopsy result.

Three studies evaluated surgical enucleation for renal cell carcinoma. Novick and associates of Rochester, Minnesota (Abstract 14–3) found local recurrence in 2 of 33 patients (6%). Bazeed and associates of Mainz, West Germany (Abstract 14–4) found no local recurrences in 49 patients. Both of these series were highly selective, the patients having small low-grade and stage I lesions. Marshall and associates of Baltimore (Abstract 14–5) enucleated in vitro 16 radical nephrectomy specimens and with enucleation, residuual tumor was left in seven. Tumors in this group were 5–12 cm in size.

There were several noteworthy studies concerning testis tumors. Loehrer and associates of Indianapolis (Abstract 34–8) evaluated 51 patients who underwent resection of teratoma after chemotherapy for disseminated non-seminomatous germ cell tumor. Nine patients died. Recurrences were usually local, thus meticulous dissection is essential. Patients with nongerm cell elements, increased tumor burden, and primary mediastinal tumors have a worse prognosis.

Böhle and associates of Berne, Switzerland (Abstract 34–3) found that 10 of 12 patients with "primary" retroperitoneal tumors had primary testicular tumors on follow-up examination. None of the four patients with primary mediastinal tumors had a later primary testicular tumor. Tiffany and associates of Memorial Hospital in New York City (Abstract 34–9) studied 23 patients with germ cell tumors who had surgical excision of retroperitoneal, mediastinal, and neck masses after chemotherapy. Four of 11 patients with fibrosis or necrosis in the thoracic or neck specimens had malignancy in the retroperitoneal tissue.

Hellström and associates of Oulu, Finland (Abstract 28–6) did a prospective randomized study to compare findings in 11 patients treated with bladder neck incision with those in 13 patients having transurethral resection (TUR) of the prostate. Symptomatic response was compared. Urodynamically, the TUR group did better. None of the bladder neck incision group had retrograde ejaculation, whereas 62% of the TUR group did have retrograde ejaculation. Sinha and associates of Minneapolis (Abstract 28–7) reported the successful use of local anesthesia (bupivacaine and lidocaine) for performing TURs of the prostate in 100 patients.

Fitzpatrick and Reda of Dublin (Abstract 26–1) found that the prognosis of bladder carcinoma among patients aged 30–40 years is no different from that of the older population. The prognosis for the group younger than 30 years of age was more favorable. Prout and associates of Boston

(Abstract 26–2) report the 5-year follow-up of 160 patients with grade 1 transitional cell carcinoma of the bladder. There was a 67% recurrence rate. In 20% the disease progressed in grade; in 4% invasive transitional cell carcinoma developed; five patients underwent cystectomy, and one died of metastatic disease.

Herr and associates of Memorial Hospital in New York City (Abstract 26–5) found that in 47 patients with flat carcinoma in situ of the bladder, 68% of patients treated with bacillus Calmette-Guerin (BCG) vaccine were free of disease at 6 years compared with none of the patients managed by TUR alone. Intravesical BCG was as effective as intravesical BCG plus intradermal BCG. A single 6-week course was effective for up to 6 years. Kelley and associates of St. Louis (Abstract 30–4) also reported on their studies of BCG in superficial bladder cancer; 77% of patients whose purified protein derivative skin test converted positive were free of tumor compared with only 34% of those who did not convert. Fewer patients with a granulomatous response had recurrent superficial bladder cancer. Haaff and associates of St. Louis (Abstract 26–7) found a favorable response of 42% (8 of 19 patients) to a single 6-week course of BCG for carcinoma in situ, and 56% (5 of 9) responded to a second 6-week course.

Two cryptorchidism studies are among the most interesting pediatric papers included in the 1987 YEAR BOOK. Jarow and associates of Baltimore (Abstract 47–1) reported on 28 prepubertal patients younger than 11 years of age studied with human chorionic gonadotropin (hCG) stimulation. Twenty-one with normal testosterone response had testes at exploration. Of the seven patients with no testosterone response to hCG, the six explored had no testes. It is concluded that if a boy is prepubertal, has no response to hCG, and has elevated levels of gonadotropins, exploration is not necessary. The John Radcliffe Hospital Cryptorchidism Study Group (Abstract 47–2) reports that the true rate of undescended testes at age 1 year is 2%. This contrasts with the 0.8% figure reported by Scorer and Farrington (*Congenital Deformities of the Testis and Epididymis*, London, Butterworths, 1971, pp. 15–17) and the orchidopexy rate of 1.9%. The discrepancy is that, in some of the boys, undescended testes redeveloped between 3 months and 1 year.

As described in Abstract 47–7, Anderson and Williamson of Bristol, England, found that testes prone to torsion already show impaired spermatogenesis. Fifty-six patients with acute torsion were investigated prospectively. No correlation was found between the duration of torsion and subsequent sperm concentration. Twenty of 35 patients biopsied had histologic evidence of preexisting partial maturation arrest in spermatogenesis. Antisperm antibody formation following torsion was minimal.

Raney (Abstract 48–7), at the Philadelphia Children's Hospital, reported on 16 children with pelvic soft tissue sarcomas. The eight tumors arising from the prostate or bladder were smaller, and six of these eight patients were alive and free of tumor. The eight arising from the pelvis were larger, and only three of these patients were alive and free of tumor. All patients received chemotherapy, 81% received radiation, and many had surgery.

Livingstone and Sarembock of Cape Town (Abstract 48–5) reported on ten childhood germ cell tumors managed in a variety of ways. They think that this tumor remains localized to the testes for long periods and that metastases occur mostly by the hematogenous route. They recommend postorchiectomy surveillance. Flamant and associates (Abstract 48–4) reported on their experience with yolk sac tumors of the testis in children. Twenty-three of 24 had elevated α-fetoprotein levels that returned to normal. In this series, 85% (24·of 28 tumors) were stage I. None of the patients underwent initial retroperitoneal node dissection. The 3-year survival rate was 83%. Only one of the three in whom lymphadenopathy developed died. No value of adjuvant chemotherapy was found. The authors recommend postorchiectomy surveillance.

Roth and associates of Detroit Children's Hospital (Abstract 42–1) reported their results using the artificial urinary sphincter. Thirty-three of 47 patients had a good response; erosions developed in 2. Six had transient upper tract dilation in response to intermittent catheterization or drugs. Late deterioration of the upper tract developed in six (four had hydronephrosis and two had transient renal insufficiency). Zaontz and Firlit of Chicago (Abstract 43–1) reported the successful percutaneous antegrade ablation of posterior urethral valves in six infants with small caliber urethras. Kropp and Angwato of Toledo (Abstract 44–2) described the successful correction of neurogenic incontinence by urethral lengthening and reimplantation. The urethra is lengthened from the posterior or anterior bladder flap and reimplanted into the posterior bladder wall at the bladder neck. The patients have to use intermittent catheterization to empty the bladder. Mitchell and Kulb of Indianapolis (Abstract 46–1) reported the successful use of a splint thorugh the neourethra to allow normal voiding and drainage of the neourethra.

Exceptional articles on priapism, impotence, and infertility are included in this year's collection. Lue and associates of San Francisco (Abstract 35–1) summarized their approach to management of priapism. Intracorporeal blood gas and pressure monitoring is used to differentiate ischemic (low flow) from nonischemic (high flow) types. Priapism with pressures lower than 40 mm hg usually resolves. Those with severe ischemia are treated with a small unilateral shunt. When mild or no ischemia is present, they recommend aspiration and irrigation and instillation of diluted norepinephrine. Lue and associates (Abstract 35–6) and Delcour and associates of Brussels (Abstract 35–5) both reported on evaluation of impotence with cavernosography to detect "leaking" veins. Patients are evaluated with history, physical examination, and endocrine workup. Those with suboptimal papaverine tests should have a Doppler evaluation of arterial blood flow. Cavernosography can be used to evaluate venous leakage. In Lue's series, of the 33 patients who responded to papaverine with poor erections, five had severe venous leakage. Twenty-eight showed arterial insufficiency and venous leakage. Delcour reports venous leakage in 88 of 187 impotent men evaluated with cavernosography. Condra and associates of Kingston, Canada (Abstract 35–2) found an increased prevalence of cigarette smoking among impotent men.

Bustillo and Rajfer of UCLA (Abstract 30–2) successfully aspirated sperm from the vas deferens of two men with paraplegia and established an ongoing pregnancy in one couple. Schoysman and Bedford of Brussels (Abstract 30–3) report an 18% fertility rate in 565 patients with epididymovasostomy. There was a greater chance of pregnancy when the anastomosis was made in the corpus, rather than at the level of the caput epididymidis. Sperm motility was impaired in the more proximal anastomoses. Clarkson and associates of Winston Salem and Beaverton, Oregon (Abstract 30–7) reported that in monkeys with slight hyperlipoproteinemia induced by a moderately atherogenic diet, vasectomy led to less atherosclerosis.

A variety of other articles were selected for the YEAR BOOK. Ehrlich and associates of Los Angeles (Abstract 41–1) report successful total abdominal wall reconstruction in eight patients with prune belly syndrome. The technique consists of sharp dissection of skin and subcutaneous tissue from the musculoabdominal layer and overlapping in a double-breasted fascia closure with excision of excess medial skin.

Mohr and associates of the Mayo Clinic (Abstract 1–1) found an incidence of *asymptomatic* microhematuria in 13% of male adults and postmenopausal women. The frequency of urologic disease was 2.3%, and only 0.5% had renal or bladder cancer. The authors recommend no urologic investigation for asymptomatic microhematuria. Raman and associates of Portsmouth, England, did a controlled study in 109 patients and found that the morphology of red blood cells in either whole urine or the centrifuged urine did not provide a reliable guide to the differentiation of glomerular from nonglomerular bleeding.

Atlas of Cornell University (Abstract 13–1) reviewed the renal and systemic effects of atrial natriuretic factor (ANF), which is released by the atrium in response to mechanical stretch. The hormone increases the glomerular filtration rate (GFR) by relaxing afferent arterioles and constricting efferent arterioles. The ANF antagonizes the vasoconstrictor and aldosterone stimulation actions of angiotensin II. Blood pressure and cardiac outputs are reduced by ANF.

Klimberg and associates of Gainesville, Florida, found that they could safely use intraoperative autotransfusions in urologic oncology surgery. The autotransfusions did not appear to disseminate the cancer.

Rothenberger of Landshut, West Germany (Abstract 36–2) reported on 17 patients with penile cancer treated with local excision with a 0.5-cm margin and fulguration of the base with the neodymium-yttrium/aluminum/garnet laser. Two patients required treatment within 1 year for carcinoma in situ, and in one patient Bowen's disease of the glands developed at 59 months.

Lastly, I should mention that this year's YEAR BOOK includes 13 abstracts from articles on the subject of extracorporeal shock wave lithotripsy (ESWL), reflecting the great expansion of interest in this technique and the increasing amount of data available concerning both clinical application and the ongoing research on new ESWL devices. Also included is the most recent update on long-term follow-up of ESWL patients by Newman and associates of Indianapolis, as presented at the 1987 annual meeting of the American Urological Association. It is hard to exaggerate what ESWL technology has meant to urologists so far and interesting to reflect that the history of ESWL is still relatively short at this point and the technology still advancing.

Stuart Howards and I would like to acknowledge and thank the clinicians who helped to produce the 1987 YEAR BOOK OF UROLOGY by writing critiques in certain areas. The comments for the chapters on "Urinary Tract Infection," "Renal Infection," and "Infection and Urethritis" were written by Jackson E. Fowler, Jr., M.D., of the University of Illinois. Alan D. Jenkins, M.D., of the University of Virginia, wrote the comments for the chapters on "Calculus Formation," "Percutaneous Stone Removal," and "Ureteroscopy." Marguerite Lippert, M.D., of the University of Virginia, wrote the comments for the chapters on "Lasers" and "Cystic Disease." Alan Wein, M.D., of the University of Pennsylvania, wrote the comments on "Voiding Function" and "Voiding Dysfunction." The comments for "Renal Transplantation" were provided by Arthur Sagalowsky, M.D., of the University of Texas in Dallas. E. Darracott Vaughan, Jr., M.D., of Cornell University, commented on "Hypertension and Vascular Disease."

Jay Y. Gillenwater, M.D.

ADULT

1 Standard Diagnostic Considerations

Asymptomatic Microhematuria and Urologic Disease: A Population-Based Study
David N. Mohr, Kenneth P. Offord, Richard A. Owen, and L. Joseph Melton, III (Mayo Clinic and Found.)
JAMA 256:224–229, July 11, 1986   1–1

The prevalence of new asymptomatic microhematuria was determined in relation to age and gender in the population of Rochester, Minnesota, where more than half of the residents are seen each year at the Mayo Clinic. About 85% of all persons had at least one urinalysis. The overall prevalence of asymptomatic microhematuria was 13/100 in men aged 35 years and older and in women aged 55 years and older.

Serious urologic disease was found in 2.3% of those with asymptomatic microhematuria. Only 0.5% of these patients had bladder or renal cell carcinoma. Malignant urologic lesions were more frequent in elderly persons. More serious disease tended to occur in those with higher grades of hematuria and was more prevalent in men than in women. Ten men in the study had prostatic cancer. The three uroepithelial cancers were in patients aged 75 years or older. In only 10% to 20% of the patients did the presence of hematuria lead to further workup within 1 month, apart from repeat urinalysis. Of the patients without preexisting or subsequent urologic disease, about two thirds of those having urinalyses exhibited hematuria again in the next 3 years.

Microhematuria is very prevalent if defined as one or more red blood cells per high-power field. Complete workup of all of these patients is not warranted because the predictive value for serious urologic disease is low and early discovery of serious disease will not often alter the patient outcome. Age may help in deciding whether to evaluate the patient further. Persistent hematuria also may suggest the need for further workup. A more specific screening measure for urologic malignancies is needed.

▶ This is a nice population-based study showing that asymptomatic microscopic hematuria occurred in 13% of adult men and postmenopausal women. The frequency of urologic disease was 2.3%, and only 0.5% had renal or bladder cancer. The authors recommend no urologic investigation for asymptomatic microhematuria. This article is important because it will be oft quoted. The important factor is the word asymptomatic. All patients having any genitourinary symptoms, proteinuria, or pyuria were excluded. I do not agree with the authors' conclusions. I usually get follow-up urinalyses and urine cytology, and look for red blood cell casts or distortion characteristic of glomerular disease.

With persistent microscopic hematuria I obtain an intravenous pyelogram and usually do cystoscopy.—J.Y. Gillenwater, M.D.

A Blind Controlled Trial of Phase-Contrast Microscopy by Two Observers for Evaluating the Source of Haematuria
G. Venkat Raman, Linda Pead, H.A. Lee, and Rosalind Maskell (St. Mary's Hosp., Portsmouth, England)
Nephron 44:304–308, December 1986   1–2

In 1979 investigators first reported that examination of red blood cells (RBCs) in the uncentrifuged deposit of fresh urine by phase-contrast microscopy could discriminate between glomerular bleeding and bleeding from the renal pelvis or the lower urinary tract. Although this technique is of clear usefulness in clinical medicine, only two blind trials of the technique have been published. An attempt was made to determine whether morphological changes could be detected by examination of whole urine under an inverted microscope, whether morphological changes correlated well with diagnosis, whether there was agreement between two different observers, and how the findings compared with those obtained using phase-contrast microscopy.

Two observers, unaware of each other's findings and of the diagnosis, examined RBCs in the urine of 109 patients by phase-contrast microscopy. In addition, all specimens were examined uncentrifuged by inverted microscopy, and 48 of the 109 were also examined under a light microscope after centrifugation. The observers were unable to confirm with either method the close correlation between RBC morphology and diagnosis that had been suggested by previously published studies. Furthermore, the two observers differed in their interpretations on 38% of occasions.

The morphology of RBCs in either whole urine or the centrifuged deposit did not provide a reliable guide to the diagnosis of renal disease. Although the test did prove useful in some individual cases, the high degree of sensitivity and specificity reported in previously published studies could not be confirmed. The combination of proteinuria and the presence of cellular casts detected by an experienced observer using inverted microscopy was a more sensitive indicator of renal parenchymal disease.

▶ The authors of this article could not duplicate the work of Burch and Fairley in which dysmorphic RBCs in the urine indicated glomerular renal disease. In addition, there was no agreement between the observers. This study used two observers, neither aware of the diagnosis nor of the other's findings. Obviously, other studies will be needed to clarify the situation.—J.Y. Gillenwater, M.D.

The following review articles are recommended to the reader:

Copley, J.B.: Isolated asymptomatic hematuria in the adult. *Am. J. Med. Sci.* 291:101, 1986.

Cubelli, V., Smith, A.D.: Current progress in endourology. *NY State J. Med.* 86:527–530, 1986.

Gordon, D.H., Macchia, R.J., Koser, M.W., et al: Endourology: an overview of a new subspecialty. *NY State J. Med.* 86:522–526, 1986.

Olin, T.: Adverse reactions to intravascularly administered contrast media. *Acta Radiol. (Diagn.) (Scand.)* 27:257, 1986.

O'Reilly, P.H.: Diuresis renography 8 years later: Update. *J. Urol.* 136:993, 1986.

Newhouse, J.H. (ed.):*Special Issue: Nuclear Magnetic Resonance Imaging. Urol. Radiol.* 8:119–166, 1986.

2 Wound Healing

Repair of Chronic Radiation Wounds of the Pelvis
Stephen J. Mathes and Dennis J. Hurwitz (Univ. of California at San Francisco, and Univ. of Pittsburgh)
World J. Surg. 10:269–280, April 1986   2–1

Irradiation is currently used as primary or adjuvant therapy for pelvic tumors. Late wound complications of this technique still occur and can result in complex pelvic wounds, which often fail to heal with local wound management.

Twenty-four patients with chronic pelvic wounds were treated by muscle, musculocutaneous, and fasciocutaneous flaps, resulting in successful wound repair. Flap selection was based on wound location. An independent source of circulation separate from the wound was necessary for well-vascularized flaps. Frequently used flaps were the rectus femoris, rectus abdominis, gracilis, and gluteus maximus muscle, musculocutaneous flaps, and the gluteal thigh skin fascial flap. Wound débridement and coverage with well-vascularized flaps is a useful and reliable method for repair of complex wounds resulting from pelvic radiation therapy.

▶ Previous radiation impairs wound healing because of impaired circulation resulting from radiation-induced obliterative endarteritis. The addition of new vascularized tissue allows delivery of components of the host defense mechanism, oxygen, and systemic antibiotics to the wound and subsequent healing. In discussing wound breakdown from radiation, the authors point out that initial management consists of correction of nutritional deficiencies, wound biopsy for possible tumor recurrence, topical antibiotic therapy with sulfadiazine, and systemic specific antibiotics after the vascularized flap is brought into the area. We have had remarkable success in repair of radiation-induced fistulas with the help of plastic surgeons using myocutaneous flaps. Recently, a vesicorectal radiation-induced fistula was repaired using a pedicled large bowel flap (Bricker, E.M., et al.: *Surg. Gynecol. Obstet.* 148:499, 1979; Bricker et al.: *Ann. Surg.* 193:555, 1981).—J.Y. Gillenwater, M.D.

3 Urinary Tract Infection

▶ ↓ The comments for this chapter were written by Dr. Jackson E. Fowler, Jr., Clarence C. Saelhof Professor of Urology, University of Illinois College of Medicine, Chief of the Division of Urology at University of Illinois Hospital.— J.Y. Gillenwater, M.D.

Bacterial Adherence to Bladder Uroepithelial Cells in Catheter-Associated Urinary Tract Infection
Richard Daifuku and Walter E. Stamm (Harborview Med. Ctr., Seattle, and Univ. of Washington)
N. Engl. J. Med. 314:1208–1213, May 8, 1986   3–1

Changes in bacterial adherence seen during bladder infection in 55 catheterized patients were studied prospectively. Such changes are important in the pathogenesis of community-acquired urinary tract infections, but their significance for catheterized patients has not been appreciated. Similar changes in both groups may influence the subsequent risk of bacteriuria. The bacterial species used for the study were *Escherichia coli, Klebsiella pneumoniae, Proteus mirabilis, Serratia marcescens,* and *Pseudomonas aeruginosa;* all were isolated from patients with urinary tract infections. All were fimbriated; *K. pneumoniae* and *P. aeruginosa* had a glycocalix at the cell surface, and *P. aeruginosa* and *P. mirabilis* produced glucan in sucrose broth.

Bacteriuria or candiduria developed in 38% of the 55 patients during prospective observation. Infections in women were more frequent and lasted longer than those in men. Bacterial adherence was assessed in three categories: gram-negative rods, gram-positive coccal infections, and candidal infections. Mixed infections were excluded. Data on 17 infections were analyzed. Significant changes in adherence were limited to the period just before onset of bacteriuria. Adherence was significantly higher before gram-negative rod infections than before gram-positive coccal infections. In the 48–96 hours before infection up to the time of the first positive culture, adherence in patients with gram-negative rod infections declined, but adherence with gram-positive coccal infections increased. Cells from patients with candidal infections showed increases in adherence of *E. coli* and *P. mirabilis* in this period. By the Cox proportional hazard model, it was discovered that the bacterial adherence data from the period just before bacteriuria predicted the risk of gram-negative rod and gram-positive coccal infections. The coefficients of adherence were positive for gram-negative rods and negative for gram-positive cocci, indicating that the risk of gram-negative rod infection rose but the risk of gram-positive coccal infection decreased with increased adherence. Women were 12.7 times more prone to gram-negative rod infections than men for a given value of adherence. In patients who were uninfected during catheterization, no significant changes in uroepithelial cell adherence were observed.

Bacterial infection from catheterization is thought to occur by migration of bacteria from the rectum or up the column of urine in the catheter when the collecting system is contaminated. Presumably, adherence to the uroepithelial cells initiates colonization. Interestingly, *P. aeruginosa* and *S. marcescens* showed the greatest adherence, and these two species are most often associated with nosocomial urinary tract infections. Different bacteria may have different adhesins, and epithelial cell adhesiveness may be increased in women with a history of recurrent cystitis. The changes observed in adhesiveness were transient, occurring just before the onset of bacteriuria. Better understanding of this phenomenon may aid development of strategies for early intervention and prevention of catheter-associated bacteriuria. Various species may share receptors on uroepithelial cells or may share less specific mechanisms of adherence. Such receptors might be satturated, or the expression of bacterial adhesins could be suppressed. Vaccines against the adhesins are also a possibility. Further study of the interactions between bacteria and bladder epithelium are warranted.

▶ This is an intriguing study that expands upon previous observations concerning bacterial adherence to epithelial cells in the pathogenesis of bacteriuria. In contrast to studies of vaginal epithelial cells, where susceptibility to bacterial adherence appears to be relatively constant for a given individual, this study demonstrates that susceptibility to adherence may be transient. Illumination of the reasons for this phenomenon would enhance greatly our understanding of host epithelial factors important to bacterial adherence and susceptibility to bacteriuria.—J.E. Fowler, Jr., M.D.

Relationships Between Human Blood Groups, Bacterial Pathogens, and Urinary Tract Infections

Joan J. Ratner, Virginia L. Thomas, and Marvin Forland (Univ. of Texas at San Antonio)

Am. J. Med. Sci. 292:87–91, August 1986   3–2

Antibodies against blood group antigens cross-react with certain gram-negative enteric bacteria, and it has been suggested that the cross-reacting bacterial antigens might promote rapid phagocytosis in persons possessing the corresponding antibodies. In addition, bacteria unreactive with host isohemagglutinins might selectively colonize and initiate infection. Serum and urine specimens were obtained from 137 patients with acute pyelonephritis, chronic upper urinary tract infection, cystitis, or asymptomatic bacteriuria. Serums from 68 healthy controls were used to determine blood groups.

The diagnosis of chronic upper tract infection was significantly associated with blood group B. More patients than expected with blood group B had infections by *Pseudomonas* species, *Klebsiella pneumoniae*, or *Proteus* species. Fewer than the predicted number of patients with blood group A had infections with *Pseudomonas*. An increased number of patients with blood group AB had infections caused by *Escherichia coli* and *K. pneumoniae*.

The finding that blood group B is present more often in patients having chronic upper urinary tract infection suggests that isoagglutinins have a role in host susceptibility to infection. It is possible that some special trait of invasiveness or virulence is carried by the particular organisms implicated, which is unchecked when the anti-B isoagglutinin is absent. Isoagglutinins could be protective when the invading organisms produce the appropriate blood group antigen. Either anti-A isoagglutinins may be less protective, or fewer strains of uropathogens may have blood group A antigens on their surfaces.

▶ Recognized and yet to be identified host factors undoubtedly contribute to susceptibility and resistance to bacteriuria in general and to renal infection in specific. For the reasons summarized in the abstract, these investigators focused on blood type as a parameter that might confer susceptibility to urinary tract infection. A significant association between the diagnosis of "chronic" upper tract infection and blood type B compared with a control population was found, but the power of the association ($p<.05$) was not overwhelming. Whether the findings are spurious or reflect a significant physiologic phenomenon that is partially obscured by other host or bacterial factors is difficult to determine.—J.E. Fowler, Jr., M.D.

Evaluation of Rapid Methods for the Detection of Bacteriuria (Screening) in Primary Health Care

Hans O. Hallander, Anders Kallner, Arne Lundin, and Eva Österberg (Natl. Bacteriological Laboratory, Karolinska Hosp., Stockholm, and Sollentuna Health Care Ctr., Sweden)
Acta Pathol. Microbiol. Immunol. Scand. Sect. B, 94:39–49, February 1986

3–3

The diagnostic value of six methods of bacteriuria testing was assessed in 781 urine specimens obtained at a primary health care center. Conventional culture was used as a reference method. To achieve the highest possible efficiency, the cutoff limit for classification of test results into positive and negative was set at $\geq 10^5$ colony-forming units per ml.

The following diagnostic efficiencies were obtained: bacterial ATP, 0.94; bacterial count in sediment, 0.93; nitrite test, 0.92; dipslide test, 0.92; white blood cell (WBC) count in sediment, 0.87; and granulocyte esterase, 0.83. The dipslide most closely resembled the reference method. The counting of bacteria in sediment was highly specific but poorly sensitive. The counting of WBCs and the granulocyte esterase test strip had low specificity and poor sensitivity. The nitrite test strip had the disadvantage of low sensitivity, because it could yield false negative results for pathogens lacking nitrate reductase and with urine insufficiently incubated in the bladder. The ATP test resulted in the highest diagnostic efficiency by carefully optimizing the discrimination limit.

By combining the ATP and dipslide tests the highest diagnostic efficiency (0.96) was obtained. The often used combination of the dipslide and nitrite test did not improve diagnostic efficiency. A rapid primary test could obtain high diagnostic efficiency in conjunction with other tests for follow-up testing of specimens with intermediate or uninterpretable primary results.

By using ATP as the primary test, with follow-up testing of specimens with 3–25 nmole/L of ATP (12% of specimens), the most promising results were obtained. An overall diagnostic efficiency of 0.98 was seen with follow-up testing by conventional culture. A total of 81% of the patients with urinary tract infections could be classified without culture by performing the nitrite test on specimens with intermediary ATP results. A final diagnosis based on conventional culture was necessary for 10% of the total because of findings of intermediary ATP and negative nitrite results.

The major advantages of the ATP test are that it is rapid and simple, it provides an objective numerical result, and it can be done while patients wait. Also, it is not influenced by adhesion of bacteria to somatic cells.

▶ Two aspects of this investigation are noteworthy for the clinician. First, the diagnosis of bacteriuria based on the microscopic visualization of bacteria in the urinary sediment was associated with high specificity but low sensitivity. A similar finding was made for the diagnosis of bacteriuria based on identification of more than 20 leukocytes per high-power field in the urinary sediment. Therefore, a large proportion of patients without bacteriuria will be treated unnecessarily if therapeutic decision making is based solely on these parameters. These data provide further fuel for the argument that urine culture is critical when knowledge concerning the presence or absence of bacteriuria is necessary for optimal patient management.—J.E. Fowler, Jr., M.D.

Streptococci as Urinary Pathogens
Lynn E. Collins, Rosemary W. Clarke, and Rosalind Maskell (St. Mary's Hosp., Portsmouth, England)
Lancet 2:479–481, Aug. 30, 1986   3–4

Much pyuria goes unexplained by overnight aerobic urine culture on primary isolation media, and fastidious species of streptococci may be part of the reason. A prospective study of streptococcal urinary infection was performed, including that caused by all catalase-negative, gram-positive cocci and coccobacilli. Of the 11,725 urine specimens examined during the 2-month study period, 2,486 isolates (21%) were considered to be important.

Substantial numbers of catalase-negative, gram-positive cocci or coccobacilli were isolated in 242 instances, comprising about 10% of significant isolates. Seventy-four of these isolates (30%) were species other than *Streptococcus faecalis* and *Streptococcus agalactiae*. One third of isolates were not detected on cysteine-lactose-electrolyte-deficient agar after overnight incubation in CO_2. Twenty of 24 isolates of coccobacilli were *Gardnerella vaginalis*. Many isolations of fastidious species were accompanied by pyuria.

More streptococcal species can be detected if cysteine-lactose-electrolyte-deficient agar is used and cultures are incubated overnight in a 7% CO_2 atmosphere. Cultures leaving symptoms or pyuria unexplained are reincubated for another 24 hours. If fastidious species are expected, specimens also are inoculated onto chocolate blood agar and blood agar containing nalidixic acid.

▶ This study demonstrates that fastidious gram-positive cocci or coccobacilli may be isolated from the urine of patients with unexplained voiding symptomatology or pyuria if the specimen is incubated for an additional 24 hours on selective media in a carbon dioxide environment. As a laboratory rather than a clinical investigation, the significance of these microbiologic findings with respect to the actual etiology of the patient's symptomatology is unclear.—J.E. Fowler, Jr., M.D.

World-Wide Clinical Experience With Norfloxacin: Efficacy and Safety
C. Wang. J. Sabbaj, M. Corrado, and V. Hoagland (Merck Sharp & Dohme Res. Labs., Rahway, N.J.)
Scand. J. Infect. Dis. (Suppl. 48):81–89, 1986   3–5

Norfloxacin is a quinolone carboxylic acid derivative with excellent in vitro activity against many gram-negative bacilli, gram-positive cocci, and other microorganisms. Review was made of clinical trials conducted worldwide, comprising 2,346 patients. Doses ranged from 800 mg daily to 400 mg twice or three times a day. More than half of the patients were treated for urinary tract infections. Less frequent indications were gastrointestinal tract infections, including prophylaxis of travelers' diarrhea, gonorrhea, and prevention of infections in granulocytopenic patients.

Norfloxacin was 96% effective in patients having uncomplicated cystitis. The drug was as effective as co-trimoxazole or nalidixic acid. Nearly 90% of patients with chronic or complicated urinary tract infections, treated for longer periods, had a favorable clinical and bacteriologic outcome. Less favorable results were obtained in these cases using co-trimoxazole. Norfloxacin was consistently effective in patients with gonorrhea when used in a dose of 600 mg every 4 hours. A single 800-mg dose eradicated infection in 95% of the patients. Norfloxacin also proved effective against gastroenteritis and in preventing travelers' diarrhea. Adverse clinical and laboratory effects each were observed in about 12% of treated patients. Serious adverse effects occurred in fewer than 0.5%, but they were much more frequent in granulocytopenic patients given multiple-day treatment.

Norfloxacin offers advantages over available antibiotic regimens because of its safety and in vitro spectrum of activity. Extended coverage of gram-negative organisms, including *Pseudomonas aeruginosa*, makes the drug an excellent choice for treating complicated urinary tract infections, such as those in patients with renal stones or neurogenic bladder. The drug also is an effective short-term treatment for uncomplicated urinary tract infections. The activity of norfloxacin against penicillinase-producing strains of *N. gonorrhoeae* makes it preferable to oral agents (e.g., ampicillin) in treating gonorrhea.

Norfloxacin Versus Co-Trimoxazole in the Treatment of Recurring Urinary Tract Infections in Men
J. Sabbaj, V.L. Hoagland, and T. Cook (MSD Res. Labs., Woodbridge, N.J.)
Scand. J. Infect. Dis. [Suppl.] 48:48–53, 1986   3–6

Norfloxacin is a lipid-soluble weak organic acid antibiotic that is bound to a low extent to plasma proteins. It has a wide spectrum of activity against bacteria isolated from patients with urinary tract infections. A multicenter clinical study was performed to compare norfloxacin with co-trimoxazole in the treatment of men with urinary tract infections caused by susceptible organisms. The open, randomized study included 129 patients who received either 400 mg of norfloxacin twice daily or co-trimoxazole in a dose of 160/800 mg twice daily, given orally. Sixty norfloxacin-treated patients and 49 given co-trimoxazole were evaluable.

Norfloxacin had a broader spectrum of in vitro activity than co-trimoxazole had. The infecting organism was eradicated by norfloxacin in 93% of the patients and by co-trimoxazole in 80%, a significant difference. The difference was more marked in patients having positive pretreatment prostatic fluid or ejaculum cultures. Three co-trimoxazole-treated patients, but none in the norfloxacin group, had drug-related adverse clinical experiences. There was only one adverse drug-related laboratory effect in the norfloxacin group and none in the co-trimoxazole group.

Norfloxacin was significantly more effective than co-trimoxazole in the treatment of urinary tract infections in men in this study. Further experience is needed to determine the long-term results of norfloxacin therapy in men with recurrent urinary tract infections and prostatitis, but the available results are encouraging.

▶ The first of these two articles (Abstract 3–5) concerning norfloxacin, an oral antimicrobial with activity against most gram-negative enteric bacteria including *Pseudomonas, Neisseria gonorrhoeae,* and a variety of gram-positive cocci, provides important information about the compound. The peak concentration of norfloxacin in the urine is approximately 250 times that in the serum, adverse side effects are infrequent, activity against anaerobes is minimal, and activity against *N. gonorrhoeae* is maintained even if the organism produces penicillinase. As was observed with nalidixic acid, the forerunner of norfloxacin, neuropsychiatric adverse reactions have been noted. These reactions (e.g., hallucinations, euphoria, depression, and dizziness) are not common but unusual for antimicrobials. The physician who prescribes this drug should be aware of these potential side effects.

The second paper (Abstract 3–6) examines the efficacy of norfloxacin among men with bacteriuria and in some cases presumed prostatic infection. Because of the lipid solubility of the agent, as well as low binding to plasma proteins, diffusion into the prostatic ducts and fluid might be anticipated. Unfortunately, appropriate culture documentation of prostatic infection was not carried out, and the duration of bacteriologic surveillance following treatment was only 4–6 weeks. As such, the true efficacy of norfloxacin in the treatment of chronic bacterial prostatitis is not established. Nonetheless, the agent proved as efficacious as trimethoprim-sulfamethoxazole in the patients treated. At this time it is reasonable to recommend norfloxacin for the treatment of males with bacteriuria or chronic bacterial prostatitis caused by organisms resistant to trimethoprim-sulfamethoxazole. It is encouraging that the side effects during 4–6 weeks of treatment with conventional dosage were no greater than those associated with trimethoprim-sulfamethoxazole.—J.E. Fowler, Jr., M.D.

Nosocomial Urinary Tract Infections Due to Enterococcus: Ten Years' Experience at a University Hospital
Allan J. Morrison, Jr., and Richard P. Wenzel (Univ. of Virginia)
Arch. Intern. Med. 146:1549–1551, August 1986   3–7

From 1975 through 1984, 473 enterococcal nosocomial urinary tract infections were identified at the University of Virginia Hospital. The overall rate of patients with hospital-acquired urinary tract infections caused by enterococcus was 21.1/10,000 discharges (annual range, 17.3–32.2). The proportion of nosocomial UTIs caused by this organism was 9.3% (annual range, 5.3% to 15.7%).

Risk factors associated with fatal outcome included age older than 50 years, concurrent diagnosis of acute respiratory failure, gastrointestinal tract hemorrhage, and hospitalization on the internal medicine service. There were 72 fatalities, and the crude mortality was 15.2%. Of 124 patients with neurogenic bladder, 7.3% died. Among patients without neurogenic bladder mortality was 18.1%. Patients with neurogenic bladder (compared with those without neurogenic bladder) were younger (mean age, 39 years vs. 50 years), more often male (64% vs. 52%), and more likely to have had a nosocomial UTI during that same admission (29% vs. 17%).

Mixed infections were found in 19% of all patients. However, there was no statistically significant difference in the proportion of mixed infections among those who died, compared with survivors (21% vs. 19%). Overall, 95% had previous urethral catheterization; this proportion remained unchanged when survivors were compared with nonsurvivors (95% vs. 96%).

Enterococcal infections reflect endemic as opposed to epidemic events. Previously, nosocomial outbreaks were reported at this hospital by the authors without inclusion of the enterococcus. During the last 5 years of the present study, a constant antibiotic susceptibility pattern of the enterococcus to ampicillin was demonstrated by more than 98% of the urine isolate strains. Also, the use of cephalosporin antibiotics increased at the hospital, perhaps allowing for the selective pressure of the emergence of a cephalosporin-resistant pathogen. However, antibiotic treatment data for all study patients prior to enterococcal infection were not uniformly recorded and the interpretation and risk factor analysis that was used may not be organism-specific. Further studies are needed to define attributable morbidity and mortality for the enterococcus and other urinary pathogens that cause the most frequent nosocomial infections at the hospital.

▶ This epidemiologic investigation demonstrates that, in one university hospital, enterococcus has become the second leading cause of nosocomial urinary tract infections. It is speculated that the wide use of cephalosporin antibiotics, which generally are not active against the organism, has led to this endemic. The take-home message for the practicing urologist is that enterococcal infections, whether hospital or community acquired, remain susceptible to ampicillin therapy.—J.E. Fowler, Jr., M.D.

Bacteriuria and Mortality in an Elderly Population
Gunnar R. Nordenstam, C. Åke Brandberg, Anders S. Odén, Catharina M. Svanborg Edén, and Alvar Svanborg (Vasa Hosp., Sahlgren's Hosp., and the Univ. of Göteborg, Sweden)
N. Engl. J. Med. 314:1152–1156, May 1, 1986   3–8

The association between bacteriuria and mortality in adult and elderly populations may result from increased mortality as a result of bacteriuria alone or from a factor that increases both mortality and bacteriuria. Both bacteriuria and mortality increase with age, so that an overestimation of the mortality caused by bacteriuria is easily made. A study was designed to eliminate age differences and the influence of concomitant disease on the association between bacteriuria and death.

The first group studied included 521 men and 627 women aged 70 years who were examined at ages 70, 75, 79, and 81 years, annually thereafter. A second group of persons aged 70 years was reexamined only at age 75 years. The participants answered questionnaires dealing with all types of urinary tract diseases and gave specimens for bacteriuria screening. Cancer statistics came from the official Swedish population registries.

The 5-year mortality for women with bacteriuria was 13.4%, whereas control women had a mortality rate of 9.4%. If women with indwelling catheters were excluded from the two groups, the mortality after 5 years was 9.0% and 9.2%. After 9 years, the mortality was 23.9% and 23.3% in the groups comprising all women, irrespective of indwelling catheters. Men with bacteriuria had a rate of cancer nearly five times higher than that in control men, and higher 5-year mortality. Among men with bacteriuria but without cancer, mortality was not increased. Apparently, it is the fatal diseases associated with bacteriuria rather than the bacteriuria itself that accounts for the increased mortality among elderly patients with bacteriuria.

▶ This is probably the best study to date concerning the association between bacteriuria and mortality in the elderly. The bottom line is that fatal diseases associated with bacteriuria account for the increase in mortality among elderly patients with bacteriuria. Interesting peripheral observations include the finding that enterococcus followed *Escherichia coli* as the second most common cause of bacteriuria, that 9% of women and 2.4% of men had bacteriuria during the period of study, that approximately 50% of all the women had either documented bacteriuria or a history of bacteriuria, that diabetes mellitus did not apparently predispose to bacteriuria, and that only 6% of women with bacteriuria, but 2% of those without bacteriuria, experienced dysuria.—J.E. Fowler, Jr., M.D.

Lack of Association Between Bacteriuria and Symptoms in the Elderly
Jerome A. Boscia, William D. Kobasa, Elias Abrutyn, Matthew E. Levison, Adele M. Kaplan, and Donald Kaye (Med. College of Pennsylvania, Philadelphia)
Am. J. Med. 81:979–982, December 1986   3–9

A high prevalence of bacteriuria exists in the geriatric population, with at least 20% of women and 10% of men older than 65 having this problem. Most elderly persons with bacteriuria do not have symptoms of urinary tract infection; rather, they have asymptomatic bacteriuria. Nevertheless, elderly individuals with and without bacteriuria occasionally experience urinary symptoms such as incontinence, frequency, and urgency, as well as symptoms such as anorexia, insomnia, fatigue, malaise, and weakness. It was hypothesized that some of these urinary symptoms in the elderly (as well as symptoms indicating a lack of well-being) may be associated with bacteriuria. An attempt was made to determine whether apparently asymptomatic elderly patients with bacteriuria actually are asymptomatic.

The study population consisted of 59 women and 13 men aged 69–101 who did not have dysuria. The patients were questioned about other urinary symptoms (incontinence, frequency, urgency, suprapubic pain, flank pain, fever) and symptoms indicating a lack of well-being (anorexia, difficulty in falling asleep, difficulty in staying asleep, fatigue, malaise, weakness) when they were with and without bacteriuria. Twenty-two had bacteriuria that resolved spontaneously, bacteriuria developed subsequently in 24 nonbacteriuric patients, and 26 had bacteriuria that resolved without antimicrobial therapy. Patients occasionally reported urinary symptoms indicating a lack of well-being when they were with or without bacteriuria. However, there were no reported differences in symptoms found if bacteriuric patients were compared with themselves when they were nonbacteriuric. It would appear that bacteriuria without dysuria in the elderly is in fact asymptomatic.

▶ In my experience, the significance of voiding symptomatology that might possibly be caused by bacteriuria has been difficult to assess in elderly patients. This study provides personal reassurance that my clinical acumen has not as yet been ravaged by premature senility. The incidence of symptoms suggestive of bacteriuria (excluding dysuria) were the same among patients during and before or after bacteriuric episodes. Although controversy exists about the necessity for treatment of "asymptomatic" bacteriuria among the aged, this study clearly implies that urinalysis and urine culture are necessary to identify elderly bacteriuric patients.—J.E. Fowler, Jr., M.D.

Detection of Papillomavirus DNA in Human Semen

Ronald S. Ostrow, Karen R. Zachow, Michihito Niimura, Takashi Okagaki, Sigfrid Muller, Mitchell Bender, and Anthony J. Faras (Univ. of Minnesota, Jikei Univ., Tokyo, and Mayo Clinic and Found.)
Science 231:731–733, Feb. 14, 1986   3–10

Human papillomavirus (HPV) DNA was detected in semen, indicating the potential of sexual transmission of the virus. Examinations were made in two groups of patients, those with epidermodysplasia verruciformis, a chronic and familial condition characterized by flat warts and pigmented papules that progress to squamous cell carcinoma after sun exposure in one of every three patients, and veterinarians and meat handlers, who have a high incidence of wart disease and frequent recurrence after treatment. The total DNA was extracted from semen samples obtained from three patients from these groups and analyzed by the Southern blot hybridization technique.

Initially, semen was examined from an HPV-5-infected patient with epidermodysplasia verruciformis and from a former meat handler with a debilitating wart disease of the hands and chronic lymphatic leukemia. In both patients the semen contained HPV DNA. To determine if progeny of the patient with epidermodysplasia verruciformis also had HPV DNA, a DNA extract from the son's semen was analyzed; it was positive for the virus.

Centrifugation of the semen samples obtained from the two adults followed by an isotonic saline wash showed that about 95% of the HPV DNA was associated with the wash extracts. This suggested that the HPV DNA was not associated with sperm, but rather was present as either free viral particles or HPV DNA. Yet the presence of free viral particles could not be detected by electron microscopy. Ten additional semen specimens obtained from normal donors were negative for HPV DNA.

Although no clinical evidence existed for urinary papillomas in the patients studied, tests were made to determine whether exfoliated HPV-infected cells or virions shed by an undetected urethral lesion might be responsible for the initial results. No HPV DNA was detected. This suggested that the positive hybridization results obtained from the semen samples did not reflect HPV shedding from urinary or bladder lesions. No clinical evidence of genital neoplasia was observed in spouses, although subclinical infections could not be ruled out. The transmission of HPV

DNA via semen to sexual partners could not be demonstrated, but the presence of the viral genome in these patients suggests that sexual transmission by this route could occur.

The following review articles are recommended to the reader:

Arego, D.E., Koch, S.J.: Bacteriuria in paitents with spinal cord injury. *Hosp. Pract.,* 21:87, 1986.

Block, B.: Urinary tract infections. *Am. Fam. Physician* 33:172, 1986.

Holder, C.D., Craig, C.P.: Complications of urinary tract infections. *Hosp. Pract.* 21:110C, 1986.

Jenkins, R.D., Fenn, J.P., Matsen, J.M.: Review of urine microscopy for bacteriuria. *JAMA* 255:3397, 1986.

Mulholland, S.G.: Controversies in management of urinary tract infection. *Urology* 27 (Suppl. 2):3, 1986.

Parsons, C.L.: Bladder surface glycosaminoglycan layer: Efficient mechanism of environmental adaptation. *Urology* 27 (Suppl. 2):9, 1986.

Shortliffe, L.M.: Asymptomatic bacteriuria: Should it be treated? *Urology* 27 (Suppl. 2):19, 1986.

Svanborg Edén, C.: Bacterial adherence in urinary tract infections caused by *Escherichia coli. Scand. J. Urol. Nephrol.* 20:81, 1986.

4 Pain Management

Central and Peripheral Motor Effects of Morphine on the Rat Urinary Bladder
U. Sillén and A. Rubenson (Östra sjukhuset, Göteborg, Sweden)
Acta Physiol. Scand. 126:181–187, February 1986   4–1

The peripheral and central influence of morphine on detrusor activity was evaluated in an experimental animal model. Intravesical pressure recordings were obtained in anesthetized rats. Morphine activity was registered as its influence on bladder hyperactivity induced by central catecholaminergic stimulation with l-dihydroxyphenylalanine (L-DOPA) after peripheral inhibition of decarboxylase, and as its action on the response to regional injection of the receptor agonists acetylcholine and substance P, and to peripheral motor nerve stimulation.

The bladder response to L-DOPA was inhibited by the intracerebroventricular administration of 10 µg of morphine and by the systemic administration of 1–5 mg of the drug. The intravenous injection of morphine during the time of maximal L-DOPA response also completely inhibited the detrusor contractions, but increased amounts of the drug were necessary. There was slight depression of the bladder response to peripheral nerve stimulation, acetylcholine, and substance P. Depression of the detrusor reactivity to these substances was insignificant with all dose ranges of morphine. The intra-arterial injection of morphine (0.01–5.0 mg) elicited only a weak bladder contraction. The intravenous and intracerebroventricular administration of naloxone antagonized the inhibitory actions of intravenous and intracerebroventricularly administered morphine.

The inhibitory effect of morphine appears to be of central origin, because low intracerebroventricular doses were effective but peripherally administered doses were not. Also, intracerebroventricular injections did not influence peripheral detrusor reactivity to regional intra-arterial administration of receptor agonists and to postganglionic motor nerve stimulation. Opioid receptors appear to mediate the observed action because it could be antagonized by naloxone after systemic and intracerebroventricular administration. The intracerebroventricular distribution of methylene blue suggests that morphine may act in the area of the fourth ventricle. The main effect of morphine on the rat bladder appears to be centrally elicited inhibition of detrusor activity mediated by opioid receptors.

▶ Epidural morphine is more frequently being used for postoperative pain relief. One of the potential side effects is urinary bladder retention. In this study the authors conclude that the cause of urinary retention is CNS stimulation in the area of the fourth ventricle through opioid receptors.—J.Y. Gillenwater, M.D.

5 Lasers

▶ ↓ The comments for this chapter were written by Dr. Marguerite Lippert, Assistant Professor of Urology, University of Virginia School of Medicine.—J.Y. Gillenwater, M.D.

Treatment of Urological Tumors by Neodymium-YAG Laser

A. Hofstetter (Med. Univ. of Lübeck, West Germany)
Eur. Urol. 12:21–24, September 1986

5–1

The neodymium:yttrium/aluminum/garnet (Nd:YAG) laser is used both endoscopically and at open surgery to destroy benign and malignant tumors of the urethral, vesical, and ureteral mucosa. Bulky bladder tumors first undergo resection of the exophytic portion with the electric snare deep in the bladder wall after coagulation of the tumor margins. The tumor base and edges are then postcoagulated with the Nd:YAG laser. Smaller bladder tumors are destroyed primarily with the laser after irradiating the surrounding tissue to seal afferent vessels. The treated tumor is removed with biopsy forceps. A transurethral catheter generally is not required, lowering the risk of nosocomial infection. Intestinal perforation has not occurred when the radiation dose has been limited to 45 W.

Since 1976, more than 600 patients have been treated for bladder tumor using the Nd:YAG laser, with local relapse rates of 1% to 5%. Sedation has replaced anesthesia in most cases. A prospective trial comparing laser treatment with transurethral resection showed the former to result in a lower relapse rate, whether or not adjuvant chemotherapy with mitomycin was administered. There were almost no local relapses after laser treatment, in contrast to results after transurethral resection. In addition, no change from local to multiple tumor growth was observed after laser irradiation, unlike transurethral resection.

Ureteral tumors have also been treated in patients not suitable for radical operation. Only 1 of 5 such patients experienced relapse. Two renal pelvic tumors were treated with the Nd:YAG laser. Close monitoring is necessary after laser treatment of urothelial tumors, and new ureteroscopic methods are useful for this purpose. Laser treatment of urethral and genital condyloma acuminata has succeeded in 97% of 493 patients. One of 17 patients with penile cancer died of metastatic disease that has been understaged at the time of treatment. The laser application continues to be the most effective means of treatment in benign genital tumors.

A Prospective Randomized Study on Neodymium-YAG Laser Irradiation Versus TUR in the Treatment of Urinary Bladder Cancer

Hans Olav Beisland and Per Seland (Aker Hosp. and the Deaconess Hosp., Oslo)

Scand. J. Urol. Nephrol. 20:209–212, 1986   5–2

There is some evidence from previous studies that treatment of bladder tumors with the neodymium:yttrium/aluminum/garnet (Nd:YAG) laser compares favorably with transurethral resection (TUR) and electrocoagulation. A prospective randomized study was carried out to compare laser irradiation with TUR in 122 patients having transitional cell bladder carcinoma up to stage T2; the 95 men and 27 women had a mean age of 68 years. Thirty-eight patients previously had TUR or electrocoagulation. Forty patients had multiple tumors, with a mean of 3.5 tumors. Sixty patients were randomized to TUR and 62 were randomized to laser treatment.

Rates of recurrence in the treated area were 5% in the laser group and 32% in the TUR group, a highly significant difference. Small tumors did not recur in either group, and larger stage T1 tumors recurred only in the TUR group. Six of 10 stage T2 tumors in the TUR group and 3 of 15 in the laser group recurred. The median time to recurrence was 3 months. Comparable numbers of patients in the two groups had new disease in untreated areas.

It was concluded that irradiation with the Nd:YAG laser is the best approach to stage T1 urinary bladder tumors. Tumor size determines whether laser treatment should be used alone or combined with TUR. Further studies are needed to compare combined laser/TUR treatment of T2 tumors with other methods.

▶ Both of these articles by Hofstetter and by Beisland and Seland provide convincing data that bladder tumor patients are less likely to have local recurrence if treated with laser irradiation as opposed to TUR. However, Beisland and Seland's data don't agree with Hofstetter's data that the recurrence rate is also lower in the nontreated areas of the bladder after laser irradiation as opposed to TUR. Furthermore, Beisland and Seland show no difference in local recurrence rates for those patients who had T1 tumors less than 6 mm in diameter (the width of the diathermy loop), whether treated with laser or TUR. We have found Nd:YAG laser treatment of bladder tumors to be ideal for patients who have multiple recurrent superficial tumors, because it can be done without regional or general anesthesia, without urethral catheters, and in an outpatient setting. Our use of disposable laser fibers has allowed us greater flexibility in scheduling multiple bladder tumor procedures without the technical delay of repolishing fibers.—M.C. Lippert, M.D.

Laser Treatment of Condylomata Acuminata

Barry S. Stein (Brown Univ.)

J. Urol. 136:593–594, September 1986   5–3

The CO_2 or neodymium:yttrium/aluminum/garnet (Nd:YAG) laser was used to treat condylomata acuminata in 45 patients. At first, the laser was used when podophyllum or 5-fluorouracil therapy had failed, but subsequently patients with large or meatal-urethral lesions were treated initially with the laser. Smaller lesions and those on the glans are best treated with the CO_2 laser, and larger lesions, especially those on the penile shaft or in the perianal region, are best treated with the more penetrating Nd:YAG laser. Intraurethral lesions are also treated with this device. Treatment of perianal and intraurethral lesions required regional or general anesthesia.

Seven patients with small, flat lesions or condylomata on the glans had excellent cosmetic results after treatment with the CO_2 laser. None of 22 patients treated with the Nd:YAG laser for condylomata of the penile skin or scrotum had persistent disease. One large skin defect followed treatment of a large penile shaft lesion. None of seven perianal lesions treated under regional or general anesthesia persisted locally. Of nine patients with urethral meatal lesions who were examined urethroscopically under general anesthesia after laser treatment, five had intraurethral condyloma that were then treated urethroscopically. Two of them had persistent meatal disease, but no complications developed during follow-up for as long as 1 year after treatment.

Laser treatment of condylomata acuminata has consistently provided local control of disease. Lesions larger than 1–2 cm should be treated in stages. Pain is relatively lacking postoperatively, even if extensive disease is treated. Urethroscopy is suggested for meatal lesions and anoscopy for perianal lesions to rule out urethral or rectal disease that will lead to recurrences. Laser treatment is now preferred for all but the smallest condylomata.

▶ This is a summary of everyday urologic use of lasers for condyloma acuminata. Practical guidelines are given with regard to proper choice of laser type, laser settings, anesthesia, and route of delivery. For intraurethral lesions, we have used the rounded contact probe (sapphire tip) through the urethroscope at a 15-W setting. This technique has simplified the treatment of distal urethral condyloma without decreasing treatment effectiveness.—M.C. Lippert, M.D.

Use of the Neodymium-YAG Laser in the Treatment of Ureteral Tumors and Urethral Condylomata Acuminata: Clinical Experience
A. Schilling, R. Böwering, and E. Keiditsch (Municipal Hosp., Munich-Bogenhausen, Munich, West Germany)
Eur. Urol. 12:(Suppl.1)12:30–33, September 1986   5–4

Irradiation with the neodymium:yttrium/aluminum/garnet (Nd:YAG) laser was performed on seven males and five females who had a total of 16 ureteral tumors. The mean age was 67.3 years. All tumors were located in the lower ureter and were nonmetastatic. Also treated were 48 patients with more or less pronounced condylomatous involvement of the urethra. Seven patients with extensive involvement of the entire urethra (bulbar urethra to the external meatus) were selected for follow-up assessment; their mean age was 32 years (range, 21–62 years).

Laser irradiation of the ureteral tumors was well tolerated. During a mean follow-up period of 23 months (range, 3–31 months), no local tumor recurrences were observed. After 14 months, a heterotropic recurrence developed distal to the original tumor site. In patients with condylomata acuminata, the mean follow-up period was 1.9 years (range, 6 months to 5 years). After an average of three laser sessions, four patients remained free of condylomata. Two patients needed another treatment after 3 months, as did one patient after 12 months. These two patients remained free of recurrences for 7 and 9 months, respectively.

Radical measures (e.g., nephroureterectomy) as a first step are no longer necessary. After tumor classification, laser irradiation does not preclude subsequent surgery. No nearby organs were injured and no strictures developed as late complications. The defect appeared to be reepithelialized after 2–3 weeks. Although the low incidence of perforation was probably the result of tangential irradiation, this means that only the tumor's distal side is immediately accessible. Thus, effective treatment requires tumor removal after coagulation so that shadow areas are exposed.

The extent that the urethral condylomas studied were true recurrences or overlooked primary condylomas is uncertain, as repeated movement of the instrument shaft might mechanically flatten small condylomas, making them unrecognizable. Adequate treatment of deep urethral condyloma includes circumcision, orientating cystoscopy with the laser on standby, no catheterization, short-term follow-up examinations, and treatment of the partner for prevention of reinfection.

▶ Treatment of ureteral tumors in a manner similar to bladder tumors is intriguing. These authors obtained biopsy specimens through the ureteroscope before irradiating the tumor. Only if the tumor was of low malignancy grade and low infiltration stage on permanent pathology did they consider laser irradiation as definitive treatment. Pretreatment staging included CT as well as infusion urography and retrograde ureterography. Indwelling ureteral catheters were left in only five patients, who had an extensive coagulated area.—M.C. Lippert, M.D.

The following review article is recommended to the reader:

Council on Scientific Affairs: Lasers in medicine and surgery. *JAMA* 256:900, 1986.

6 Malignancy

Intraoperative Autotransfusion in Urologic Oncology
Ira Klimberg, Ronald Sirosis, Zev Wajsman, and James Baker (Univ. of Florida, Gainesville)
Arch. Surg. 121:1326–1329, November 1986   6–1

Autologous blood transfusion has become progressively safer and more effective, and it presently is used routinely with cardiopulmonary bypass. Autotransfusion with the Haemonetics Cell Saver was used in 49 patients having major urologic cancer operations in the past 2 years. Patients were followed for at least 1 year after operation. The 47 men and 2 women in the series had a median age of 63.5 years. The most frequent operations were radical cystoprostatectomy for bladder cancer, radical retropubic prostatectomy with pelvic node dissection for prostatic adenocarcinoma, and radical nephrectomy for renal cell carcinoma.

Four patients died and 88% are alive without evidence of disease. Mean intraoperative blood loss was 1,633 ml and the median volume of autotransfused blood was 566 ml. A mean of 665 ml of homologous blood was transfused. The mean hematocrit at hospital discharge was 35%. The total transfusion requirement for 45 surviving patients was 219 units, of which 102 units were autologous blood taken at the time of surgery. At least 500 ml of blood was salvaged and transfused in 23 of 26 patients who lost more than 1 liter of blood intraoperatively. No complications were directly related to autotransfusion, and no patient had evidence of posttransfusion hepatitis.

Autotransfusion may be used safely in surgery for patients with genitourinary malignancy. The need for homologous blood transfusion is thereby minimized and in some cases it is avoided. Further studies of the safety of autotransfusion in oncologic surgery are indicated.

▶ This paper addresses an important question: Can you safely use intraoperative autologous transfusions in urologic cancer surgery without causing systemic dissemination of cancer? The series is small and follow-up short, but the conclusion that autotransfusion did not disseminate cancer seems justified. In elective surgery the use of predeposited blood and autotransfusion is becoming more popular and works well.—J.Y. Gillenwater, M.D.

Pelvic Complications After Interstitial and External Beam Irradiation of Urologic and Gynecologic Malignancy
Paul F. Schellhammer, Gerald H. Jordan, and Anas M. El-Mahdi (Eastern Virginia Med. School, Norfolk)
World J. Surg. 10:259–268, April 1986   6–2

Most pelvic malignancies are irradiated, placing the pelvic organs at risk of radiation damage. The incidence and management of such damage were reviewed.

The most frequent and severe complications are associated with cystectomy performed for carcinoma of the bladder after radiation therapy has failed and with radiotherapeutic and surgical treatment of cervical carcinoma. There is an 11% incidence of bowel injury after radiotherapy before cystectomy. Bowel and urinary tract complications after external beam irradiation or ^{125}I brachytherapy for prostate carcinoma are similar. A triple-course fractionation protocol can reduce the morbidity of external beam radiation therapy. Rectal ulceration requiring colostomy occurs in 3% of patients receiving external beam irradiation or interstitial ^{125}I therapy. Surgical correction of rectal fistulas with vascularized flaps can be successful after ^{125}I injury, but it has not been successful after external beam injury. Urethral complications are associated with transurethral resection before external beam radiation therapy for prostastic carcinoma. This complication can be reduced significantly by withholding irradiation for 4–6 weeks after resection.

Although the goal of radiation therapy is destruction of the tumor without affecting the surrounding tissue, it is unrealistic to expect total tumor destruction without some damage to adjacent tissue. Therefore, radiation injury to healthy tissue is a risk accepted to obtain the benefits of this therapy, but it must be minimized during treatment.

▶ Recently, one of our surgeons and I repaired a large rectovaginal fistula by using a pedicled graft of proximal nonirradiated colon and interposing omentum between the bladder and rectum. There are a variety of clever ways in which one can use the nonirradiated bowel loop, illustrated in the articles published by Bricker (*Surg. Gynecol. Obstet.* 148:499, 1979; *Ann. Surg.* 193:555, 1981).—J.Y. Gillenwater, M.D.

Ablation of Tumor and Inflammatory Tissue With Absolute Ethanol
R. Uflacker, R. M. Paolini, and M. Nobrega (Hosp. Beneficencia Portuguesa and Instituto do Coracao da Universidade de Sao Paulo, Sau Paulo, and Hosp. Osvaldo Curz, Recife, Brazil)
Acta Radiol. [Diagn.] 27:131–138, March–April 1986   6–3

There are several techniques for vascular occlusion and tumor ablation that are effective for preoperative management and palliative treatment. Although the particulate occluding agents are the most widely used, absolute ethanol was introduced recently as an effective method of producing permanent tissue ablation and vascular occlusion. Absolute ethanol is useful in the treatment of renal tumors and esophageal varices. A review was made of experience using absolute ethanol for ablation of tumor and inflammatory tissue.

The study population consisted of 38 patients examined by angiography via a percutaneous femoral approach whose lesions were ablated with absolute ethanol. Thirty patients had various types of renal tumors, three had chronic end-stage renal failure with malignant hypertension, one had a fibrosarcoma of the right leg, and one had a metastasis in the humerus from a renal carcinoma. In addition, one patient had a large adrenal carcinoma, one had metastatic liver disease, and another had an extensive hypervascular inflammatory lesion of the right upper pulmonary lobe. The amount of ethanol used ranged from 5 ml to 50 ml. Twenty-two patients experienced substantial transient pain during ethanol injection, but sedation was necessary in only three of them. Two patients experienced skin necrosis, and one of these patients required plastic reconstruction. Two patients died within 5 days of the procedure; these deaths were unrelated to the ablation. Two patients had upper gastrointestinal tract bleeding within 2 days of the ethanol injection, and one of these died in acute renal failure. In another patient left colonic infarction developed after left renal tumor ablation. Absolute ethanol is a useful, efficient sclerosing agent that causes extensive tumor destruction and marked reduction in tumor vascularity and inflammatory lesions. Absolute ethanol caused an 18% complication rate.

▶ After an initial enthusiasm, we have not been using percutaneous infarction of tumors with the expectation that it makes the surgical procedure easier. We do not believe that it makes the surgery that much easier. Also, the patients experience pain from the infarction. In this series there was one case of left colon infarction after renal ablation with absolute ethanol. Renal infarction and later nephrectomy with hopes of some miracle immunologic response have not been effective in causing regression of metastatic renal cell cancer.—J.Y. Gillenwater, M.D.

The following review articles are recommended to the reader:

Garnick, M. B. (ed.): Proceedings from a workshop symposium of the 14th international congress of chemotherapy. *Urology* 27 (Suppl. 1):1–32, 1986.

Peehl, D., Stamey, T. A.: Oncogenes: A review with relevance to cancers of the urogenital tract. *J. Urol.* 135:897, 1986.

7 Calculus Formation

▶ The comments for this chapter were written by Dr. Alan D. Jenkins, Assistant Professor of Urology, University of Virginia School of Medicine.—J.Y. Gillenwater, M.D.

Renal Calcium Deposition in Children: Sonographic Demonstration of the Anderson-Carr Progression
H. Patriquin and P. Robitaille (Hôpital Ste-Justine, Montreal)
AJR 146:1253–1256, June 1986   7–1

The Anderson-Carr theory of calculus formation, based on cadaver studies, states that microaggregates of calcium form at the tips and margins of the renal pyramid and may fuse to form plaques ("Randall's plaques"), which may perforate through the calix to form a nidus for further stone formation. Fifty children with diseases predisposing to nephrocalcinosis were examined with sonography and CT to determine the patterns of calcium deposition in the kidney in vivo and to correlate them with the Anderson-Carr progression of calculus formation. In seven patients high-resolution CT was performed.

At sonography, 24 patients had hyperechoic pyramids. Four patterns of hyperechogenicity were identified: hyperechogenic rim around the sides and tips of the pyramid; intense echogenic rim with echoes faintly filling the entire pyramid; intense echoes throughout the entire pyramid; and solitary focus at the tip of the pyramid near the fornix. These patterns appeared to follow the Anderson-Carr progression theory: The first three patterns represented increasing stages of calcium deposition beginning in the periphery of the renal pyramids, and the fourth showed stone formation at fornices. The sonographic pattern appears to provide an in vivo demonstration of the Anderson-Carr progression of renal stone formation.

▶ One neglected aspect of clinical urinary stone formation is particle retention. Healthy individuals often have urine that is supersaturated for calcium oxalate or calcium phosphate, and crystals of these salts may be seen in a fresh urine specimen. These particles are usually washed out of the urinary tract while they are very small, but retention of these crystals, possibly by attachment to the renal papilla, would permit the growth of clinically significant stones. Carr (*Br. J. Urol.* 26:105, 1954) speculated that these crystals were picked up by forniceal lymphatics, where they could grow until they eroded through the urothelium. Randall (*Surg. Gynecol. Obstet.* 64:201, 1937) found areas of subepithelial papillary calcification that could provide a nidus for macroscopic stone formation. Intracellular crystallization followed by epithelial erosion is a possible mechanism for the genesis of Randall's plaques.

Meticulous work by Cifuentes-Delatte (*J. Urol.*, May 1987) found that small calcium oxalate stones are not uniformly round, but have one surface with a concave depression. A small crystalline aggregate of calcium phosphate was sometimes found in this depression. Clinically significant growth of calcium oxalate stones may be initiated by epithelial precipitation of calcium phosphate that is subsequently overgrown with calcium oxalate.—A.D. Jenkins, M.D.

Immunochemistry of Urinary Calcium Oxalate Crystal Growth Inhibitor (CGI)
Michelle Lopez, Yasushi Nakagawa, Frederic L. Coe, Cheng Tsai, Alfred F. Michael, and Jon I. Scheinman (Univ. of Minnesota, Univ. of Chicago, and Duke Univ.)
Kidney Int. 29:829–833, 1986   7–2

Renal stone disease appears to involve breakdown of the normal balance between urinary supersaturation of calcium oxalate and urinary inhibitors of crystal nucleation and growth. A glycoprotein crystal growth inhibitor (CGI) was isolated from human urine and kidney that seems to account for most urinary macromolecular crystal growth. Antibodies to CGI suitable for immunoassay are available; they have been used along with CGI isolated from human urine in monomeric form, Tamm-Horsfall protein from human urine, and an antibody to this protein.

The anti-CGI, raised in rabbits, reacted on immunodiffusion, as determined by enzyme-linked immunoassay (ELISA) and by Western blotting of polyacrylamide gel electrophoresis-separated antigen. Immunofluorescence study localized CGI in the distal renal tubules in the same distribution as Tamm-Horsfall protein. Isolated Tamm-Horsfall protein bound CGI, and the bound inhibitor was only partially removed with ethylenediamine tetraacetic acid. The ELISA with anti-CGI detected inhibitor complexed to Tamm-Horsfall protein.

Whereas CGI in human urine possesses 90% of urinary macromolecular crystal growth inhibitory activitiy, Tamm-Horsfall protein does not alter crystal growth despite bound CGI. The balance between free and bound CGI may influence the overall balance of urinary macromolecules and the development of nephrolithiasis. Various urinary ionic constituents may affect the binding equilibrium of CGI.

▶ Urinary crystal growth inhibitors are usually classified according to the crystalline salt whose growth they inhibit: calcium phosphate or calcium oxalate. Traditional inhibitors of calcium phosphate crystal growth are pyrophosphate, citrate, and magnesium. Pyrophosphate and citrate also inhibit calcium oxalate crystal growth, but most of the calcium oxalate crystal growth inhibition in urine is provided by large molecular weight polyanions, e.g., glycoaminoglycans and RNA fragments. From human urine, Coe and his colleagues have isolated acidic glycoproteins that are potent inhibitors of calcium oxalate crystal growth. Patients with idiopathic calcium urolithiasis appear to have a functionally poor glycoprotein CGI.

This study localized CGI to the distal renal tubules, and the distribution of

CGI was the same as that of Tamm-Horsfall protein. Tamm-Horsfall protein alone appears to have no effect on crystal growth, but binding of CGI by this protein appears to reduce the inhibitory activity of CGI. The balance between free and bound CGI, not total CGI, may determine net inhibitory activity.— A.D. Jenkins, M.D.

Inhibitors of Urinary Stone Formation in 40 Recurrent Stone Formers
B. François, R. Cahen, and B. Pascal (Centre Hospitalo-Universitaire Lyon Sud, Pierre-Bénite, France)
Br. J. Urol. 58:479–483, October 1986   7–3

Recurrent urolithiasis may result from an increased concentration or output of lithogenic substrates, an increase in factors promoting nucleation, or a decrease in those physiologic factors that inhibit lithogenesis. Excretion of various inhibitors of urinary stone formation was estimated in 20 controls and 40 stone formers. The study group included 31 men and 9 women aged 21–66 years who had a history of recurrent stone formation, calcium-salt stones, and no established nephropathy or renal failure. A strict 800-mg calcium diet containing low levels of oxalic acid and purines was administered. The inhibitors studied were zinc, magnesium, citrates, and glycosaminoglycans (GAG).

No abnormality in excretion of zinc, magnesium, or GAG was apparent, but 11 patients had a low level of urinary citrate, usually in association with a urinary pH above 6. The citrate concentration was lower than control values in 19% of determinations and the 24-hour citrate output was lower in 33% of determinations. The ratio of average urinary citrate concentration in the patient and control groups was 0.56.

Hypocitraturia was observed in more than one fourth of the patients with recurrent urolithiasis in this study. In a few cases it was an isolated abnormality, but it usually was associated with hyperuricuria and a tendency to alkaline urine. None of the patients had renal tubular acidosis or gastrointestinal tract problems. There is evidence that oral citric acid administration can prevent experimentally produced stones, but it may induce alkalinization of the blood and urine. It might prove useful to determine urinary citrates systematically using a specific technique, e.g., the enzyme assay with citrate lyase.

▶ This and the following paper examine the popular topic of idiopathic hypocitraturic calcium urolithiasis. Urinary citrate is easily measured with a commercially available enzymatic kit. Low urinary citrate levels in the presence of an active urinary tract infection may underestimate true renal citrate excretion, because bacteria can metabolize citrate. These authors excluded patients with struvite stones, but they should have documented the absence of bacteriuria with formal urine cultures.

No difference between stone formers and healthy controls was found for 24-hour urinary citrate excretion, but the citrate concentration was significantly lower in the metabolically active stone formers. Volume data for the 24-hour urine collections were not reported, but the volumes had to be greater in the stone formers (if both groups had the same excretion, but the stone formers had a lower concentration). The "hypocitraturia" could be explained, at least in part, by a more avid fluid intake in the stone-forming patients. Nevertheless, true hypocitraturia is present in a subset of patients with idiopathic calcium urolithiasis, but its role as an isolated or critical factor in the pathogenesis of calcium stone formation is not known.—A.D. Jenkins, M.D.

Idiopathic Hypocitraturic Calcium-Oxalate Nephrolithiasis Successfully Treated With Potassium Citrate

Charles Y.C. Pak and Cindy Fuller (Univ. of Texas at Dallas)
Ann. Intern. Med. 104:33–37, January 1986   7–4

Hypocitraturia is frequent in nephrolithiasis and is important in calcium stone formation because of the inhibitory action of citrate in reducing urinary saturation of stone-forming calcium salts through formation of calcium complexes. Treatment with potassium citrate would seem to be logical in patients with "idiopathic" hypocitraturic calcium oxalate nephrolithiasis. Thirty-seven adults with a history of recurrent calcium oxalate stone formation were studied. Seventeen had hypocitraturia as the only abnormality; the others had absorptive hypercalciuria or, in two instances, hyperuricosuric calcium oxalate nephrolithiasis. Twenty-five patients took potassium citrate alone in daily doses of 30–80 mEq to restore a normal urinary citrate concentration. Twelve patients also received thiazide, allopurinol, or both.

Potassium citrate therapy consistently produced sustained increases in urinary citrate and potassium excretions and pH. Urinary calcium excretion did not change significantly in patients given potassium citrate alone. Potassium citrate therapy led to a sustained reduction in the urinary relative saturation ratio of calcium oxalate. The amount of undissociated uric acid decreased, but the relative saturation ratio of brushite was unchanged. The permissible increment in oxalate increased to the normal range. Only four patients continued to form stones, for a remission rate of 89%. Treatment was well tolerated except for minor gastrointestinal tract symptoms that were minimized by taking the drug with meals.

Potassium citrate is a rational treatment of patients with idiopathic hypocitraturic calcium oxalate nephrolithiasis. It restores normal urinary citrate excretion and inhibits new stone formation. Stone formation ceased in nearly 90% of patients in this study.

▶ Urinary citrate can retard stone formation in two ways. Citrate is a weak inhibitor of calcium oxalate crystal growth, but its major effect is a reduction of calcium oxalate supersaturation through complexation of calcium. Dr. Pak and his colleagues have championed the use of potassium citrate for the treatment of metabolically active calcium oxalate urolithiasis. The availability of potassium citrate tablets has rendered this an easy, safe approach. Unfortunately, hypocitraturia is found as an isolated abnormality in a minority of patients. Most patients with hypocitraturia have additional metabolic abnormalities, such as hypercalciuria, hyperuricosuria, or even mild hyperoxaluria. One third of the patients in this study were treated with thiazide, allopurinol, or both, in addition to potassium citrate.

Potassium citrate is useful in patients with renal tubular acidosis or uric acid lithiasis, and may be beneficial in patients with isolated hypocitraturia and metabolically active stone formation. Potassium citrate may be safer than allopurinol in patients with hyperuricosuric calcium oxalate nephrolithiasis, but patients prefer the single daily dose of allopurinol. To minimize the number of medications, potassium citrate could be used as a secondary drug in patients with concurrent hypercalciuria and hypocitraturia.—A.D. Jenkins, M.D.

Rice-Bran Treatment for Calcium Stone Formers With Idiopathic Hypercalciuria
S. Ebisuno, S. Morimoto, T. Yoshida, T. Fukatani, S. Yasukawa, and T. Ohkawa (Wakayama Med. College, Japan)
Br. J. Urol. 58:592–595, December 1986   7–5

The lithogenic and lithoinhibitory substances in the urine are thought to be important factors in urolithiasis. A high urinary calcium level is common in patients with renal calcium stones, and most of these patients probably have intestinal hyperabsorption of calcium. Because of this, a reduction in urinary calcium excretion may prevent stone formation, and several reports have provided evidence to support this claim. Rice-bran has effectively reduced urinary calcium excretion in patients with idiopathic hypercalciuria, and the hypocalciuric effect of rice-bran has been confirmed experimentally and clinically. A review was made of further experience in the treatment of patients with idiopathic hypercalciuria; the effect of rice-bran therapy on the recurrence rate of renal calcium stones was assessed, as was its influence on certain trace elements.

The study population consisted of 138 male and 26 female hypercalciuric patients with calcium-containing urinary stones. They were given rice-bran, 10 gm twice daily after meals, for 1–43 months. Blood and 24-hour urine specimens were collected and analyzed at regular intervals before and after treatment. The frequency of stone episodes was reduced dramatically, especially in "active recurrent stone formers." Urinary calcium excretion was also considerably reduced, and that of urinary phosphate and oxalate was slightly increased. There were no changes in serum levels of iron, copper, and zinc even when patients were treated for long periods. In general, the treatment was tolerated well and there were no serious side effects. Rice-bran therapy is particularly useful in patients with hyperabsorptive hypercalciuria and appears to be effective in the prevention of recurrent urinary stone disease.

▶ Hypercalciuria in most stone-forming patients is caused by intestinal hyperabsorption of dietary calcium. The hypercalciuria can be reduced by restricting the dietary calcium intake or by decreasing gastrointestinal tract absorption with a calcium-binding agent, e.g., sodium cellulose phosphate. The hypocalciuric effect of certain cereals was demonstrated 50 years ago. Subsequent studies showed that the mechanism was binding of dietary calcium in the gastrointestinal tract by nonabsorbable sodium phytate (inositol hexaphosphate). Sodium cellulose phosphate is a more modern drug that has the same mechanism of action. One problem with this class of drugs is that urinary excretion of magnesium increases and that of oxalate decreases. As expected, rice-bran treatment produced a mild hyperoxaluria. Urinary magnesium levels were normal, because this rice-bran preparation had a high magnesium content.—A.D. Jenkins, M.D.

Clinical Results of Allopurinol Treatment in Prevention of Calcium Oxalate Stone Formation
Hans-Göran Tiselius, Lasse Larsson, and Erik Hellgren (Univ. Hosp., Linköping, Sweden)
J. Urol. 138:50–53, July 1986   7–6

Allopurinol, 300 mg daily, was given to 76 male and 23 female patients with calcium oxalate stone disease. Treatment was started irrespective of the biochemical findings in blood or urine. Of the total, 65 were free of recurrent stone formation at the latest follow-up, 28 had new stones, and 6 demonstrated residual concrement growth. For those patients who had recurrent stone formation, 62% had been treated for more than 5 years, compared with 21% who were free of recurrent stones. Treatment was interrupted within the first 2 years by 46% of the patients who had further stone formation.

With increasing length of follow-up, the number of patients without recurrences decreased. Of 29 patients treated for an interval equal to or longer than that anticipated for new stone formation, only 12 remained free of stones. About 60% of the patients had new stones. Of 35 patients treated for more than 5 years, 20 continued to have stones and 15 did not. There was no difference among patients with recurrent and nonrecurrent stones with regard to urate excretion. Urinary urate excretion was decreased by about 30%, whereas all other urine variables were unaffected by treatment. Patients with recurrent stone formation had a urine composition that suggested a higher risk for crystallization.

Despite allopurinol treatment, the recurrence rate was substantial in patients followed for at least 5 years. The mean rate of stone formation was reduced in patients in whom the treatment period exceeded the interval anticipated for a new stone to develop. Only 43% of the patients treated for 5 or more years remained free of further stone formation.

It is believed that, possibly with the exception of hyperuricosuria or hyperuricemia, allopurinol treatment for recurrent calcium oxalate stone disease is weak. For valid conclusions to be reached, however, a larger number of allopurinol-treated patients with hyperuricosuric calcium oxalate stones need to be followed for long intervals. Also, it is difficult to draw conclusions as to the effects of different forms of treatment, especially because of the unpredictability of patients with calcium oxalate stone disease.

▶ Many patients with idiopathic calcium urolithiasis do not understand the chronic nature of their disease and the commitment required for a treatment program to be effective. Fluid and diet therapy is simple to comprehend but difficult to follow. A single daily dose of thiazide or allopurinol is very appealing and much less bother than multiple doses of orthophosphate or citrate.

These Swedish investigators found that empiric allopurinol is ineffective in the treatment of recurrent calcium oxalate stone disease in the absence of hyperuricosuria or hyperuricemia. Dr. Ettinger and his colleagues, in the following paper (Abstract 7–7), concluded that allopurinol could provide clinically significant protection to recurrent calcium oxalate stone formers who had hyperuricosuria as an isolated defect.—A.D. Jenkins, M.D.

Randomized Trial of Allopurinol in the Prevention of Calcium Oxalate Calculi
Bruce Ettinger, Anne Tang, John T. Citron, Barbara Livermore, and Thomas Williams (Kaiser Permanente Med. Ctrs., San Francisco, Walnut Creek, and Sacramento, and Univ. of Texas at San Antonio)
N. Engl. J. Med. 315:1386–1389, Nov. 27, 1986   7–7

Hyperuricosuria is the only metabolic abnormality in up to a fifth of patients with recurrent calcium oxalate calculi, and some studies have shown allopurinol to prevent recurrent calculi in these patients. The efficacy of allopurinol was examined in a double-blind study of 60 hyperuricosuric, normocalciuric patients with a history of calculi. Two or more stones consisting of more than 79% calcium oxalate had formed in the preceding 5 years, and at least one stone had formed in the preceding 2 years. Patients were assigned to either 100 mg of allopurinol three times daily or placebo tablets. The 29 allopurinol-treated patients and the 31 given placebo were clinically comparable.

Compliance neared 90% in both the treated and placebo groups. A hypouricosuric effect of allopurinol was evident after 3 months. Serum and urinary calcium levels were unchanged in both groups. New stone events occurred in 58% of the placebo group and in 31% of allopurinol-treated patients. Rates of events declined in both groups, compared with baseline rates. Actuarial analysis showed a significantly longer interval before recurrence of calculi in the allopurinol-treated patients.

Allopurinol can provide clinically significant protection in calcium oxalate stone formers who have hyperuricosuria as an isolated metabolic defect. Allopurinol presently is recommended in place of thiazides for such patients. Combined treatment is not recommended, however, as the risk of allergic reaction may be increased.

▶ This and the preceding paper examine the effectiveness of allopurinol in the care of patients with metabolically active idiopathic calcium urolithiasis. Between 10% and 20% of patients with idiopathic calcium urolithiasis have hyperuricosuria as an isolated metabolic abnormality. Dr. Ettinger and his associates found that allopurinol (100 mg three times daily) effectively prevented recurrent calcium oxalate stone formation in this subset of patients. They currently recommend allopurinol instead of thiazides for patients with isolated hyperuricosuria, even though thiazides can be as effective. There is an increased risk of allergic reactions with the simultaneous administration of thiazides and allopurinol.—A.D. Jenkins, M.D.

Anticystinuric Effects of Glutamine and of Dietary Sodium Restriction
Philippe Jaeger, Luc Portmann, Alda Saunders, Leon E. Rosenberg, and Samuel O. Thier (Univ. of Lausanne, Switzerland, and Yale Univ.)
N. Engl. J. Med. 315:1120–1123, Oct. 30, 1986   7–8

Glutamine reportedly can induce a marked reduction in cystine excretion in patients with cystinuria. However, these findings have not been confirmed by other investigators. To clarify this discrepancy, four patients with cystinuria were studied to assess the effects of glutamine and dietary sodium on the urinary excretion of dibasic amino acids.

Patient 1 had an ad libitum dietary sodium intake of about 300 mmole daily. Glutamine, administered orally in a dosage of 2.1 gm/day in three divided doses for 3 weeks, caused a marked decrease in urinary excretion of cystine and ornithine, but had no effect on excretion of lysine and arginine. Patient 2 had ad libitum dietary sodium intake of about 150 mmole daily. A similar dose of glutamine had no significant effect on the excretion rates of any amino acids studied. The most striking difference between patients 1 and 2 was their dietary intake of sodium. Patient 3, therefore, was given glutamine during dietary sodium intakes of 150 mmole and 300 mmole per day. Cystine and ornithine excretions, as well as lysine and arginine excretions, were significantly increased after a high sodium intake. Glutamine had a significant anticystinuric and antiornithinuric effect during high sodium intake but had no effect when sodium intake was 150 mmole per day. In the fourth patient, the effect of a further reduction in sodium intake was studied. A sodium intake of 50 mmole per day decreased urinary excretion of cystine markedly within 17 days, as well as the excretion of lysine, arginine, and ornithine.

These findings indicate that oral doses of glutamine can induce a marked decrease in urinary excretion of cystine. The reduced excretion of dibasic amino acids occurs at a high sodium intake but not at an intake of 150 mmole per day. However, because a sodium-dependent excretion of the dibasic amino acids occurs at an intake down to about 50 mmole per day, dietary sodium restriction may be a safe approach to patients with cystinuria.

▶ The ability of glutamine to reduce urinary cystine excretion was reported 8 years ago but never confirmed. The present inquiry found that cystine excretion increased significantly with a high sodium intake. Glutamine decreased cystine excretion only after an elevation associated with a high sodium intake and, therefore, would not be a practical treatment for cystinuria. Restriction of dietary sodium may be beneficial in cystinuric patients, especially if they cannot tolerate other agents such as D-penicillamine.—A.D. Jenkins, M.D.

Management of Cystine Nephrolithiasis With Alpha-Mercaptopropionylglycine

Charles Y.C. Pak, Cindy Fuller, Khashayar Sakhaee, Joseph E. Zerwekh, and Beverley V. Adams, with investigators from collaborating units (Univ. of Texas at Dallas)
J. Urol. 136:1003–1008, November 1986   7–9

Although effective in the treatment of cystinuria, the use of D-penicillamine is often accompanied by severe side effects that cause its withdrawal in about half of the patients treated. To determine the therapeutic role of α-mercaptopropionylglycine (α-MPG) as an alternative to D-penicillamine, 66 patients with cystine nephrolithiasis were studied, including 49 who had taken D-penicillamine before treatment with α-MPG and 17 who had not.

Treatment with D-penicillamine was associated with adverse side effects in 83.7% and α-MPG in 75.5% of patients who took both drugs. Symptoms were severe enough to stop D-penicillamine therapy in 69.4% and α-MPG in 30.6% of patients. Among those who discontinued taking D-penicillamine, 64.7% could be maintained with α-MPG. Among patients without a history of D-penicillamine therapy, 64.7% had adverse reactions to α-MPG. However, only 1 (5.9%) had serious side effects precluding cessation of α-MPG. During long-term treatment with α-MPG in an average dose of 1,193 mg per day, urinary cystine levels were maintained at 350–560 mg daily and urinary saturation of cystine was kept undersaturated. In addition, α-MPG produced remission of stone formation in 63% to 71% of patients and reduced individual stone formation rate in 81% to 94%.

α-Mercaptopropionylglycine has a definite therapeutic role in cystinuric patients with toxicity to D-penicillamine. Although overall side effects are frequent with α-MPG, serious side effects requiring cessation of therapy are uncommon and occur less frequently than with D-penicillamine. Moreover, α-MPG exhibits a biochemical action similar to that of D-penicillamine and is effective in inhibiting cystine stone formation.

▶ D-Penicillamine is used with increased oral fluids and alkali for the treatment of cystinuria. The drug undergoes a disulfide exchange reaction with cystine to form the soluble mixed disulfide of penicillamine and cysteine. Several analogues of D-penicillamine have been tested in the hope that fewer side effects would occur, but all have the same mechanism of action.

α-Mercaptopropionylglycine (or Thiola) is one such agent. The present authors found that adverse side effects occurred in three fourths of the patients who received either α-MPG or D-penicillamine. D-Penicillamine administration was halted in 70% of the patients. Most of these patients subsequently tolerated α-MPG, even though two thirds had adverse reactions. One third of the patients did not tolerate initial treatment with α-MPG.

Treatment with α-MPG does not appear to be significantly better than that with D-penicillamine, but it may be worthwhile in those individuals who have had a serious reaction to the latter drug. Some patients may still tolerate D-penicillamine if it is restarted slowly after a drug-free interval.—A.D. Jenkins, M.D.

Glucagon and Ureteric Calculi

David R. Webb, Ian N. Nunn, Donald McOmish, and William S.C. Hare (Univ. of Melbourne and The Royal Melbourne Hosp.)
Med. J. Aust. 144:124, Feb. 3, 1986   7–10

Glucagon was administered intravenously to five men and five women with severe ureteric colic. The average age was 39 years (range, 29–60 years), and the average stone diameter was 4.5 mm (range, 2–5 mm). Treatment consisted of 2 L of 5% dextrose intravenously in a 3-hour period, 1 mg of glucagon given intravenously after 30 minutes, and administration of pethidine, 100 mg, and prochlorperazine, 12.5 mg, for pain or nausea, if necessary. Progress was monitored radiographically and clinically.

Initially, seven patients received glucagon and three received placebo. A successful therapeutic result could not be obtained regardless of whether patients received glucagon, placebo, or glucagon after placebo. All placebo recipients and four of the seven given active medication required analgesia parenterally. Four patients required basket extraction of the stone, four passed the stone spontaneously more than 24 hours after hospital admission, and two underwent ureterolithotomy.

Because of a marked spasmolytic effect on smooth muscle, it was believed that glucagon could assist in the passage of ureteric calculi and diminish ureteric colic. This study was undertaken in the hope that hospital admission could be avoided and successful treatment obtained on an outpatient basis. Despite the small sample size, the 100% failure rate does not justify further investigation of this compound for short-term treatment.

▶ The spasmolytic effect of glucagon has been used to aid cannulation of the ampulla of Vater during endoscopic retrograde pancreatography. This study found that glucagon did not relieve renal colic or speed the spontaneous passage of ureteral calculi. There is no reason to think that glucagon would speed ureteral stone passage even if it did inhibit ureteral peristalsis. Patients in whom an obstructing steinstrasse develops after extracorporeal shock wave lithotripsy usually pass the sand after placement of a percutaneous nephrostomy. The effectiveness of peristalsis seems to improve after relief of the hydraulic ureteral distention. Inhibition of peristalsis by any agent, and the resultant ureteral dilatation, may delay spontaneous passage of a ureteral stone.—A.D. Jenkins, M.D.

The following review article is recommended to the reader:

Special Issue: Stone Diseases. *Urol. Int.* 41:325–396, 1986.

8 Pre- and Post- Operative Management

Osmotic Demyelination Syndrome Following Correction of Hyponatremia
Richard H. Sterns, Jack E. Riggs, and Sydney S. Schochet, Jr. (Univ. of Rochester and West Virginia Univ.)
New Engl. J. Med. 314:1535–1542, June 12, 1986   8–1

The need rapidly to correct severe hyponatremia to prevent death is tempered by concern that rapid correction may lead to central pontine myelinolysis. Eight patients treated at two centers in the past 5 years had serious neurologic complications from hyponatremia. Each became worse after relatively rapid correction of hyponatremia at a rate exceeding 12 mmole of sodium per L per day. The 5 patients at one hospital accounted for all neurologic complications in 60 patients with a serum sodium concentration of less than 116 mmole/L. No patient having less rapid correction of hyponatremia had neurologic sequelae. Only one patient became hypernatremic.

These findings are consistent with experimental evidence that pontine and extrapontine myelinolysis can result from rapid correction of hyponatremia, rather than from hyponatremia itself. Clinically evident neurologic injury is not observed when chronic hyponatremia is corrected slowly. Review of other series confirmed an association between rapid correction of hyponatremia and neurologic sequelae. Uneventful recovery is the rule when the rate of correction is less than 13 mmole/L/day.

There is no proved advantage to correcting hyponatremia rapidly. The convincing evidence that rapid correction may be hazardous suggests that chronically hyponatremic patients be managed chiefly by water restriction and withdrawal of thiazide diuretics. This may prevent further instances of osmotic demyelination syndrome.

Hyponatremia, Convulsions, Respiratory Arrest, and Permanent Brain Damage After Elective Surgery in Healthy Women
Allen I. Arieff (Univ. of California and VA Med. Ctr., San Francisco)
N. Engl. J. Med. 314:1529–1535, June 12, 1986   8–2

Hyponatremia may be the most frequent electrolyte disorder in general hospital patients, but permanent brain damage from this cause appears to be rare. Fifteen previously healthy women experienced severe hyponatremia after elective operations, independent of serious underlying medical disorders, and subsequently died or lived with permanent brain damage. The mean age was 41 years and the mean preoperative serum sodium concentration was 138 mmole/L.

All of the patients sustained grand mal seizures and respiratory arrest requiring intubation about 50 hours after operation, when the mean plasma sodium concentration was 108 mmole/L. The urinary sodium concentration averaged 68 mmole/L and osmolality, 501 mOsm/kg. Suspicion of cerebral vascular disorder resulted in delayed treatment in ten patients. Saline, with or without furosemide, was given after hyponatremia was diagnosed. Four patients died, three without regaining consciousness. Seven patients recovered consciousness but subsequently had impaired alertness and progressive obtundation, followed by recurrent seizures and coma. The six who survived remained in a vegetative state on follow-up for 2 years or longer. Histologic study in five patients showed no evidence of central pontine myelinolysis. Possible contributory factors included thiazide diuretics in three and phenothiazines in two others. All patients but two had received at least 6 L of hypotonic fluid postoperatively and had a urine output of less than 650 ml/24 hours.

Severe symptomatic hyponatremia can develop rapidly after elective operations in generally healthy women and can lead to death or a persistent vegetative state. Hyponatremia may interfere with glial metabolism or influence neurotransmitter release. The brain damage may also result in part from hypoxia with postanoxic encephalopathy after respiratory arrest.

▶ These two papers (8–1 and 8–2), taken together, are both disturbing and fascinating. Arieff defines a syndrome of postoperative hyponatremia in relatively young women that has devastating consequences. For unknown reasons this syndrome does not seem to appear in men and thus has not been described in patients after transurethral resection of the prostate. It seems to be caused by inappropriate intravenous fluid therapy and antidiuretic hormone secretion.

Sterns and associates describe eight new patients with central pontine myelinosis (CPM), an entity first described in 1959 (Wright, D. G., et al.: *Arch. Neurol. Psychiatry* 81:154, 1959). Sterns and associates argue from their data and the literature that rapid correction of hyponatremia (more than 12 mmole/L/day) results in CPM. It should be noted that their patients had chronic hyponatremia, whereas Arieff's patients had acute hyponatremia. None of the latter women had CPM, and Arieff believes that correction of 0.5 mmole/hour is indicated. He states that CPM occurs only when hyponatremia is corrected to more than 132 mmole/L. It would seem that his recommendations are reasonable, particularly for acute-onset hyponatremia. In the chronic hyponatremia patient slightly slower correction would seem appropriate. These papers provide new insight into a rare but extremely serious complication of a metabolic problem that all of us encounter from time to time.—S.S. Howards, M.D.

9 Kidney Trauma

Fate of Functionless Post-Traumatic Renal Segment
Norman E. Peterson (Univ. of Colorado)
Urology 27:237–242, March 1986   9–1

When a renal segment is found to be without function, the tendency is to remove it surgically and repair the viable part of the kidney. However, this may not always be necessary. A review was made of 209 blunt renal injuries treated between 1973 and 1983, 50 of them major, and of 131 penetrating injuries, 61 major. Functionless renal parenchymal segments were demonstrated urographically and managed conservatively in 13 instances. One patient subsequently became hypertensive and underwent partial nephrectomy, with a good outcome. Another required renal arterial embolization because of significant delayed hematuria. The other patients, and two with complications, were asymptomatic and normotensive after 5–10 years. Function was normal in the intact parenchyma but did not return in the initially functionless segments.

The surgical significance of renal injuries resulting in a functionless parenchymal segment depends on the clinical sequelae of injury to the collecting system and of interruption of major branch vessels. Extravasation generally resolves spontaneously in the absence of urinary tract obstruction. Perinephric abscess, which is rare, may be drained percutaneously or incisionally. Angiography is necessary if there is persistent, delayed, or intermittent posttraumatic hematuria. Selective embolization may be used to control bleeding vessels. Hypertension is often delayed for some time after trauma. Routine nonoperative management is not suggested if segmental infarction is present, but operation sometimes is best delayed, especially if the diagnosis is made in the subacute stage, the patient is in stable condition, and there is doubt as to the need for operation to salvage renal parenchyma or prevent complications.

▶ The approach to renal trauma is gradually changing. This paper provides interesting information regarding the long-term outcome of kidneys with nonfunctioning segments. Only 2 of 13 such kidneys treated nonoperatively required further therapy. It has become clear over the past few years that many renal trauma patients can be handled with careful observation. Operative intervention frequently results in nephrectomy in inexperienced hands; however, Dr. Jack McAninch reported at the 1987 meeting of the American Association of Genitourinary Surgeons that he has saved between 80% and 90% of the kidneys on which he has operated for trauma. He also mentioned that the decision whether or not to intervene in patients with stab wounds can be made from a CT scan, and slightly less than 50% of these patients require surgical intervention. The CT scan is now accepted by most authorities as the best initial diagnostic study for patients with significant renal trauma.—S.S. Howards, M.D.

10 Ureteral Injuries

Iatrogenic Ureteral Injury
Robert A. Dowling, Joseph N. Corriere, Jr., and Carl M. Sandler (Univ. of Texas at Houston)
J. Urol. 135:912–915, May 1986   10–1

Information on 27 patients treated for iatrogenic ureteral injury between 1979 and 1984 was reviewed. Nearly two thirds of the 20 women were younger than age 45 years, whereas all but 1 of the 7 men were older. About half of the injuries were incurred during gynecologic procedures and nearly a third during urinary tract operations.

Four injuries were recognized and treated at primary operation. In most of these patients a ureter was transected in the course of a difficult pelvic dissection, and primary anastomosis over an indwelling stent was performed. In the delayed cases, flank pain and fever were the most common symptoms. Four patients were seen 10–30 days after hysterectomy with a ureterovaginal fistula. Five others had a ureterocutaneous fistula. The diagnosis was made by excretory urography, and the nature and level of injury were confirmed by retrograde ureterography in most cases. Percutaneous nephrostomy was not considered in six patients (table). Successful percutaneous nephrostomy was carried out in 11. Both ureteral ligations and ureteral fistulas were included in this group. Four patients required operation after attempted percutaneous nephrostomy drainage. Complications attended two thirds of prolonged percutaneous nephrostomy drainage procedures. Six patients were treated for pyelonephritis.

RESULTS IN 23 PATIENTS WITH DELAYED PRESENTATION
OF IATROGENIC URETERAL INJURY

	No./Total
Percutaneous nephrostomy not considered:	6/23
Nephrectomy, 1	
Ureteroneocystostomy, 2	
Retrograde ureteral catheter, 1	
Surgical deligation, 2	
Percutaneous nephrostomy not established:	2/17
Spontaneous resolution, 1	
Nephroureterectomy, 1	
Percutaneous nephrostomy successful:	11/15
Ureteral ligations, 6	
Ureteral fistulas, 5	
Percutaneous nephrostomy established but failed:	4/15
Ureteroneocystostomy, 2	
Ureteroureterostomy, 1	
Nephrectomy, 1	

The ureter may be injured in 10% or more of radical hysterectomies. Percutaneous nephrostomy, with or without stenting, is a useful approach to iatrogenic ureteral injuries recognized late in the postoperative period. Ureteral fistulas must be stented. The nephrostomy catheter is removed after contrast study has shown resolution of the injury. However, complications, including pyelonephritis, may occur. The rare instance of ureteral ligation that is discovered within 3 days of operation may be managed best by immediate operation.

Iatrogenic Ureteral Injury: Aggressive or Conservative Treatment
S. Witters, M. Cornelissen, and R. Vereecken (Catholic Univ. of Leuven, Belgium)
Am. J. Obstet. Gynecol. 155:582–584, September 1986   10–2

Most ureteral injuries in women having pelvic surgery occur at the level of the infundibulopelvic ligament, and they are especially likely to occur when the course of the ureter is abnormal or when the ureter is inadequately identified. Twenty-eight ureteral injuries in 23 women and 3 men were treated in 1980–1984. Most injuries occurred during gynecologic surgery. There were 13 partial or complete ligations and 10 transections in the series.

Seven injuries in six patients were recognized at initial operation, and ureteroureterostomy or ureteroneocystostomy was carried out successfully. Fourteen other patients underwent operative reconstruction in the first 3 weeks. Percutaneous nephrostomy succeeded in only two of six patients; the other four required delayed ureteroneocystostomy. Eighteen patients in all underwent ureteroneocystostomy. Four had ureteroureterostomy, and three had a Boari bladder flap procedure. All but one of the patients having ureteroneocystostomy or a Boari bladder flap operation had a good outcome. The 25 patients evaluated after 1 year were free of symptoms and had normal findings at intravenous urography. A patient having pelvic flap reconstruction also had a good outcome.

Ureteroneocystostomy has given excellent results in patients with iatrogenic ureteral injuries, and it is indicated for use whenever feasible. If a lower ureteral injury is present and the defect is too long for ureteroneocystostomy, with or without a psoas hitch maneuver, construction of a bladder flap will provide sufficient length for anastomosing the ureter to the bladder.

▶ Ureteral injuries are not uncommon, occurring in approximately 2% of gynecologic procedures and 3.5% of abdominal perineal resections. Most are recognized at the time of surgery, although this was not the case in the above reviews, which came from referral centers.

Intraoperative injuries should be repaired immediately. Whenever possible, a ureteral neocystostomy should be done because the success rate is very high. We think that, barring special circumstances, all ureteral injuries can be repaired when discovered. Prompt resolution of the problem benefits the patient and also the physician who caused the injury, because he is usually concerned about possible litigation.

The Houston group (Abstract 10–1) is much more predisposed to use percutaneous nephrostomy than are the surgeons in Belgium (Abstract 10–2). We agree that fistulas that can be bypassed with a double-J catheter should be treated nonoperatively, but we prefer surgical intervention for the obstructed ureter. This resolves the problem more quickly and with a higher success rate. The data above support this approach. Witters and associates had success in only two of six patients treated with percutaneous nephrostomy. Although Dowling and associates avoided surgery in six of ten patients with obstructed ureters, the average duration of nephrostomy drainage was 55 days and in one patient the procedure failed after 165 days.—S.S. Howards, M.D.

11 Lower Tract Trauma

Management of the Ruptured Bladder: Seven Years of Experience With 111 Cases
Joseph N. Corriere, Jr., and Carl M. Sandler (Univ. of Texas at Houston)
J. Trauma 26:830–833, September 1986   11–1

The 111 patients seen in a 7-year period with bladder rupture represent the largest series of patients with extraperitoneal bladder rupture managed conservatively. Iatrogenic bladder injuries and injuries caused by migrating internal objects were excluded. Blunt trauma was responsible for 86% of injuries. More than 81% of patients were 40 years or younger. There were 63 males and 48 females in the series. All but 1 of 55 patients with extraperitoneal bladder rupture resulting from blunt trauma had a pelvic fracture. Thirty-two injuries of other genitourinary organs occurred, including 11 posterior urethral injuries in males. No deaths resulted from urologic injuries or other treatment.

All penetrating injuries were managed by débridement of the missile tract, closure of the defect, and suprapubic or Foley catheter drainage. No complications occurred, and all patients had normal cystograms after 10 days. Forty-eight patients with blunt injuries had formal closure of the bladder wound and cystotomy or Foley catheter drainage for at least 10 days, and all of them did well without complications (table). Thirty-nine other patients were managed by bladder drainage alone, usually Foley catheter drainage. Extravasation persisted at 10 days in five patients, in whom tube drainage was continued until the bladder wound healed. None of these patients had complications.

Noniatrogenic bladder injuries generally may be managed successfully by conservative means. If a bone spicule perforates the bladder, however,

MANAGEMENT OF BLADDER RUPTURES DUE TO BLUNT TRAUMA	
Intraperitoneal injuries (35)	
Exploration, closure, cystotomy	34
Died before therapy	1
Extraperitoneal injuries (55)	
Exploration, closure, cystotomy	9
Foley catheter or SP tube only	39
Died before therapy	7
Combined intra- and extraperitoneal injuries (5)	
Exploration, closure, cystotomy	5

(Courtesy of Corriere, J.N., Jr., et al.: J. Trauma 26:830–833, September 1986. © by Williams & Wilkins, 1986.)

surgical removal clearly is indicated. Extraperitoneal bladder ruptures may be treated by simple catheter drainage and close observation; antibiotics have not been used routinely. If a patient is to be explored for associated injuries and is not very ill, the dome of the bladder is opened, the rupture repaired intravesically, and suprapubic drainage instituted.

▶ Drs. Corriere and Sandler unequivocally establish with this paper that extra-peritoneal nonpenetrating injuries of the bladder can be treated by urethral catheter drainage alone. Several points should be emphasized. They still recommend open repair of intraperitoneal injuries, penetrating injuries, and injuries in which bone punctures the bladder. Fourteen percent of their patients required long-term drainage before they healed. Dr. Jack McAninch, who discussed this paper at the annual meeting of the American Association for the Surgery of Trauma, believes that, in spite of these results, the treatment of choice for these injuries is open repair to avoid infected hematomas, pseudo-diverticulas, and persistent drainage. We usually explore these patients but do on occasion treat them with catheter drainage. The latter approach requires very careful observation.—S.S. Howards, M.D.

12 Adrenals

Difficulties in the Prospective Diagnosis of Functional Adrenal Diseases by CT
P.J. Kenney, D.P. Streeten, and G.H. Anderson (SUNY, Upstate Med. Ctr.)
Urol. Radiol. 8:184–189, 1986   12–1

The widespread availability of CT has greatly improved radiologic detection of adrenal abnormalities. Computed tomography is valuable in detecting functional adrenal disorders including cortical adenoma, pheochromocytoma, adrenal carcinoma, and adrenocortical hyperplasia. Nevertheless, CT images of adrenal masses are nonspecific, and nonfunctioning masses are often seen as incidental findings. An evaluation was made of the accuracy of prospective CT interpretation in patients suspected of having functional adrenal disorders. The technique was also compared with intensive radiologic methods, i.e., selective adrenal venography and venous sampling.

Sixty-five patients who were strongly suspected of having functional adrenal disorders underwent CT evaluation; 37 of these also underwent adrenal venography and selective adrenal venous sampling. Of the 65 patients, 21 had a hyperfunctioning cortical adenoma, 25 had cortical or medullary hyperplasia, 11 had pheochromocytoma, and 10 had no functional adrenal disease. Diagnosis by CT alone was correct in 66%; diagnosis by CT and venous sampling was correct in 89%. Incorrect prospective CT diagnosis was most often the result of a normal appearance of functionally hyperplastic glands (nine patients), nodular hyperplasia simulating a focal adenoma (eight), or an incidental nonfunctioning mass (3).

It is necessary to correlate CT findings with biochemical evaluation, and it is useful to carry out venous sampling in selected patients to avoid inappropriate surgery. When CT is interpreted in correlation with complete biochemical analysis, the correct diagnosis can usually be made, although in a small number of patients adrenal venous sampling may still be required.

▶ This study documents that CT alone is not very accurate for the evaluation of adrenal disease. This information is neither new nor surprising. Anyone who treats adrenal pathology soon realizes that the evaluation is complex and time consuming and requires a sophisticated diagnostic team. Computed tomography is usually very good for pheochromocytomas, which are usually large, and for adrenal carcinoma. As confirmed by Kenney and associates, CT often misses adrenal hyperplasia and the adenomas associated with primary aldosteronism. In these patients careful biochemical workup, radionuclide scanning, and venous sampling are often necessary.—S.S. Howards, M.D.

Fifty Cases of Primary Hyperaldosteronism in Hong Kong Chinese With a High Frequency of Periodic Paralysis: Evaluation of Techniques for Tumor Localization

J.T.C. Ma, C. Wang, K.S.L. Lam, R.T.T. Yeung, F.L. Chan, John Boey, P.S.Y. Cheung, J.P. Coghlan, B.A. Scoggins, and J.R. Stockigt (Queen Mary Hosp., Hong Kong, and Alfred Hosp., Melbourne)

Q. J. Med. (New Series) 61:1021–1037, November 1986   12–2

Various methods of localizing adrenal aldosteroma were assessed in a series of 50 consecutive patients seen in 1969–1985. An adrenocortical adenoma was excised in 46 instances. Adrenal venous sampling and venography were carried out at the same time, with estimates of aldosterone and cortisol levels. Computed tomography also was performed.

The mean age was 40 years. Muscle weakness and periodic paralysis were the most frequent presenting features. Twenty-one patients had 33 episodes of periodic paralysis. The leg muscles were the most frequently affected. The mean duration of known hypertension was about 4 years. One fifth of the patients had significant vascular complications. The mean presenting serum potassium level was 2.1 mmole/L. Plasma renin activity usually was below the limit of detection. Adrenal venography was an unreliable localizing procedure and it was misleading in two instances; adrenal venous sampling for steroid analysis was much more helpful. The side of the adenoma was predicted in 97% of the patients based on estimates of left adrenal venous and vena caval aldosterone levels. High-resolution CT was 100% accurate in 18 surgically treated patients. The smallest tumor detected was 0.8 cm in diameter. Hypokalemia was corrected in all patients treated surgically, and 37 of the 46 patients required no further antihypertensive therapy.

Episodic paralysis is not the rule in patients with primary hyperaldosteronism. Chinese patients appear to have especially low serum potassium levels. At present, CT is the first-line study method. Adrenal venous sampling is reserved for those in whom CT does not show a tumor despite biochemical findings indicating an aldosterone-producing adenoma. A unilateral loin approach to excision of the adenoma is most useful. If surgery is not feasible, spironolactone therapy is effective in the management of hypertension and hypokalemia.

▶ We agree that venography is not very useful in patients with primary hyperaldosteronism. Indeed, it can be dangerous, resulting in injury to the normal glands. Our experience and that of others (please see above) with CT is not as good as that reported by Ma and associates. Two interesting aspects of their experience are the high incidence of hypokalemia and paralysis, and the fact that left adrenal plus caval sampling was so accurate. This is important because right adrenal sampling is often technically very difficult.—S.S. Howards, M.D.

The Value of the Clonidine-Suppression Test in the Diagnosis of Pheochromocytoma

Bengt E. Karlberg, Lisbeth Hedman, Sten Lennquist, and Thomas Pollare (Univ. Hosp., Linköping, and Academic Hosp., Uppsala, Sweden)
World J. Surg. 10:753–761, October 1986   12–3

The clinical diagnosis of pheochromocytoma is simple when typical signs and symptoms are associated with biochemical evidence of increased catecholamine production. Nevertheless, in the presence of small tumors and/or less characteristic clinical symptoms, the diagnosis may be difficult. Because of this, there is a need for more specific biochemical markers in the safe and accurate diagnosis of pheochromocytoma. In normal individuals, administration of clonidine (which acts by stimulating central α-adrenergic receptors and thereby decreases sympathetic nerve stimulation at the peripheral receptors) suppresses plasma catecholamine activity. But in pheochromocytoma patients, however, clonidine administration should not suppress plasma catecholamines.

Assessment was made of the value of the clonidine-suppression test in the diagnosis of pheochromocytoma in three different groups: Group I, 10 patients with surgically verified catecholamine-secreting tumors; group II, 34 patients with "neurogenic" hypertension; and group III, 14 normotensive, healthy persons. Clonidine, 300 μg given orally at time 0, significantly reduced the mean systolic/diastolic blood pressure in all three groups, with the maximum fall occurring between 2 and 3 hours after administration of the drug. The mean plasma concentrations of noradrenaline/norephinephrine (NA) decreased in groups II and III, but the plasma concentrations of adrenaline/epinephrine (A) were low and remained unchanged throughout the test. In contrast, in patients with pheochromocytoma (group I), NA and A mean plasma concentrations were high before clonidine and remained high or somewhat elevated during the 3 hours of observation. In none of the patients was a decrease in plasma catecholamines observed during the test. After successful surgery for catecholamine-secreting tumors, all ten patients in group I had normal blood pressure and normal basal plasma catecholamine concentrations with normal suppression of NA after clonidine therapy.

The clonidine-suppression test is a safe, simple diagnostic method for verification or exclusion of pheochromocytomas, especially in patients with normal resting catecholamine levels. There was no significant or clinically relevant side effects during the test apart from sedation and dry mouth.

▶ The diagnosis of pheochromocytoma is usually not difficult. We still prefer to screen patients with urinary tests for catecholamines, vanillylmandelic acid determinations, and metanephrines. Results of serum tests can be misleading and require a good laboratory. There are patients with pheochromocytomas who have normal serum levels of catecholamines between hypertensive episodes. Karlberg and associates have confirmed the observation of Bravo et al. (*N. Engl. J. Med.* 305:623, 1981) that the clonidine suppression test is simple, safe, and accurate. For the occasional patient in whom the diagnosis is difficult, it appears to be a useful addition.—S.S. Howards, M.D.

Incidentally Discovered Mass of the Adrenal Gland

Arie Belldegrun, Sarwat Hussain, Steven E. Seltzer, Kevin R. Loughlin, Ruben F. Gittes, and Jerome P. Richie (Brigham and Women's Hosp., Boston, and Harvard Univ.)

Surg. Gynecol. Obstet. 163:203–208, September 1986
12–4

The wider use of high-resolution CT has led to the incidental discovery of increasing numbers of asymptomatic adrenal masses. However, these incidental adrenal masses pose a dilemma in terms of clinical significance and the need for further evaluation or treatment. A review was made of experience with 88 adrenal abnormalities detected incidentally on some 12,000 abdominal CT scans performed in an 8-year period, for an incidence of 0.7%.

Of the 61 patients available for follow-up, 28 had no known primary malignant condition and were evaluated for symptoms unrelated to adrenal pathology. The remaining 33 patients had a known primary malignant condition and CT was obtained as part of a staging workup or for tumor monitoring. Overall, adrenal lesions were detected in 53 patients and involved 59 glands; 8 patients had symmetrically enlarged adrenals. All 17 adenomas, except for 2 (4 cm and 6 cm), measured 1.0–3.5 cm on CT scanning. All carcinomas of the adrenal cortex were at least 6 cm in diameter. One striking feature was the high percentage of malignant masses discovered by CT: 39% of the group without known malignancy, including 18% with carcinoma of the cortex, and 21% with metastatic tumors, and 73% of those whose malignancy was known. Adrenalectomy, performed in 23 patients (26%), included three adenomas measuring 2.5 cm, 3.0 cm, and 6.5 cm; five carcinomas of the adrenal gland measuring 6–20 cm; two hyperplasias; and three adenocarcinomas of unknown origin. The remaining 38 patients had nonfunctioning masses. Follow-up scans, performed an average of 25.1 months (range, 3–60) after detection, revealed no change in size. All silent primary (nonmetastatic) masses measuring 3.5 cm or less manifested benign behavior.

All solid metabolically inactive lesions in the adrenal glands larger than 3.5 cm on CT abdominal scan deserve exploration. Smaller lesions may be followed safely with serial CT scans.

▶ Adrenal "incidentalomas" have been discussed in the 1983, 1985, and 1986 Year Books. This series is the largest of which we are aware. Of course, more than half of the lesions were found in patients with known primary malignancies. The authors conclude that lesions smaller than 3.5 cm on CT can be followed and those larger than 3.5 cm should be explored. This is not very different from our policy stated in the 1986 Year Book that one should first rule out a functioning lesion with the usual endocrine workup; then, for nonfunctioning lesions smaller than 3 or 4 cm, follow with serial sonograms; with lesions between 4 and 5 cm, do fine-needle aspiration biopsy (FNAB); for lesions 6 cm or larger, operate. The Brigham group thinks that FNAB is not useful, but we disagree. We do concur that the patient's age and other variables need to be considered in any decision.—S.S. Howards, M.D.

Comparison of Adrenal Cortical Tumors in Children and Adults

Philip T. Cagle, Aubrey J. Hough, T. Jeffrey Pysher, David L. Page, Ed H. Johnson, Rebecca T. Kirkland, John H. Holcombe, and Edith P. Hawkins (Baylor College of Medicine and Texas Children's Hosp., Houston, Univ. of Arkansas, Univ. of Oklahoma, and Vanderbilt Univ.)
Cancer 57:2235–2237, June 1, 1986   12–5

Various morphological features were examined as predictors of malignant behavior in a series of 23 adrenocortical tumors resected from children in 1953–1983. The 19 girls and 4 boys had a mean age of 5.5 years. Comparison was made with findings in 42 adult patients. Six children and 13 adults had malignant tumors.

Five children died of disease a median of 6 months after resection, and another had pulmonary metastasis. Seventeen patients lived for 2–25 years without disease. All six carcinomas in pediatric patients displayed hormonal, usually virilizing, effects. Ten benign tumors produced Cushing's syndrome and six, virilization. Tumor size was the only reliable predictor of malignant behavior in the pediatric series (table); both 100 gm and 500 gm were useful cutoff values. Benign tumors in children were more likely than those in adults to exhibit mitoses, necrosis, broad fibrous bands, and moderate to severe pleomorphism.

Adrenocortical neoplasms in pediatric patients are much more likely to be benign than was previously thought. The morphological criteria for predicting biologic behavior differ for pediatric and adult tumors. Tumor size is the only reliable predictor in children. Tumors weighing less than

COMPARISON OF MORPHOLOGICAL PATTERNS OF ADRENAL CORTICAL
TUMORS IN CHILDREN AND ADULTS*

	Childhood tumors (N = 23)		Adult tumors (N = 42)	
	Benign	Malignant	Benign	Malignant
Total	17	6	29	13
Size				
>100 g	5	6	6	10
>500 g	0	5	3	6
Necrosis	12	6	4	11
Moderate to severe pleomorphism	11	5	7	13
Mitoses	10	4	2	3
Abnormal mitoses	4	3	NS	NS
Broad fibrous bands	8	3	2	10
Capsular invasion	4	3	6	6
Vascular invasion	3	3	3	4
Calcifications	7	1	NS	NS

*NS, not stated.
(Courtesy of Cagle, P.T., et al.: Cancer 57:2235–2237, June 1, 1986.)

100–150 gm tend to be benign, whereas those heavier than 500 gm consistently exhibit malignant behavior.

▶ The definition of "malignant" that these authors use is "producing metastases and/or resulting in death . . . ." Because it is self-evident that a malignant tumor can be excised surgically and cured, the authors' conclusions are not valid. The major conclusion should be rephrased to state that pediatric adrenal cortical neoplasms are much more likely to be benign or *surgically curable* than previously thought.—S.S. Howards, M.D.

Immunohistochemical Evidence for the Vascular Origin of Primary Adrenal Pseudocysts
Pamela A. Groben, Joseph B. Roberson, Jr., Sally R. Anger, Frederic B. Askin, William G. Price, and Gene P. Siegal (Univ. of North Carolina)
Arch. Pathol. Lab. Med. 110:121–123, February 1986   12–6

Pseudocysts are the most common symptomatic, nonfunctioning cystic adrenal lesions. Tissue from two patients with adrenal pseudocysts was examined by immunohistochemical analysis of paraffin sections with antibodies directed against laminin and type IV collagen to determine the origin of these cysts.

The antibody staining pattern showed intense linear staining surrounding the cystic spaces and at the adrenal cortex-pseudocyst interface, suggesting that these lesions are vascular. Therefore, they are related to adrenal cysts of endothelial origin.

13 Kidney and Ureter

Atrial Natriuretic Factor: Renal and Systemic Effects
Steven A. Atlas (Cornell Univ.)
Hosp. Pract. 21:67–77, July 15, 1986

13–1

Observations that atrial tachyarrhythmias and atrial distention are associated with renal sodium and water loss were followed by the isolation of an active factor in atrial extracts, i.e., atrial natriuretic factor (ANF). It is a small polypeptide hormone that appears to reside predominantly, if not solely, in the heart. Atrial natriuretic factor-like immunoreactivity has been described in the salivary glands as well as in the pituitary and many brain regions, particularly the hypothalamus.

In addition to inducing natriuresis, ANF inhibits release of renin, aldosterone, and vasopressin, and has prominent hemodynamic effects when infused, including a decrease in blood pressure. The latter apparently results from reduced cardiac output, but a direct vasorelaxant effect is a possibility. Atrial natriuretic factor antagonizes the vasoconstrictive effect of angiotensin II, and the distribution of ANF receptors in the brain overlaps that of angiotensin II receptors. The effects of ANF on renin secretion may be related to its renal hemodynamic actions. Infusion of ANF inhibits vasopressin release in dehydrated dogs. Atrial natriuretic factor inhibits adenylate cyclase in certain tissues, e.g., adrenal cortex and vascular smooth muscle.

Deficiency of ANF has not been described clinically, but its abnormal release could have a role in idiopathic edema and other disorders of volume regulation. The use of ANF as a therapeutic agent is attractive, because it is a naturally occurring diuretic that causes only minimal potassium loss. It must be given parenterally, however, and it might conceivably have adverse effects, e.g., a decrease in cardiac output.

▶ This is an excellent summary of current knowledge about ANF. The existence of such a hormone has long been postulated by DeWardener, and one of the first papers showing that a humoral substance that inhibited renal tubular reabsorption of sodium was released in volume overload was by Howards et al. (*J. Clin. Invest.* 47:1561, 1968). Atrial natriuretic factor is released by the atrium in response to mechanical stretch. The hormone increases the glomerular filtration rate by relaxing afferent arterioles and constricting efferent arterioles. It antagonizes the vasoconstrictor and aldosterone stimulation actions of angiotensin II. Blood pressure and cardiac outputs are reduced by ANF. Future studies of ANF will undoubtedly show diseases with increased or decreased production of ANF, and it will perhaps be used as a clinical diuretic.—J.Y. Gillenwater, M.D.

Proteinuria in Benign Nephrosclerosis

Gabriel Morduchowicz, Geoffrey Boner, Mina Ben-Bassat, and Joseph B. Rosenfeld (Beilinson Med. Ctr., Petah Tikva, and Sackler School of Medicine, Tel Aviv, Israel)

Arch. Intern. Med. 146:1513–1516, August 1986   13–2

Proteinuria and renal failure are uncommon in benign nephrosclerosis. A retrospective study was made of the clinical course of 12 patients aged 24–59 years with hypertension, proteinuria in excess of 1 gm/day, and findings of benign nephrosclerosis in renal biopsy specimens. Hypertension and proteinuria were diagnosed during pregnancy in three patients. Eleven patients were followed for 5–21 years (mean, 14.5 years) after onset of hypertension.

Four patients were nephrotic, with proteinuria of more than 3.5 gm/1.73 m/day at biopsy, and five others became nephrotic in the course of their disease. Renal function deteriorated in 7 of 12 patients, 2 of them reaching end-stage renal disease and requiring maintenance dialysis. Histopathologic findings in all biopsy specimens, obtained a mean 7.7 years after onset of hypertension, were indicative of benign nephrosclerosis.

The combination of hypertension, proteinuria, and benign nephrosclerosis is predictive of a poor prognosis, with renal failure developing in a high percentage of patients. This observation is supported by another study in which 75% of 16 patients with benign nephrosclerosis and nephrotic syndrome progressed to end-stage renal disease during a period of 1–4 years.

▶ In hypertension, two different pathologic and clinical courses have been described: malignant nephrosclerosis and benign arteriolar nephrosclerosis. In this report 7 of 12 patients with benign nephrosclerosis associated with hypertension and proteinuria of more than 1 gm/day had a decrease in renal function.—J.Y. Gillenwater, M.D.

Focal Glomerulosclerosis and Proteinuria in Patients With Solitary Kidneys

Victor Gutierrez-Millet, Javier Nieto, Manuel Praga, Gabriel Usera, Miguel A. Martinez, and Jose M. Morales (1 de Octubre Hosp., Madrid)

Arch. Intern. Med. 146:705–709, April 1986   13–3

Glomerulosclerosis in the presence of a reduced renal mass has been ascribed to compensatory increases in renal blood flow and the glomerular filtration rate (GFR). Studies were done in ten normotensive patients (nine men) aged 28–51 years with a solitary functioning kidney and proteinuria. Six patients had unilateral nephrectomy previously, three because of tuberculous pyelonephritis, and four had unilateral renal agenesis. Pyelography showed one functioning kidney with compensatory hypertrophy in each patient.

Six patients had chronic renal failure at biopsy. Proteinuria was in the nephrotic range in three. The degree of proteinuria could not be related to the GFR. Immunologic findings were normal except in two patients. Two became hypertensive and required treatment on follow-up for 4–8 months after renal biopsy. Focal glomerulosclerosis was found in all seven surgical biopsy specimens. Six lesions were classified as focal and segmental glomerulosclerosis and one was classified as focal and global glomerulosclerosis. Tubulointerstitial lesions were seen in five cases and minimal arteriolar wall thickening in four. Variable deposition of IgM and C3 was seen in the focal and segmental lesions. Ultrastructural studies showed diffuse foot process fusion and detachment of podocytes from the glomerular basement membrane in regions of altered loops. Sclerotic areas exhibited basement membrane-like material and hyaline deposits occluding the capillary lumen.

The glomerular lesions seen in patients with a solitary kidney could result from chronic glomerular hyperfiltration that is maintained for a sufficient time. Males with a high protein intake in early life may be at increased risk.

▶ Most urologists believe that a patient with a solitary kidney does not have an increased risk of morbidity and mortality from renal disease. In one study, animals with about 84% of the functioning renal mass removed became proteinuric and hypertensive, and progressive renal failure ensued associated with glomerulosclerosis. Brenner et al. (*N. Engl. J. Med.* 307:652, 1982) suggested that the progressive sclerosing glomerulopathy could be a consequence of the increased GFR and renal blood flow in the remaining glomeruli. In this paper, ten patients with a solitary kidney and proteinuria were evaluated. Renal biopsies in seven patients showed glomerulosclerosis. It must be pointed out that six of the ten patients presented with chronic renal failure and three with nephrotic syndrome. This is a highly selected group of patients and does not prove that patients with a solitary kidney are at a higher risk for the development of glomerulosclerosis.—J.Y. Gillenwater, M.D.

Percutaneous Ablation in Patients With End-Stage Renal Disease: Alternative to Surgical Nephrectomy
Frederick S. Keller, Maurice Coyle, Josef Rosch, and Charles T. Dotter (Univ. of Alabama at Birmingham and Oregon Health Sci. Univ.)
Radiology 159:447–451, May 1986   13–4

Bilateral percutaneous renal ablation by transcatheter infarction has been performed successfully in patients with end-stage renal disease (ESRD). A review was made of an 11-year experience with percutaneous transcatheter ablation performed in 18 kidneys in ten patients with ESRD who were either on hemodialysis or had undergone renal transplantation. Indications for renal ablation included nephrotic syndrome with massive protein loss in seven patients (13 kidneys), poorly controlled posttransplantation hypertension in the absence of transplant renal artery stenosis in two (3 kidneys), and diabetic nephropathy with persistent urine leak from ureterocutaneous fistulas after pelvic irradiation in one (2 kidneys).

In the earlier years, the embolic materials used were isobutyl-2-cyanoacrylate and Gelfoam mixed with sodium tetradecol sulfate either alone or in combination with Gianturco coil springs. Absolute ethanol was used thereafter. Prior to ethanol injection, an occlusion balloon catheter was placed in the main renal artery to avoid reflux of the ethanol into the aorta. Perfusion of the inferior adrenal artery was prevented by placing the tip of the catheter and the occluding balloon distal to its origin. Ethanol, 3–10 ml, was injected. The occlusion balloon was left inflated for 10 minutes and, after deflation, a test injection of contrast medium was performed under fluoroscopy to check for arterial flow. Embolization was complete if there was stasis in the major renal arteries and no flow of contrast material in the distal branches.

Total renal infarction was achieved in all 18 kidneys. Complete ablation of renal function, except in one patient in whom only one kidney was ablated, was also achieved. Both patients with posttransplantation hypertension became normotensive after renal ablation. Only one complication occurred, i.e., thrombosis of the femoral artery at the catheter entry site. All patients had flank pain, fever, leukocytosis, and serum elevations of lactic dehydrogenase, the severity of which correlated with the amount of tissue infarcted. Percutaneous renal ablation is an effective alternative to surgery in patients with ESRD who require nephrectomy.

▶ In patients with end-stage renal disease the kidneys are usually left in to perform functions of water excretion, synthesis of vitamin D_3, and production of erythropoietic stimulating factor. This study shows that percutaneous renal ablation is safe and effective. The indications for renal ablation in the end-stage renal disease patients were uncontrollable hypertension and massive proteinuria.—J.Y. Gillenwater, M.D.

Phenazopyridine (Pyridium) Poisoning: Possible Toxicity of Methylene Blue Administration in Renal Failure

Michael Sharon, George Puente, and Lawrence B. Cohen (City Univ. of New York)

Mt. Sinai J. Med. 53:280–282, April 1986   13–5

The full spectrum of toxic effects of phenazopyridine poisoning were observed in a patient, possibly complicated by methylene blue administration.

Man, 46, with a history of schizophrenia and polypharmacy abuse complained of yellow skin. He had self-administered 30–40 tablets of phenazopyridine daily (100 mg/tablet) for 1 week prior to his admission because of urinary hesitancy, frequency, and nocturia.

Findings included methemoglobinemia (26%) and cyanosis, acute renal failure (blood-urea-nitrogen, 84 mg/dl, and serum creatinine level, 9.2 mg/dl), and skin and urine pigmentation. The patient was oliguric (15 ml/hour) during the first 18 hours after admission, for which he was treated with furosemide intravenously,

400 mg in a 4-hour period, and one oral dose of metolazone, 10 mg, as well as hydrocortisone sodium succinate, 100 mg every 6 hours. One 70-mg dose of methylene blue was administered intravenously to correct the methemoglobinemia.

Urine output increased to 200–300 ml/hour, and the creatinine level decreased to 1.8 mg/dl in the next 10 days. The methemoglobin level decreased from 10% 8 hours later to 3% 10 days later. Skin and urine pigmentation gradually returned to normal. The patient was asymptomatic on day 7, with a hemoglobin value of 9.2 gm/dl, hematocrit of 27%, uncorrected reticulocyte count of 5%, and lactate dehydrogenase level of 437 μ/ml. Upon discharge he was given a daily oral folate supplement for his hemolytic episode. At 2 months' follow-up, pigmentation and creatinine level were normal. The hemoglobin value was 14.2 gm/dl, the reticulocyte count was 1.0%, glucose-6-phosphate dehydrogenase activity was normal, and the methemoglobin level was 0.3%.

The observed hemolysis after intake of methylene blue for methemoglobinemia possibly gave rise to an erythrocytotoxic effect, which could have resulted from impaired renal clearance of this compound. Physicians should be aware of the toxic effects of phenazopyridine. Methylene blue treatment in patients with methemoglobinemia and renal failure should be undertaken only for symptoms other than cyanosis, or if rapid oxidized hemoglobin levels occur. Dosage adjustments are recommended for patients with diminished renal clearance.

▶ This is an interesting case report that describes toxicity to very large doses of pyridium. The authors point out that the dose of methylene blue needs to be reduced in patients with renal failure.—J.Y. Gillenwater, M.D.

Aluminum and Renal Disease
Alan B. Gruskin (Wayne State Univ.)
NKF Newsletter 2:6–7, 1986   13–6

Hemodialysis patients have been observed to have deteriorating brain function as well as extremity jerks, difficulty in walking, seizures, and progressive cognitive impairment. Some become unresponsive, comatose, and die, and are found subsequently to have increased blood aluminum levels and deposits of aluminum in bone and brain. Other patients have experienced severe pain from nonhealing fractures, and these also may be associated with brain involvement. Anemia has been reported in these patients as well.

Similar disorders were found in predialysis patients given aluminum-containing drugs to control bone disease related to renal failure. Certain aluminum-containing drugs, used to bind phosphorus in the gut, are available without prescription and are the most prominent source of aluminum exposure. Water used for dialysis also contains aluminum, which may enter the body across dialysis membranes. Intravenous solutions may contain aluminum. Little ingested aluminum is actually absorbed, but aluminum deposited in bone interferes with appropriate calcium deposition. Some of the effects of aluminum resemble those of lead.

Calcium-containing phosphate binders are now being used in place of products containing aluminum. Deferoxamine, which binds nonprotein-bound aluminum, can be added to dialysis solutions to bind aluminum during peritoneal dialysis. Further studies are needed of acute and chronic aluminum exposure and how aluminum alters intracellular chemistry.

▶ This is a nice review of aluminum toxicity in patients with end-stage renal disease. The aluminum, taken to decrease the serum phosphate content, causes heavy metal poisoning in the brain and bone marrow. Patients should be treated with a calcium-containing phosphate binder instead of a product containing aluminum.—J.Y. Gillenwater, M.D.

The Immediate and Delayed Effects of Marathon Running on Renal Function

R.A. Irving, T.D. Noakes, G.A. Irving, and R. Van Zyl-Smit (Univ. of Cape Town, South Africa)
J. Urol. 136:1176–1180, December 1986   13–7

Acute renal failure associated with rhabdomyolysis has been described in marathon runners, but renal responses to endurance running, especially in the recovery phase, remain incompletely defined. Renal function was studied in six healthy male marathon runners by obtaining blood and urine specimens for 2 days before and 5 days after a standard marathon run. The race was held over a hilly course in cool, rainy conditions. Five runners had previously completed at least one marathon or longer event, and one was essentially untrained. All of the men completed the run successfully in a mean time of 3 hours 31 minutes.

A mean weight loss of 1.75 kg occurred during the race. The serum creatine kinase, serum urea, and creatinine levels increased. Renal function appeared to be unchanged, but fractional sodium excretion was significantly decreased. Osmolar clearance remained unchanged. The plasma renin activity was within normal limits after the race. Creatinine clearance was increased the day after the race whereas fractional sodium and potassium excretion remained reduced. Creatinine clearance peaked on day 3. Fractional sodium excretion returned to baseline on postrace day 2. The creatinine production rate was significantly increased on postrace day 3, and urea production was decreased within 3–5 days after the race.

Renal function was well maintained during the marathon race in these men, but certain changes in function accompanied recovery. Sodium retention was noted for 24–48 hours after the race, followed by sustained diuresis of a more dilute urine. Persistent glomerular proteinuria was not observed. The rise in creatinine clearance probably reflects an increasing glomerular filtration rate secondary to effects of products of muscle damage on the kidney.

▶ As a jogger I am interested in what happens to renal function during exercise. Severe exercise acutely reduces renal blood flow and the glomerular filtration rate (from stimulation of the sympathetic nervous system) and causes sodium retention and mild proteinuria (from increased glomerular filtration and decreased tubular resorption). In this study, renal function was well maintained during the marathon race because the athletes did not become dehydrated, as a result of cool and wet racing conditions. In the postrace follow-up, there was increased sodium retention for the first 24–48 hours. Decreased urea excretion and production from days 3–5 suggested an anabolic state. Creatinine clearances increased from day 2 to day 5 postrace. No long-term effects were noted. A good review of postexercise proteinurea was included in the 1986 YEAR BOOK (Poortmans, J. R.: *JAMA* 253:236, 1985; abstract 1–1).—J.Y. Gillenwater, M.D.

The Long-Term Effect of Cisplatin on Renal Function
Paul Fjeldborg, Jesper Sørensen, and Poul E. Helkjaer (Aalborg Hosp., Denmark)
Cancer 58:2214–2217, Nov. 15, 1986   13–8

Cisplatin therapy has produced high complete remission rates in patients with testicular cancer, but acute renal dysfunction may occur. Long-term nephrotoxicity from cisplatin was examined in 31 patients treated for disseminated nonseminomatous testicular cancer in 1980–1983. One patient died of septicemia and acute renal failure. Twenty-two patients having a median age of 23 years at diagnosis were evaluated 16–52 months after completion of cisplatin therapy when there was no evidence of disease. Ten healthy men and ten men with suspected urologic disorders served as controls. Cisplatin, bleomycin, and vinblastine were used in the study patients. Cisplatin was given intravenously in a dose of 20 mg/sq m in the first 5 days of each course. The median cumulative dose was 452 mg/sq

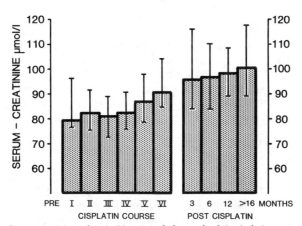

Fig 13–1.—Serum creatinine values in 22 patients before each of six cisplatin treatment courses and in the months after treatment. The *bars* are the median values and the *vertical lines* connect the first and the third quartiles. (*) P < .05, compared with pretreatment value. (**) NS, compared with 3 months postcisplatin. (Courtesy of Fjeldborg, P., et al.: Cancer 58: 2214–2217, Nov. 15, 1986.)

m. A uniform hydration procedure was followed, maintaining diuresis above 100 ml/hour with furosemide.

The serum creatinine level rose significantly during and after treatment (Fig 13–1). Four patients had an increase of more than 30% at some time during treatment, and the glomerular filtration rate (GFR) fell by 13% in these patients. The rise in creatinine level could not be related to the cumulative dose of cisplatin. The change in the GFR was related to the concomitant change in serum creatinine level, but not to the time since completion of cisplatin therapy.

A presumably permanent reduction in the GFR is observed in cisplatin-treated patients with testicular cancer but without signs of persistent tubular damage. The fall in the GFR is moderate and asymptomatic, and it would not appear to be of great clinical import. However, some patients might become uremic in conjunction with a progressive fall in GFR or the expected fall in glomerular filtration with advancing age; future nephrotoxic drug therapy might increase the risk.

▶ This study documents a long-term decrease of 13% in renal blood flow and the GFR in 22 patients who received cisplatin chemotherapy. No renal tubular injury was identified. The mechanism of renal damage is not known.—J.Y. Gillenwater, M.D.

Nephrotoxicity Induced by Cancer Chemotherapy With Special Emphasis on Cisplatin Toxicity
F. Ries and J. Klastersky (Institut Jules Bordet, Brussels, Belgium)
Am. J. Kidney Dis. 8:368–379, November 1986   13–9

The kidneys are highly susceptible to toxic injury by antineoplastic agents. Methotrexate-associated renal failure may be secondary to precipitation of drug in the renal tubules, a direct antimitotic effect on tubular cells, or possibly a change in glomerular filtration. Leucovorin rescue may counter the cytotoxic effects of methotrexate in patients with established nephrotoxicity. Semustine may produce a slowly rising serum creatinine level with progressive, irreversible renal failure. The nephrotoxicity of this drug is cumulative. Dose-related renal toxicity is the major limitation to steptozotocin therapy. Mithramycin produces renal failure and proteinuria in a cumulative manner, and the renal toxicity may be irreversible. Toxicity from mitomycin C is not dose related. Immune complexes have been found in some affected patients. Tubular abnormalities have been described in association with the pyrimidine analogue 5-azacytidine.

Dose-related nephrotoxicity is a major consideration in cisplatin therapy. The drug apparently interacts with the nucleophilic sites of pyrimidines in DNA, producing cytotoxic hydroxyl radicals. Epithelial cell degeneration, proximal tubular necrosis, interstitial edema, and lymphocytic infiltration all are dose-related effects of cisplatin. Glomerular changes generally are not seen. Hydration regimens are of demonstrated efficacy. Forced diuresis, combining hydration with furosemide or mannitol administration, has had beneficial clinical effects in numerous studies. Drugs studied for possible detoxifying actions include probenecid, sodium thiosulfate, acetazolamide, and radioprotective agents. In addition, selenium may prove useful as a cisplatin-precipitating agent.

▶ This is an excellent review of the nephrotoxicity caused by several cancer chemotherapeutic agents. The one of most interest to urologists is cisplatin. The authors point out that renal cisplatin toxicity is related to the tubular urine concentration. Urine dilution by forced hydration and diuretic-induced diuresis reduces renal toxicity. Urologists should avoid the concomitant administration of nephrotoxic drugs such as the aminoglycoside antibiotics. Newer platinum complexes being evaluated for antitumor activity showed little or no nephrotoxicity.—J.Y. Gillenwater, M.D.

Cyclosporine Nephrotoxicity: Pathogenesis, Prophylaxis, Therapy, and Prognosis
B.D. Kahan (Univ. of Texas at Houston)
Am. J. Kidney Dis. 8:323–331, November 1986   13–10

Cyclosporine A, an immunosuppressive agent that is selective for T-cell-related immune responses has improved the success of renal allografting. However, an optimal therapeutic index remains to be defined. Nephrotoxicity, the most significant complication, is only indirectly related to dosage. Typically, creatinine clearance is reduced and the serum creatinine level is elevated with a disproportionate increase in blood urea nitrogen. Hyperkalemia and hypertension characteristically are present, and there may be hyperuricemia and renal tubular acidosis. Nephrotoxicity has been described in from one third to three fourths of renal transplant recipients. It may be acute, subacute, or chronic.

Cyclosporine A nephrotoxicity has been ascribed to increased intra-proximal tubular pressure, activating glomerulotubular feedback, as well as a decreased filtration coefficient and vasoconstriction. Tubular injury takes place, but for reasons that are not clear, and the tubular effect appears not to be the chief mechanism of nephrotoxicity. Altered renal hemodynamics have been suggested, and an arteriolopathy may be responsible for nephrotoxic effects.

Nephrotoxicity may be avoided by changing to azathioprine therapy after 3 months, but the risk of rejection and graft loss may be increased. The author prefers cautious dose reduction with concomitant institution of full-dose azathioprine therapy. More precise drug administration minimizes injury. More sensitive tests will allow quantification of the risk of renal impairment sooner after allotransplantation.

▶ This article reviews cyclosporine nephrotoxicity. Cyclosporine A has improved the survival of patients having renal transplantation. Nephrotoxicity is the most serious complication. The mechanism of nephrotoxicity is not well defined, but several mechanisms seem to be important, including increased intratubular pressure, a decreased filtration coefficient, and renovasoconstriction. It is important to avoid tubulotoxic drugs, e.g., the aminoglycosides, amphotericin B, and trimethoprim.—J.Y. Gillenwater, M.D.

The following review articles are recommended to the reader:

Cronan, J.J., Zeman, R.K.: Renal mass imaging: The internist's role. *Am. J. Med.* 81:1026, 1986.

De Broe, M.E., Porter, G.A.: Drug-induced nephrotoxicity: An international symposium. *Am. J. Kidney Dis.* 8:283–383, 1986.

Fine, L.: The biology of renal hypertrophy. *Kidney Int.* 29:619, 1986.

Kahan, B.D.: Cyclosporine nephrotoxicity: Pathogenesis, prophylaxis, therapy, and prognosis. *Am. J. Kidney Dis.* 8:323, 1986.

Stillwell, T.J., Kramer, S.A., Lee, R.A.: Endometriosis of ureter. *Urology,* 28:81, 1986.

Tegtmeyer, C.J., Sos, T.A.: Techniques of renal angioplasty. *Radiology* 161:577, 1986.

14 Renal Neoplasms

Renal Oncocytoma
H.J.E. Lewi, C.A. Alexander, and S. Fleming (Western Infirmary, Glasgow)
Br. J. Urol. 58:12–15, February 1986   14–1

Renal oncocytoma is an uncommon renal parenchymal tumor consisting of oncocytes, or well-differentiated granular eosinophilic cells in a tubular, alveolar, or papillary pattern. Findings in 22 patients with renal oncocytoma seen between 1965 and 1984 were reviewed. The 11 males and 11 females had a mean age of 15 years. Nine patients were asymptomatic. The others had hematuria or loin pain. Urography showed a mass or renal tumor in 18 of 21 patients, and ultrasonography was usually confirmatory. There were no distinctive radiologic appearances.

Eleven patients had grade 1 tumors, with only uniformly well-differentiated cells and minimal pleomorphism, whereas the other 11 had grade 2 tumors lacking mitosis and necrosis. Lesions that were more pleomorphic were excluded. Three patients had stage III disease at operation, and one had metastatic disease. Three patients died shortly after nephrectomy. Four patients had metastases; two were seen initially with grade 1 tumors. Cumulative survivals were 86% at 1 year, 65% at 5 years, and 37% at 10 years.

Renal oncocytoma is not a benign or premalignant tumor, and its potential for metastasis appears to be unrelated to histologic appearances. The finding of renal oncocytoma should not alter the postoperative management of a renal tumor patient. There is no role for partial nephrectomy in renal oncocytoma patients unless bilateral tumors are present or the tumor is found in a solitary kidney.

▶ The 18% incidence of metastasis in this series of patients with oncocytoma is impressive and certainly bears out the authors' conclusion that oncocytomas cannot be treated as benign renal tumors. It is noteworthy that even the tumors that were grade 1 histologically could also metastasize.—J.Y. Gillenwater, M.D.

Local Excision of Urothelial Cancer of the Upper Urinary Tract
M.A. Bazeed, T. Schärfe, E. Becht, P. Alken, and J.W. Thüroff (Johannes Gutenberg Univ., Mainz, West Germany)
Eur. Urol. 12:89–95, March–April 1986   14–2

Nine of 93 patients (9.6%) were operated on for urothelial cancer by local tumor excision in the upper urinary tract. Absolute indications for conservative surgery included solitary kidney or nonfunctioning contralateral kidneys (four patients), bilateral tumors (one), low-stage tumors (three), and a high-risk patient (one). Five patients were women and four were men. The average age was 63.2 years (range, 39–80 years). The tumor was located in the renal pelvis in six patients; three patients had ureteral tumors.

Surgical procedures for renal pelvis and caliceal tumors included renal pelvis resection in six patients (seven kidneys) combined with partial resection of the kidney because of widespread caliceal involvement in two, and replacement of the resected renal pelvis by a peritoneal autotransplant in five patients. In three patients with ureteral cancer, partial ureteral resection was done with an Anderson-Hynes pyeloplasty in one case and a ureterovesical reimplantation in two.

Follow-up ranged from 5 months to 65 months (mean, 23 months). Three patients had local recurrences in four kidneys within 1–3 years postoperatively, having grade 2 and grade 3 primary lesions. All were treated successfully by repeated local excision. With a normal contralateral kidney, local tumor excision was done electively in four patients (three low-grade/low-stage lesions, one high-risk patient). None had recurrence. One patient died 8 months after operation of cardiac infarction, and another died 26 months after operation of urosepsis; tumor recurrence was not found at autopsy in either patient. The remaining seven patients have not had further recurrences. One patient who had been receiving dialysis because of tumor obstruction of a solitary kidney did not require further dialysis.

Local excision of urothelial cancer of the upper urinary tract is indicated for tumors in solitary kidneys or nonfunctioning contralateral kidneys, for bilateral tumors, in patients with chronic renal failure, and for localized low-stage/low-grade tumors when treatment by radical nephroureterectomy or a more conservative approach has the same prognosis. Peritoneal autotransplant allows generous renal pelvis excision with a wide safety margin and facilitates reoperation if recurrence develops.

▶ The prognosis of urothelial cancer of the upper urinary tract is mostly dependent on the stage and grade of the tumor at the time of therapy. It must be remembered that the entire upper tract urothelium is at risk and is the site of multifocal abnormalities. Local recurrences developed in four of six kidneys, which were managed successfully by local excision. More experience with local excision and a longer follow-up, are needed before its routine use can be advocated.—J.Y. Gillenwater, M.D.

Surgical Enucleation for Renal Cell Carcinoma
Andrew C. Novick, Horst Zincke, R.J. Neves, and H. Michael Topley (Cleveland Clinic Found. and Mayo Clinic and Found.)
J. Urol. 135:235–238, February 1986   14–3

Long-term disease-free survival is achieved by partial nephrectomy in many patients with localized renal carcinoma. Enucleation is especially appealing because it is a relatively simple, rapid procedure, but a possible risk of leaving disease behind has been a concern. Information on 33 patients undergoing enucleation of renal carcinoma between 1970 and 1983 was reviewed. The 24 men and 9 women had a mean age of 59 years. Five patients had Hippel-Lindau syndrome. None had evidence of metastatic disease. Twenty patients had bilateral renal cancer and 13 had cancer in a solitary kidney. The mean postoperative follow-up was 45 months.

Enucleation was performed in situ in 27 patients and extracorporeally with autotransplantation in the other 6. All excised tumors were of low grade and well encapsulated. Three patients with bilateral cancer had extension of disease into the contralateral perinephric fat or intrarenal veins. There were no operative deaths, but five patients had a urinary fistula and one had deep vein thrombosis. Excellent renal function was preserved in all. Eight-five percent of patients are tumor free. Four patients had recurrent cancer; three died, one of unrelated causes. Two patients had local recurrences in the kidney that was operated on.

Tumor encapsulation can be documented preoperatively by combined angiography and CT. Operative bleeding is reduced when the surrounding normal tissue is left in place and as much functioning parenchyma as possible is preserved. Multiple tumors can be enucleated from nearly any part of the kidney.

Conservative Surgery of Renal Cell Carcinoma

M.A. Bazeed, T. Schärfe, E. Becht, C. Jurincic, P. Alken, and J.W. Thüroff (Johannes Gutenberg Univ., Mainz, West Germany)
Eur. Urol. 12:238–243, July 1986   14–4

Between 1967 and 1985, 25 women and 32 men aged 31–77 years (mean, 54.8 years) underwent conservative surgery of renal tumors. In 25 patients the tumor was found during medical examination performed for other reasons. In 25 patients specific urologic symptoms led to diagnosis. In the remaining seven, tumor discovery resulted from unspecific symptoms, e.g., weight loss and weakness.

In 29 patients the indication for conservative surgery included chronic renal failure, benign pathology of the contralateral kidney, a functional or anatomical solitary kidney, and bilateral tumors. In 28 patients, elective surgery was done for small, peripherally located lesions, in cases of uncertain malignancy, and, in one instance, when tumor was detected by chance during stone surgery. Tumors removed for imperative indications measured 2–11 cm (mean, 5.8 cm) in size. In the elective group, tumor size ranged from 1 cm to 7 cm (mean, 3.3 cm). The operative procedure was tumor enucleation in 49 patients and partial kidney resection in seven; in one case kidney resection was combined with resection of suprarenal metastases.

All 28 patients who underwent elective conservative surgery are alive with no cancer evidence. In the imperative surgery group, six patients died, one postoperatively, two from previously known metastases, and three from unrelated reasons. One patient was lost to follow-up; the remaining 50 were followed for 6–103 months (mean, 35.8 months). Eighteen of 29 patients are alive without evidence of cancer and two have metastases (known preoperatively in one of these). Two patients had local tumor recurrence but not at the previous tumor site.

Results in the group with imperative indications support the concept of conservative surgery. Technical ease of tumor removal and preservation of function of the affected kidney were observed. Five simultaneous bilateral tumors were seen, and in four others the contralateral tumor developed as late as 15 years after radical nephrectomy. Another advantage results from preoperative uncertainty of malignancy of some small tumors; four of six benign lesions were unsuspected and would have been subjected to radical nephrectomy according to classic concepts. Conservative surgery is recommended, especially for small peripherally located tumors.

The Feasibility of Surgical Enucleation for Renal Cell Carcinoma

Fray F. Marshall, Jerome B. Taxy, Elliot K. Fishman, and Richard Chang (Johns Hopkins Univ.)
J. Urol. 135:231–234, February 1986   14–5

Partial nephrectomy is the current treatment of choice for renal cell carcinoma. Surgical enucleation has been suggested as an alternative, especially for patients with multiple tumors or those who are at high risk. To examine the efficacy of surgical enucleation, 16 radical nephrectomy specimens were dissected and investigated pathologically.

Well-circumscribed, low-grade tumors could be enucleated successfully. Venous invasion, tumor heterogeneity, occult metastases in lymph nodes, satellite tumor nodules in the kidney, and extrinsic spread through the renal capsule could present problems in this type of operation. Computed tomography did not always predict which patients were possible enucleation candidates.

Partial nephrectomy, rather than enucleation, remains the treatment of choice as a parenchymal-sparing operation for renal cell carcinoma.

▶ The preceding articles (Abstracts 14–3, 14–4, and 14–5) describe large series of patients who underwent surgical enucleation for renal cell carcinoma. Two report excellent results: 6% local recurrence (Novick et al.) and 0% local recurrence (Bazeed et al.). It must be remembered that both of these series were highly selective, with small, low-grade and stage I lesions. Marshall and associates studied 16 radical nephrectomy specimens and found that with enucleation residual tumor was left in seven. Preoperative CT scans did not separate into categories those patients who could and could not be enucleated. Tumors in this group were large, ranging from 5 cm to 12 cm. Rosenthal et al. (*Eur. Urol.* 10:222, 1984) found the pseudocapsule to be sometimes infiltrated by tumor cells, with occasional infiltration into adjacent renal parenchyma. Bennington (*Cancer* 32:1017, 1973) found that between 5% and 10% of renal cell carcinomas are multifocal. Because the three series above have only short follow-ups, I think final conclusions cannot be reached. Renal cell carcinoma is notorious for delayed activity. In my opinion, radical nephrectomy is still the treatment of choice for most renal cell carcinomas, and partial nephrectomy, when technically possible, is a better cancer operation than enucleation.—J.Y. Gillenwater, M.D.

Surgical Management of Renal Cell Carcinoma With Vena Cava Tumor Thrombus
Luciano Giuliani, Claudio Giberti, Giuseppe Martorana, and Salvatore Rovida (Univ. of Genoa, Italy)
Eur. Urol. 12:145–150, May–June 1986   14–6

Of patients with renal cell carcinoma that has spread, approximately 10% will have inferior vena cava involvement. Surgery for caval tumor thrombus is an important part of radical nephrectomy to control renal cell carcinoma. To assess the prognosis of patients with inferior vena cava involvement who underwent surgery, a retrospective study was conducted of patients who were followed for up to 14 years.

Twenty-eight patients aged 34–84 years who had involvement of the inferior vena cava by renal cell carcinoma underwent radical ablative surgery. Seven patients had caval wall tumor infiltration and nine patients had metastases. The patients with caval involvement alone had a 2-year survival of 69%, whereas those with caval infiltration had a 2-year survival of 0%. Those with distant metastases had a 2-year survival of 27%. The location of caval tumor thrombus extension had no effect on survival.

Caval involvement associated with renal cancer has a very negative impact on survival. However, as no effective adjuvant therapy is available, radical ablative surgery is the only treatment.

Cancer of the Kidney Invading the Vena Cava and Heart: Results After 11 Years of Treatment
C.D. Vaislic, P. Puel, P. Grondin, A. Vargas, A. Thevenet, F. Fontan, C. De-ville, A. Leguerrier, B. Touchot, A. Piwnica, and D. Maiza (Rangueil Hosp., Toulouse, France, St. Francis Hosp., Miami Beach, Centre Hospitalier Univ., Montpellier, France, Haut Levêque Bordeaux, France, Centre Hosp., Rennes, France, Hôpital Broussais, Paris, and C.H.U. Côte de Nacre, Caen, France)
J. Thorac. Cardiovasc. Surg. 91:604–609, April 1986   14–7

The prognosis for cancer of the kidney that invades the vena cava is grave. This situation is found in 3% to 10% of cancers of the kidney, and 40% of these reach the heart. Extracorporeal circulation, deep hypothermia, and circulatory arrest are used during operation to allow excision of the carcinoma. A multicenter study was conducted to examine the safety and efficacy of this technique in 18 patients.

No deaths occurred. Survival was 6 months without operation. If there were no detectable metastases before operation, the 5-year postoperative survival was 75%.

Removal of carcinomas of the kidney that extend into the vena cava appears to provide the only chance of survival for these patients at this time. The good 5-year survival rate and the minimal operative risk should encourage systematic investigation of cancers of the kidney and their treatment, if necessary, by this procedure.

▶ These two papers (Abstracts 14–6 and 14–7) on renal cell carcinoma with caval extension offer new information about the disease. In the series by Vaislic et al. (Abstract 14–7) 11 of 18 patients had tumor thrombus extension into the heart. They used extracorporeal circulation with circulatory arrest and deep hypothermia with no operative mortality. In the patients with no detectable metastasis there was a 75% 5-year survival. In the series by Giuliani et al. (Abstract 14–6) none of the seven patients with vena caval wall infiltration lived for 12 months. Better control and visualization of the vena cava can be accomplished by rotating the liver after dividing the triangular and coronary ligaments. If the tumor extends into the hepatic veins or into the heart, we seek the help of the cardiac surgeon. For the difficult cases, extracorporeal circulation with circulatory arrest and deep hypothermia is helpful.—J.Y. Gillenwater, M.D.

Adjuvant Medroxyprogesterone Acetate and Steroid Hormone Receptors in Category M0 Renal Cell Carcinoma: An Interim Report of a Prospective Randomized Study
Giorgio Pizzocaro, Luigi Piva, Roberto Salvioni, Giovanni Di Fronzo, Enrico Ronchi, Patrizia Miodini, and The Lombardy Group (Istituto Nazionale Tumori, Milan)
J. Urol. 135:18–21, January 1986   14–8

Almost 50% of the patients with renal cell carcinoma can be cured by radical operation alone; preoperative and postoperative irradiation appear ineffective. Recently, one study reported a favorable response rate using medroxyprogesterone acetate as adjuvant therapy to a radical operation. A prospective 4 year randomized study was conducted to assess the efficacy of adjuvant therapy in patients who had undergone radical surgery and had no signs of distant metastases.

The study group, 136 patients with category M0 renal cell cancer treated by transperitoneal radical nephrectomy, received 500 mg of medroxyprogesterone three times weekly for 1 year. Control patients were given no adjuvant therapy. The excised kidneys were used for sex steroid hormone receptor studies on both the tumor and the surrounding healthy tissue; the dextran-coated charcoal technique was used.

During the follow-up period of 13–60 months, relapses occurred in 15 of 58 evaluable patients (25.8%) who received adjuvant therapy and in 15 of 63 evaluable controls (23.8%). The metastases were usually found in the lung and bones. Disease recurrence was greater in those patients with no tumor receptors (35.1%) than in those patients with tumors expressing at least one sex steroid receptor type (17.8%). Several patients experienced minor side effects, and three others discontinued the adjuvant therapy because of severe toxicity.

After a median 3-year follow-up, adjuvant medroxyprogesterone acetate proved to be of no therapeutic benefit in patients who had undergone radical nephrectomy. Further studies are needed to determine the significance of sex steroid receptors on the efficacy of steroid hormone treatment of renal cell carcinoma.

▶ In our experience, progesterone does not seem to work in metastatic renal cell carcinoma.—J.Y. Gillenwater, M.D.

Failure of Immunotherapy for Metastatic Renal Cell Carcinoma
Jackson E. Fowler, Jr. (Univ. of Virginia)
J. Urol. 135:22–25, January 1986   14–9

About 50% of patients with renal cell carcinoma will present with metastases or distant metastases will develop despite removal of the primary tumor. Various immunotherapeutic modalities for the treatment of disseminated disease have been studied, including one in which an aggregated soluble fraction of autologous tumor was reported to cause regression of pulmonary metastases in about 50% of selected patients. Autologous and allogeneic aggregated tumor antigen was used to treat 16 patients with renal cell carcinoma who had undergone nephrectomy or excision of the metastatic lesions. Seven others judged unsuitable for operation received an allogeneic tumor antigen preparation. The patients (mean age, 57 years) had histologic or radiographic evidence of renal cell carcinoma and distant metastases. Autologous antigen was prepared from the primary tumor in 15 patients and from a metastasis in 1. Allogeneic antigen was prepared by mixing 12 autologous antigens. All antigens were coinjected with *Candida albicans* antigen every 4 weeks until metastases developed.

Of the 16 receiving autologous antigen, 2 had a minimal response. Of the seven who received allogeneic antigen, none had an objective response. The lack of efficacy of this therapy led to its discontinuation. Administration of autologous or allogeneic antigens has minimal activity against metastatic renal cell carcinoma.

▶ Unfortunately, Jay Fowler, when he was in our department, could not duplicate the results of Tykkä [*Scand. J. Urol. Nephrol.* (Suppl.), 63:1,1981]. At our institution, autologous or allogeneic tumor antigen vaccine had only minimal activity against metastatic renal cell carcinoma.

At the 1987 AUA annual meeting, Schornagel (*Proceedings,* abstract 428) reported success in metastatic renal cell carcinoma using interferon α_2 and vinblastine. Belldegrun and Rosenberg (*Proceedings,* abstract 472) described a technique for isolating from fresh human renal cell cancers, tumor-infiltrating leukocytes that can be expanded in vitro in interleukin-2 for use in human therapy. No human data are available yet. Hemstreet (*Proceedings,* abstract #475) reported no complete response in 16 patients with metastatic renal cell carcinoma treated with interleukin 2.—J.Y. Gillenwater, M.D.

The following review articles are recommended to the reader:

Mundy, G.R.: The hypercalcemia of malignancy. *Kidney Int.* 31:142, 1987.
Oesterling, J.E., Fishman, E.K., Goldman, S.M., et al.: Management of renal angiomyolipoma. *J. Urol.* 135:1121, 1986.

15 Percutaneous Stone Removal

▶ The comments for this chapter were written by Dr. Alan D. Jenkins, Assistant Professor of Urology, University of Virginia School of Medicine.—J.Y. Gillenwater, M.D.

Combined Treatment of Branched Calculi by Percutaneous Nephrolithotomy and Extracorporeal Shock Wave Lithotripsy
Harald Schulze, Lothar Hertle, Jürgen Graff, Peter-Jörg Funke, and Theodor Senge (Univ. of Bochum, Herne, West Germany)
J. Urol. 135:1138–1141, June 1986   15–1

Combining extracorporeal shock wave lithotripsy (ESWL) with percutaneous nephrolithotomy may minimize the disadvantages of both. Combined treatment was used in about 6% of 1,535 patients treated for kidney stones in a 1-year period in 1984 and 1985. These 56 women and 31 men had a mean age of 54 years. Nearly one third previously had operations on the stone-bearing kidney, and about one fifth had reduced renal function. Three patients had a solitary kidney. Thirty-nine patients had complete and 38 had partial staghorn calculi; 10 had more than four renal pelvic and caliceal stones. Three fourths of the patients had evidence of urinary tract infection. Nephrolithotomy and ESWL were performed with epidural anesthesia. Residual fragments were destroyed by lithotripsy about 3 days after nephrolithotomy.

More than 80% of patients required two or three treatments. Shock wave treatment was uneventful, but six complications attended percutaneous nephrolithotomy, the most common being perforation of the collecting system. Struvite calculi were present in 80% of the patients. The mean hospital stay was 19 days. Recurrences were infrequent. Two of 16 patients discharged with nephrostomy catheters required rehospitalization.

Combined percutaneous nephrolithotomy and ESWL is a less invasive and less painful approach than open operation. Short-term results of combined treatment have been comparable with those of operation. A substantial decrease in fluoroscopy time is an important advantage of combined treatment.

Combined Percutaneous and Extracorporeal Shock Wave Lithotripsy for Staghorn Calculi: An Alternative to Anatrophic Nephrolithotomy

Richard J. Kahnoski, James E. Lingeman, Thomas A. Coury, Ronald E. Steele, and Phillip G. Mosbaugh (Methodist Hosp. of Indiana, Indianapolis, and Indiana Univ. at Indianapolis)

J. Urol. 135:679–681, April 1986 15–2

Anatrophic nephrolithotomy has been the method of choice to remove staghorn calculi. However, patients at risk for stone recurrence must undergo repeated surgery. A comparison was made of the efficacy of the noninvasive percutaneous lithotripsy and extracorporeal shock wave lithotripsy (ESWL) with the conventional method for removal of staghorn calculi.

A total of 28 patients underwent anatrophic nephrolithotripsy and 46 patients received various combinations of percutaneous lithotripsy and ESWL to remove partial or complete staghorn stones. Nephrostolithotomy access was via a lower pole posterior calix in most cases. Residual fragments were dislodged with ESWL. For lithotripsy, 2,000 shock waves of magnitude up to 24 kV were delivered at any one sitting. Gravel was washed out with secondary nephroscopy in many cases. Nephrostomy tubes remained in place until the patient was shown to be free of stones.

Fourteen kidneys were rendered free of stones with nephrostolithotomy alone. Two patients were treated successfully with ESWL alone and the remaining 36 needed a combination of the two treatments. Minute residual fragments remained in 15% of renal units, but in only 9.7% with struvite.

The treatment favored by the authors for removal of staghorn calculi is percutaneous debulking of the stone and clearing of the lower pole calices, followed by ESWL to fragment residual upper pole stones. The nephrostomy tube is especially useful in this treatment. Compared with anatrophic nephrolithotomy, this method requires a shorter hospital stay, entails less blood loss, and is equally successful in removing stones. Risks of wound infection, atelectasis, and pneumothorax are avoided by using the noninvasive technique. Only when percutaneous access is inadequate is anatrophic nephrolithotomy required.

▶ Combined percutaneous lithotripsy and ESWL has become the most popular technique for removing staghorn calculi. Blood loss and length of hospitalization associated with this new approach are less than those found with anatrophic nephrolithotomy, but the long-term rate of recurrent stone formation has yet to be determined. The lowest rate of recurrent stone formation after removal of infected staghorn calculi was reported from Stanford (Silvermen, D. E., Stamey, T. A.: *Medicine* 62:44, 1983). Dr. Stamey and his colleagues achieved a recurrence rate of only 5% using anatrophic nephrolithotomy and percutaneous chemolysis. It is doubtful that the long-term results of combined percutaneous lithotripsy and ESWL will be as good, but most patients favor this new approach over traditional open surgery. Also, ESWL alone could be used to treat any recurrent stones when the stone burden is still small.

Staged ESWL monotherapy, often with a temporary double pigtail ureteral catheter, can be used in some patients with staghorn calculi, but limited pulverization may not be possible with brittle struvite stones. The development of extracorporeal lithotripters that have a smaller focal area and require little if any anesthesia may permit more precise pulverization and lessen the burden of multiple treatments. Our approach at the University of Virginia is to use initial percutaneous ultrasonic debulking if at least half of the stone material can be removed through a single tract.—A.D. Jenkins, M.D.

Studies on Renal Damage From Percutaneous Nephrolitholapaxy
Leif Ekelund, Eric Lindstedt, S. Björn Lundquist, Torsten Sundin, and Thomas White (Univ. Hosp., Lund, Sweden)
J. Urol. 135:682–685, April 1986   15–3

Although percutaneous surgery has become an accepted procedure for renal stones, bleeding and injury to adjacent organs are commonly reported. This prospective study assesses the damage to the kidney during this procedure.

Eleven patients with kidney stones judged suitable for percutaneous nephrolitholapaxy underwent excretory urography (IVP), gamma camera renography for individual renal function measurement, and CT scanning preoperatively. Postoperatively, they received gamma camera renography, CT, antegrade pyeloureterography, and, in ten patients, selective renal angiography after removal of the nephrostomy tube. The serum creatinine level, hemoglobin value, and results of urine cultures were determined throughout the hospitalization. Percutaneous nephrostomy, dilation of the tract, and stone removal were combined into a one-stage procedure during which the patient was under epidural anesthesia.

Among 11 patients, stones were successfully removed in 10; CT examination showed small stone fragments in the remaining patient. During and immediately after surgery, bleeding was moderate and no patient required a blood transfusion. Hematuria caused the rehospitalization of two patients. Gamma camera study showed decreased renal function in all patients on day 1, but this returned to normal by day 14, except in three instances. Further, CT uncovered thickening of Gerota's fascia in nine patients and small to moderate perirenal hematomas in six. Angiography revealed discrete parenchymal scarring in some of the patients, as well as a peripheral arteriovenous fistula in one.

Percutaneous renal stone surgery is accompanied by some risk of renal damage, including peripheral fistulas and scarring that may lead to hypertension in the future. However, the damage appears transient and the long-term risks of percutaneous nephrolitholapaxy seem acceptable, considering that the alternative is open surgery.

▶ Early percutaneous nephrostomies were placed with trepidation and several days were needed for dilation of a tract before stone removal. It is now common practice to perform the initial puncture, dilate the tract, and remove the stone material in one sitting. Some investigators have even proposed not leaving a nephrostomy tube for temporary drainage! Early disasters occurred, but percutaneous nephrolitholapaxy has become a very safe and effective procedure. This paper provides evidence that the kidney tolerates this insult.

Almost 4,000 patients have been treated with extracorporeal shock wave lithotripsy at the University of Virginia. Approximately 3% have required a temporary percutaneous nephrostomy for drainage, and another 3% have undergone initial percutaneous lithotripsy. Only one arteriovenous fistula occurred. This was in a patient who inadvertently removed an 8F nephrostomy tube that had been placed for an obstructing steinstrasse. Such a complication has not been seen in those patients who had tracts dilated to 30F before endoscopic stone removal.—A.D. Jenkins, M.D.

Percutaneous Techniques for the Management of Caliceal Diverticula Containing Calculi
John C. Hulbert, Pratap K. Reddy, David W. Hunter, Wilfredo Castaneda-Zuniga, Kurt Amplatz, and Paul H. Lange (Univ. of Minnesota and VA Med. Ctr., Minneapolis)
J. Urol. 135:225–227, February 1986   15–4

Newer percutaneous techniques of intrarenal access were used to treat symptomatic calculi in 11 caliceal diverticula in seven men and three women aged 22–66 years. Four patients each had flank pain and hematuria, and two were asymptomatic. The diverticula were 1.2–2.6 cm in size. Most were adjacent to the upper or lower caliceal group. Five patients had calculi elsewhere in the kidney at presentation. Patients were managed percutaneously under local anesthesia.

Direct puncture of the diverticulum is preferred and was performed in 8 of 11 instances. Use of C-arm fluoroscopy is necessary to place the dilated tract directly onto the stone. In three cases, the guidewire initially could not be passed into the collecting system, and dilation was performed with the wire coiled in the diverticulum, a second guidewire having been coiled over which a safety catheter was passed. After removal of the calculus, the guidewire was passed under direct vision into the main collecting system. Three diverticula were approached indirectly by puncture through a different caliceal group. No major complications occurred. Three patients subsequently underwent flexible nephroscopy to remove small stone fragments. Directly punctured diverticula were absent on pyelography after 3–14 months. Percutaneous techniques may be used less invasively and more cost effectively than previous methods to treat calculi in caliceal diverticula.

▶ Open surgery was rarely contemplated for isolated caliceal stones or stones in caliceal diverticula. Percutaneous renal endoscopy, extracorporeal shock wave lithotripsy (ESWL), and worried patients are forcing urologists to reexamine their position regarding these stones. As demonstrated by these authors, percutaneous techniques permit removal of calculi from caliceal diverticula and effective obliteration of the diverticula. Although ESWL pulverizes these stones, passage of the sand cannot be predicted. We will offer ESWL to those patients with symptoms or a strong desire to have an asymptomatic stone treated, as long as they understand the uncertainty associated with this approach. The sand will pass in approximately half of these patients. Patients with retained sand are offered a second ESWL treatment session, and percutaneous extraction is reserved for those patients with retained stone material after two ESWL treatments. Removal of the crushed stone can be accomplished with pulsed water irrigation through a 20F sheath. The passage communicating with the collecting system can be dilated with a balloon.—A.D. Jenkins, M.D.

16 Ureteroscopy

▶ The comments for this chapter were written by Dr. Alan D. Jenkins, Assistant Professor of Urology, University of Virginia School of Medicine.—J.Y. Gillenwater, M.D.

Internal Ureteral Stents for Conservative Management of Ureteral Calculi During Pregnancy
Kevin R. Loughlin and Robert B. Bailey, Jr. (Brigham and Women's Hosp., Boston)
N. Engl. J. Med. 315:1647–1649, December 1986   16–1

The most common cause of severe abdominal pain during pregnancy is acute problems of the urinary tract, especially urinary calculi. The incidence of urinary calculi during pregnancy ranges from 1/715 to 1/2,247 pregnancies. Because of increasing concern about the risks of anesthetics or x-ray exposure during pregnancy, cystoscopic placement of internal ureteral tubes, or stents, between the kidney and bladder may be useful in the management of urinary calculi in pregnant women. A review was made of experience in managing ureteral calculi in eight pregnant patients by means of double-J stents.

CASE 1.—Female, 18 years, had a 1-day history of right-sided colic at 35 weeks of gestation. Urinalysis revealed microscopic hematuria, and abdominal ultrasound demonstrated hydroureteronephrosis and a presumed calculus in the distal right ureter. The patient experienced persistent pain the right flank. An indwelling double-J stent was placed under local anesthesia, after which the pain resolved without symptoms of bladder irritation caused by the stent. After a normal spontaneous delivery at term, the stent was removed cystoscopically and no stone was recovered.

CASE 2.—Woman, 30, had right-sided colic at 28 weeks of gestation. Urinalysis showed microscopic hematuria, and ultrasound revealed right hydronephrosis. Because of persistent pain, a double-J stent was placed under local anesthesia and the symptoms resolved. Normal spontaneous vaginal delivery occurred at term. At 5 days post partum, retrograde pyelography demonstrated a stone in the right ureter and ureterolithotomy was performed. Two years later, the patient again experienced right-sided colic at 35 weeks of gestation. A double-J stent was placed and symptoms resolved. After a normal spontaneous full-term vaginal delivery, intravenous pyelography showed a stone in the distal right ureter and indicated that the stent was in good position. Post partum, the stone was removed successfully with a basket at cystoscopy.

CASE 3.—Woman, 28, with Sjögren's syndrome experienced left-sided colic at 10 weeks of gestation. Urinalysis showed 10–15 red blood cells per high-power field. A double-J stent placed under local anesthesia led to resolution of symptoms. Two weeks later, pain developed in the right flank and abdominal ultrasound demonstrated mild right-sided hydronephrosis. A double-J stent was placed on the right under local anesthesia, leading to resolution of symptoms. Subsequently, flank pain recurred at 18 weeks of gestation and the stents were replaced under local anesthesia. The original stents were found to be encrusted with calcifications. At 30 weeks of gestation, the stents were again found to be encrusted and were replaced. The patient had a normal spontaneous full-term delivery and then underwent intravenous pyelography. This procedure demonstrated a stone 1.5 × 0.5 cm in size in the proximal ureter and another 0.5 × 0.6 cm in size in the pelvis, as well as a small stone in the upper ureter on the right. The stone in the right ureter passed spontaneously after the stent was removed, and those on the left were removed through a posterior lumbotomy incision.

The double-J stent permits the urologist to treat the presumed urinary obstruction without inducing general or regional anesthesia or performing percutaneous nephrostomy and without exposing the patient or fetus to irradiation. Because of the risk that the stent may become encrusted, patients should be advised to maintain good hydration. Changing the stents at regular intervals is recommended until the pregnancy is over, when the usual radiographs can be obtained and standard management of stones can be resumed.

▶ Can extracorporeal shock wave lithotripsy be used in a pregnant woman with an acute ureteral stone? Although the risk of fetal radiation injury is greatest during the first trimester, most physicians think that radiation exposure should be avoided at any time during pregnancy. The fluoroscopic localization system of the Dornier HM-3 lithotripter renders its use unacceptable during pregnancy. The effect of shock waves on placental attachment to the uterine wall is not known, but the development of lithotripters with ultrasonic localization may make this an active area of investigation.

As shown by these authors, retrograde passage of a double pigtail catheter can be done in a pregnant woman without the need for fluoroscopic guidance or major anesthesia. Relief of the obstruction allows a urologist to postpone definitive treatment until the postpartum period.—A.D. Jenkins, M.D.

Initial Experience With a Pulsed Dye Laser for Ureteric Calculi
G.M. Watson and J.E.A. Wickham (Inst. of Urology, London)
Lancet 1:1357–1358, June 14, 1986   16–2

A pulsed dye laser was developed for fragmentation of ureteric calculi. The "dye" refers to the lasing medium, a solution of coumarin dye. The laser delivers 1 μs pulses of green light, delivered through a quartz fiber only 250 μm diameter. This combination results in a very highpower density at the fiber tip, and stones are fragmented at pulse energies of 30 mJ. Fragmentation arises from formation of a plasma that is initiated when the laser energy is absorbed at the stone surface. The pulsed dye laser was used in 32 patients with 37 urinary calculi and one steinstrasse after extracorporeal lithotripsy. The calculi were located in the ureter in 33 patients, in the renal pelvis in 3, and in the bladder in 1. The mean diameter of the calculi was 7.9 mm and the mean length, 9.1 mm.

The pulsed dye laser was effective in all patients in fragmenting the stones including three calculi in which the degree of ureteric edema and large size precluded the use of the electrohydraulic probe. There was no damage to the ureteric epithelium. Continuous irrigation was achieved at flow rates of up to 120 ml/minute, thus permitting clear views as long as the catheter remained patent.

Pulsed dye laser treatment for ureteric calculi is a safe, effective procedure that allows improved flow of the irrigant and reduced damage to the ureteric wall. Because ureteroscopy is usually traumatic, laser treatment of ureteric calculi without endoscopy is being studied.

▶ The most popular technique for removal of lower ureteral calculi is ureteroscopic manipulation. Small stones can be grasped and removed whole after dilation of the distal ureter. Fragmentation of larger stones has been accomplished with ultrasonic lithotripsy or electrohydraulic lithotripsy. Pulsed dye laser lithotripsy is an advantageous development, because the quartz transmission fiber is flexible and finer than ultrasonic probes, the pulses of green light do not injure the ureter, and treatment without endoscopy may be possible with fluoroscopic control. A disadvantage is that the procedure is time consuming. At the University of Virginia, we prefer to treat all larger ureteral stones with extracorporeal shock wave lithotripsy.—A.D. Jenkins, M.D.

Complications Associated With Ureteroscopy
S. StC. Carter, R. Cox, and J.E.A. Wickham (Inst. of Urology and St. Peter's Hosps., London)
Br. J. Urol. 58:625–628, December 1986   16–3

The development of a rigid ureterorenoscope was first described in 1980, and since that time ureteric surgery has undergone a revolution. The primary indication for ureterorenoscopy is for transurethral endoscopic ureterolithotomy; however, the technique is also used for the diagnosis of ureteric filling defects, obscure positive cytology, or bleeding from the upper tract. Data were reviewed on 125 ureteroscopies performed in one unit to identify any associated complications and to detect any previously unsuspected late problems.

The study population consisted of 88 male and 23 female patients (average age, 47 years) who underwent 125 ureteroscopies in the 3 years from 1983 through 1985. Of these procedures, 119 (95%) were for stone retrieval and the rest for diagnosis. Overall, 8% of the patients sustained major complications of perforation or stricture formation and 3% required ureteric reimplantation. Clinical follow-up and imaging studies carried out more than 1 year after ureteroscopy revealed no evidence of late complications.

Ureteroscopy is a considerable improvement compared with open ureterolithotomy for lower ureteric calculi, but there is a small but significant complication rate, making it a less than satisfactory endourologic procedure. The place of ureterorenoscopy in the diagnosis and treatment of noncalculous upper tract disease is still to be defined.

▶ Ureteroscopy has been accepted enthusiastically by many urologists, but others are reluctant to use it because of the potential complications described in this paper. Ureteroscopy is safe if it is gently and patiently performed, but can be disastrous if excess force or speed is used. The ureter is more delicate and less forgiving than the urethra. Commensurately more care should be exercised when endoscoping the ureter.—A.D. Jenkins, M.D.

The following review article is recommended to the reader:

Miller, R.A., Ramsay, J.W.A., Crocker, P.R., et al.: Ureterorenal endoscopy: Which instrument, what cost? *Br. J. Urol.* 58:610, 1986.

17 Extracorporeal Shock Wave Lithotripsy

Report of the United States Cooperative Study of Extracorporeal Shock Wave Lithotripsy

George W. Drach, Stephen Dretler, William Fair, Birdwell Finlayson, Jay Gillenwater, Donald Griffith, James Lingeman, and Daniel Newman (Univ. of Arizona and other participating institutions in the United States)

J. Urol. 135:1127–1133, June 1986   17–1

Initial data are available from a cooperative study of the first 2,501 extracorporeal shock wave lithotripsy (ESWL) treatments in the United States. Of the 2,112 patients treated, males constituted 70%. Nearly half of the treated stones were in the renal pelvis. The number of shock waves used increased with stone size. Few patients had fluoroscopic exposures of longer than 7 minutes.

Stone fragments passed completely within 3 months of ESWL in 77% of the patients having single stones. The risks of obstruction, increased postoperative pain, retained fragments, and the need for further urologic operations were low in patients having stones less than 1 cm in size (Table 1). These risks increased with stone size larger than 1 cm and when multiple stones were present (Table 2). Adjunctive urologic surgical management was necessary preoperatively in 9% of the patients and postoperatively in 8% (Table 3). Fewer than 1% required open surgery after ESWL. The average length of hospitalization after treatment was 2 days; the length

TABLE 1.—OBSTRUCTIONS ON TREATED SIDE AT DISCHARGE FROM HOSPITAL BY STONE SIZE FOR SINGLE STONE

Drainage	Stone Size				
	1 Cm. No. (%)	1–2 Cm. No. (%)	2–3 Cm. No. (%)	Staghorn No. (%)	Unknown No. (%)
Lt. side treated (100%):					
Good	237 (29.4)	274 (34.5)	23 (3)	13 (1.6)	3 (0.4)
Partial obstruction	70 (8.8)	128 (16.1)	33 (4.2)	10 (1.3)	2 (0.3)
Complete obstruction	1 (0.1)	1 (0.1)	3 (0.4)	1 (0.1)	0
Unknown	20 (2.5)	20 (2.5)	2 (0.2)	5 (0.6)	1 (0.1)
Rt. side treated (100%):					
Good	178 (26.3)	223 (33)	37 (5.5)	3 (0.4)	3 (0.4)
Partial obstruction	56 (8.3)	138 (20.4)	29 (4.3)	6 (0.9)	4 (0.6)
Complete obstruction	0	4 (0.6)	0	1 (0.1)	0
Unknown	20 (3.0)	18 (2.7)	8 (1.2)	0	1 (0.1)

Omitting the unknowns, there are 794 observations for the left side and 675 observations for the right side. The probability of obstruction is significantly related to stone size class for single stones on the left side (P < .005) and on the right side (P < .005). Results for each side in all columns total 100%.

(Courtesy of Drach, G.W., et al.: J. Urol. 135:1127–1133, June 1986. © Williams & Wilkins, 1986.)

TABLE 2.—Residual Fragments at 3-Month Follow-Up by Size of Single Stone

	1 Cm.	1–2 Cm.	2–3 Cm.	Staghorn	Unknown	Totals
Residual fragments:						
Yes	45	62	19	4	4	134
No	213	231	21	9	2	476
Unknown	2	3	0	0	0	5
If yes, excretion:						
Likely	35	55	7	2	3	102
Not likely	2	1	1	2	0	6
Unknown	8	6	1	0	1	16
% free of stones at followup	81.9	78.0	52.5	69.2	33.3	77.4

(Courtesy of Drach, G.W., et al.: J. Urol. 135:1127–1133, June 1986. © Williams & Wilkins, 1986.)

TABLE 3.—Type of Additional Therapy

Therapy*	No. Pts. at Hospital Discharge	3–Mo. Followup
Percutaneous nephrostomy	51	9
Lithotomy––pelvis	0	0
Nephrolithotomy	4	2
Ureterolithotomy	4	3
Ultrasonic lithotripsy	15	4
Cystoscopic extraction attempt	96	8
Other:		
Cystoscopy	15	7
Cystoureteral catheter	9	0
Nephroscopy	2	0
Passage of wire and aspiration through nephrostomy tube	1	0
Incision of bladder neck contraction	1	0
Abdominal exploration	1	0
Nephrectomy and ureterectomy	2	0
Transurethral prostatic resection	1	0
Bladder tumor––ureteral orifice	1	0
Dissolution with tromethamine–E	5	0
Kidney irrigation	0	1
Unduplicated totals	174	31

*Patient may have more than one procedure.
(Courtesy of Drach, G.W., et al.: J. Urol. 135:1127–1133, June 1986. © Williams & Wilkins, 1986.)

of stay was directly related to stone size. Patients usually returned to work within a few days of discharge. Complications with the Dornier unit are infrequent, and some centers presently are treating significant numbers of individuals on an outpatient basis.

▶ The urologic community owes a tremendous debt of gratitude to Professors Chaussy, Schmiedt, Jocham, Brendel, Forssmann, and Walther from Munich for the careful, thorough, and systematic approach they used in investigating the Dornier HM-3 lithotripter. We also deeply appreciate the investigators and the company for insisting that urologists supervise the renal lithotripter service.

The ESWL Cooperative Study Group's report contains a large amount of information. Some of the interesting and important observations are that larger stones require more shocks, leave more retained fragments, involve more ureteral obstructions, and require more pain medication than smaller stones do. Interestingly, a significantly larger number of stones occurred on the left side (55%). Only 2% failed to show fragmentation by ESWL. No impairment of renal function could be demonstrated by renal scans and measurement of the serum creatinine level.—J.Y. Gillenwater, M.D.

Extracorporeal Shock Wave Lithotripsy: The Methodist Hospital of Indiana Experience
James E. Lingeman, Daniel Newman, Jack H.O. Mertz, Phillip G. Mosbaugh, Ronald E. Steele, Richard J. Kahnoski, Thomas A. Coury, and John R. Woods (Indiana Univ. at Indianapolis and Methodist Hosp. of Indiana, Indianapolis)
J. Urol. 135:1134–1137, June 1986   17–2

In 1984, 1,416 extracorporeal shock wave lithotripsy (ESWL) treatments were administered to 982 patients with upper urinary tract calculi. Ten percent of the patients had more than one treatment. Two thirds had a previous upper tract calculus. After initial treatments for solitary uninfected stones smaller than 2 cm in diameter that floated freely in the renal pelvis or calices, indications were expanded to all stones above the bony pelvis other than staghorn calculi. Only patients in reasonably good health were given ESWL. Antibiotics were given before lithotripsy if the urine culture was positive or a struvite stone was suspected.

The procedure lasted for 37 minutes on average. General anesthesia was used in nearly 80% of the patients, and half required no medication for pain after ESWL. Nonoperative complications were infrequent. Of the 569 patients evaluated 3 months after the procedure, 96% had a successful outcome, with no stones or only clinically insignificant residual fragments less than 5 mm in diameter. Calcium oxalate-phosphate stones were present in more than 90% of the patients.

About three fourths of these patients can be expected to be free from stones after ESWL, but a significant proportion will retain small amounts of residual stone material in their upper tracts, and the fate of these fragments is uncertain. Metabolic evaluation is important in all patients with nephrolithiasis, because a calculus is only the symptomatic expression of a more basic disorder. Costs of ESWL have been less than charges for percutaneous lithotripsy and open surgical procedures for the management of comparable stones less than 2 cm in diameter.

▶ Methodist Hospital of Indiana, in Indianapolis, received the first HM-3 model Dornier lithotripter in the United States and treated their first patient on February 23, 1984. This article is a report of their first year's results, which are excellent. At the 3-month follow-up, 72% had no stones, and an additional 24% had stone fragments of less than 5 mm in size. Five patients (0.4%) had perirenal hematoma, and seven had their hematocrit drop below the normal range. Postoperative stone basketing was necessary in 6.9% and percutaneous nephrostomy tube drainage in 1.3%. The Methodist Hospital urologists are to be congratulated on the careful use of this new technique and the manner in which they have promptly and accurately reported their results.—J.Y. Gillenwater, M.D.

Extracorporeal Shock-Wave Lithotripsy for Upper Urinary Tract Calculi: One Year's Experience at a Single Center
Robert A. Riehle, Jr., William R. Fair, and E. Darracott Vaughan, Jr. (New York Hosp.-Cornell Med. Ctr. and Memorial Sloan-Kettering Cancer Ctr., New York)
JAMA 255:2043–2048, Apr. 18, 1986   17–3

Extracorporeal shock wave lithotripsy (ESWL) offers a noninvasive means of destroying calculi in the upper urinary tract without the need for percutaneous nephroscopy or ureteroscopy. In all, 467 patients with symptomatic active stone disease were treated with ESWL. Of the 518 treatments delivered, 5% were retreatments of the same kidneys. One session sufficed for 95% of stones. Regional anesthesia was used in two-thirds of the patients. Nearly one fourth of the treatments were preceded by cystoscopy and retrograde pyelography or stent placement.

Analysis of 300 treatments indicated a stone-free rate of 75% at 3 months. The rate for patients having renal pelvic stones 20 mm or less in diameter was 91%. Apart from size, stone position, composition, and quality of disintegration were factors in stone-free rates. In 2% of attempts the targeted stone was not disintegrated. Complications were minimal, and most were related to anesthesia. Seven percent of treatments were followed by an endoscopic procedure to facilitate complete stone passage.

An overall stone-free rate of 75% was achieved in this series, with an average stone burden of 18 mm. The early stone-free rate would be improved by the more aggressive endoscopic removal of residual fragments or sand. Combined treatment with percutaneous surgery or multiple sequential ESWL treatments is necessary to treat complex stones. Distal ureteral stones are best managed by ureteroscopy or basket extraction.

▶ A 73% (224 of 300) stone-free rate at 3 months is excellent and comparable to rates reported from other centers. Six stones (2%) revealed no significant disintegration, one patient (of 467 total) had a perirenal hematoma requiring transfusion. In our experience, the stones most difficult to fragment are composed of cystine or calcium monohydrate, or are lodged in the ureter with a lot of edema.—J.Y. Gillenwater, M.D.

Extracorporeal Shock Wave Lithotripsy of Ureteral Stones: Clinical Experience and Experimental Findings
Stefan C. Mueller, Dirk Wilbert, Jochen W. Thueroff, and Peter Alken (Johannes Gutenberg Univ., Mainz, West Germany)
J. Urol. 135:831–834, April 1986   17–4

Kidney stones located above the iliac crest and visible on x-ray examination can usually be treated successfully by extracorporeal shock wave lithotripsy (ESWL). However, ureteral stones and certain impacted caliceal stones are unresponsive to ESWL.

High ureteral stones in 148 patients were treated by ESWL alone, or by ESWL after pushing the stone back into the renal collecting system with a ureteral catheter, or by ESWL after placing a catheter beside the stone. The in vitro model consisted of a Penrose drain having a diameter of 16 mm and a wall thickness of 0.13 mm into which were inserted tablets representing artificial stones. This artificial ureter was then exposed to ESWL in a medium of air or water. Under five different conditions, the artificial stones were exposed to ESWL. In an air-filled drain and in a vacuum, response to shock wave application was nil or only slight. In a gelatin-filled drain, only very high rates of shock wave application fragmented the stone. In water-filled drains with and without tension, 22–36 shock waves were needed to disintegrate the "stone."

In the clinical study, 62% of ureteral stones receiving ESWL alone resolved; 97% of stones that were pushed back disintegrated after ESWL; and 74% of stones that had catheters placed beside them during ESWL were treated successfully. Apparently, ESWL is most successful when the ureteral stone is surrounded by water. Interference from edematous mucosa or trapped air bubbles markedly reduces ESWL efficacy. To improve the success rate, ureteral stones should be pushed up into the collecting system, or a water-filled catheter placed beside the stone, before ESWL is undertaken.

▶ Most urologists treating ureteral stones with ESWL believe that the same stone would be more difficult to fragment when left in the ureter than if it is pushed back into the renal pelvis. There has been no previous scientific proof of this clinical impression. In this paper the authors show that water around the stone improves fragmentation. Edematous mucosa or extrinsic pressure holding the small fragments in place appear to prevent disintegration of the central portion of the stone. Other postulated reasons for the difficulty of fragmentation of ureteral stones are that the psoas muscle absorbs some of the energy. Water surrounding the stone permits a better transfer of energy and subsequent fragmentation of the stone. My impression is that stones located in the ureter are more difficult to fragment, and that it is more difficult to determine when the ureteral stone is fragmented.—J.Y. Gillenwater, M.D.

Extracorporeal Shockwave Lithotripsy of Distal Ureteral Calculi
K. Miller, J.R. Bubeck, and R. Hautmann (Univ. of Ulm, West Germany)
Eur. Urol. 12:305–307, July–August 1986   17–5

The use of extracorporeal shock wave lithotripsy (ESWL) has been limited to renal calculi and ureteral calculi located above the pelvic brim. For contact-free stone disintegration, distal ureteral calculi were localized and treated through modification of the patient's position on the support of the Dornier lithotripter HM3.

From January through April 1986, (16 men and 27 women) aged 21–65 years (mean, 48 years) were treated with ESWL. The current distal ureteral calculi had been symptomatic for an average of 5.1 weeks (range, 2–12 weeks). Stone size ranged from 4 mm to 10 mm.

Treatment was successful in 37 patients (86%). Successful treatment was defined as radiographically well-documented stone disintegration and discharge of stone fragments without additional measures. Stone discharge occurred within 1–6 days (mean, 1.7 days). Postoperative analgesic treatment was not required. The average hospital stay after treatment was 2.4 days (range, 1–6 days). A second ESWL session was required by six patients (14%) and was successful in two. Including these two patients, the average postoperative hospital stay for the successfully treated group was 3 days (range, 1–14 days). Four patients (10%) underwent additional ESWL when calculi failed to resolve in the first two sessions. In two patients definitive stone removal was accomplished using retrograde ureteroscopy. Open surgery was necessary in the remaining two after ureteroscopy failed. No complications or adverse side effects occurred.

The ESWL of distal calculi significantly adds to the ease and safety of upper urinary tract stone management. The advantages of ESWL, compared with ureteroscopy, include its noninvasiveness, lack of side effects, and short treatment time and time to recovery. In the authors' department, ESWL has become the choice method for distal ureteral calculi treatment, with ureteroscopy or ureterolithotomy in case of failure.

▶ To my knowledge, the first stone treated in the distal ureter by ESWL was done at our institution on November 27, 1984. This was reported at the February 1985 ESWL meeting in Indianapolis, Indiana, and at the May 1985 AUA meeting. Between November 1985 and April 1, 1987, we treated 167 distal ureteral and prevesical stones. There have been no complications noted to the bone, nerves, or intestines. All stones but one have been fragmented, although some required multiple treatments.—J.Y. Gillenwater, M.D.

Combination of Percutaneous Surgery and Extracorporeal Shockwave Lithotripsy for the Treatment of Large Renal Calculi
I.K. Dickinson, M.S. Fletcher, M.J. Bailey, M.J. Coptcoat, T.A. McNicholas, M.J. Kellett, H.N. Whitfield, and J.E.A. Wickham (London Stone Clinic, St. Bartholomew's Hosp., and Inst., of Urology, London)
Br. J. Urol. 58:581–584, December 1986 17–6

Since 1980, both percutaneous nephrolithotomy (PCNL) and extracorporeal shock wave lithotripsy (ESWL) have been in clinical use. However, treatment of large stones with ESWL alone leads to a high incidence of renal and ureteric obstruction. In addition, there is an increased incidence of complications when large stones or complex peripheral caliceal stones are treated with PCNL alone because multiple punctures and prolonged operating times are needed. An attempt was made to test the theory that, by using a combination of these two techniques, it is possible to debulk large stones using PCNL and then treat the remaining calculi with ESWL to render the remaining fragments less than 2 mm in diameter.

The study population consisted of 67 patients (71 kidneys) with large stones (more than 3 cm in diameter) or complex stones who were treated with a combination of PCNL and ESWL. Treatment was defined as successful if the patients were rendered stone free by 3 months, or if any remaining stone fragments were less than 2 mm in size without evidence of continuing obstruction, sepsis, or deteriorating renal function. It was possible to clear large stones in 71% of patients using the combination of PCNL and ESWL. Of the successfully treated patients, 24 (55%) were cleared with two procedures, 10 (23%) required one further procedure, and 9 required two or more further procedures. There was no mortality; morbidity with both procedures was low and was less than when either procedure was used alone for the treatment of complex stones.

Large and complex stones can be managed by a combination of PCNL and ESWL. If stones more suitable for open surgery are excluded (about 5% of those seen), most patients can be cleared of stones successfully in two or three procedures. Although the total hospital stay is equivalent to that after open surgery, patients experience much less discomfort and return to normal life more rapidly after PCNL and ESWL.

▶ We and most other urologists would agree with the conclusion in this article: that large staghorn renal calculi are best managed with a combination of percutaneous surgery and ESWL. However, I have had three female patients with complete staghorn calculi treated with only one lithotripter session whose stones were completely fragmented and who were stone free by 48 hours with no morbidity in passing the fragments.—J.Y. Gillenwater, M.D.

Extracorporeal Shock Wave Lithotripsy: Interventional Radiologic Solutions to Associated Problems
Charles J. Tegtmeyer, Charles D. Kellum, Allan Jenkins, Jay Y. Gillenwater, William G. Way, John Barr, George Piros, Robert Springer, Marguerite C. Lippert, and Arthur W. Wyker (Univ. of Virginia, Charlottesville)
Radiology 161:587–592, December 1986   17–7

In the past 5 years, the treatment of patients with urinary tract calculi has undergone a substantial change. In 1980 the use of extracorporeal shock wave lithotripsy (ESWL) was first described in patients with calculi, and since that time the technique has proved to be highly effective; most patients do well and require no further intervention. Nevertheless, in some patients, urinary tract obstruction develops when the tract becomes filled with small stone fragments. To manage this condition, new procedures were developed. A review was made of the techniques used in the treatment of patients who require additional interventional radiologic procedures after ESWL to facilitate removal of residual stone fragments.

When data were analyzed on the first 1,500 patients treated with ESWL at the present institution, it was found that 1,300 had calculi of less than

2.5 cm in diameter and 200 had calculi of 2.5 cm or larger. Although most patients did well and did not require further radiologic intervention, 178 interventional radiologic procedures were carried out. Urinary tract obstruction often occurred in patients with large stones when the collecting system filled with stone fragments. Nephrostomy was carried out in 5.3% of the total patient population and in 29% of the patients with stones measuring 2.5 cm or more. Only 1.8% of the patients with calculi smaller than 2.5 cm required radiologic intervention. When the obstructed collecting system could not be crossed with conventional angiographic techniques, the stone fragments were removed through a percutaneous nephrostomy tract either by flushing or by suctioning with a pulsating water jet.

Extracorporeal shock wave lithotripsy is an excellent example of modern technology successfully applied to solve a medical problem. Nevertheless, the machine is not infallible, and large stones (i.e., those at least 2.5 cm in size) are more likely to need interventional procedures. As more large stones are treated by ESWL, the need for interventional radiologic procedures will undoubtedly increase.

▶ The significant finding in this study is that of stones larger than 2.5 cm, 29% required percutaneous nephrostomy to relieve ureteral obstruction caused by the fragments. We have found that most fragments pass spontaneously after the nephrostomy tube is placed. I think that initial stone passage is aided by the increased ureteral pressure behind the stone. However, by 12–24 hours the ureter is dilated with no effective peristalsis. When the nephrostomy tube is placed the ureteral pressure becomes atmospheric and the stones must then be passing because of resumed ureteral peristalsis.—J.Y. Gillenwater, M.D.

Initial Experience With Local Anesthesia in Extracorporeal Shock Wave Lithotripsy
B. Aeikens, K.-W. Fritz, and E. Hoehne (Medizinische Hochschule, Hannover, West Germany)
Urol. Int. 41:246–247, July–August 1986   17–8

Extracorporeal shock wave lithotripsy (ESWL) involves considerable pain and requires anesthesia. General and epidural techniques have been used, but the authors performed ESWL under local anesthesia in about 30% to 40% of patients in a period of a few months. These patients are fully mobile before and after treatment. Local anesthesia is suitable for outpatient treatment and for patients transferred to outside hospitals for follow-up care.

TECHNIQUE.—The skin at the level of the twelfth rib is infiltrated intracutaneously or subcutaneously over an area of about 15 cm in diameter, using a total of 30 ml of 1% prilocaine without epinephrine. Ten to 20 adjacent superficial cutaneous wheals are made, and the anesthetized area is sealed with plastic film. Treatment usually is painless, although slight pressure may be felt in the flank region.

A few patients note light pain, which is tolerable. About 5% to 10% of patients, particularly relatively asthenic, young patients, have required epidural anesthesia. However, local anesthesia is feasible in selected patients undergoing ESWL. Epidural anesthesia is preferable for very anxious or highly pain-sensitive patients. Comparable stone destruction is achieved with both methods of anesthesia.

▶ The use of local anesthesia for ESWL has obvious advantages over general or epidural anesthesia in terms of complications and morbidity. The authors of this paper believe that 20% to 40% of lithotripter patients are candidates for local anesthesia. In 5% to 10% of these patients local anesthesia was unsuccessful because of painful internal pressure sensations. We have successfully used local anesthesia, more so on the Siemens Lithostar patients than with the HM-3 Dornier lithotripter. It is reported that the Edap and Wolf lithotripters using a piezoelectric source of shock waves do not require *any* anesthesia.— J.Y. Gillenwater, M.D.

The Effects of Extracorporeal Shock Wave Lithotripsy on Urological Prostheses and Endoprostheses
T.A. McNicholas, J.W.A. Ramsay, P.R. Crocker, D.R. Webb, and J.E.A. Wickham (St. Bartholomew's Hosp. and Devonshire Hosp. Lithotripter Ctr., London)
Urol. Res. 14:309–313, 1986   17–9

Endourologic techniques are a series of measures designed to support extracorporeal shock wave lithotripsy (ESWL) in the treatment of larger and more complex stones. They include percutaneous nephrostomy, percutaneous nephrolithotomy, and ureteroendoscopic surgery. Frequently, a plastic prosthesis is maintained in or near the area of maximal shock wave concentration during lithotripsy, raising questions concerning the effects of shock wave exposure on prostheses.

Prostheses subjected to standard lithotripsy and others removed from patients after ESWL were examined visually, biochemically, and by electron microscopy and x-ray emission spectroscopy. The fluid-filled catheter balloons tested experimentally leaked, whereas those containing air remained intact. A fluid-filled silicone balloon catheter that was exposed in vivo also was intact.

Scanning electron microscopy showed disruption of all plastic surfaces after either in vitro or in vivo exposure to shock waves. Disruption was greatest in polyvinylchloride materials, intermediate in polyethylene and polydimethylsiloxone prostheses, and least in polytetrafluoroethylene (PTFE) devices. The use of inorganic elements (e.g., barium and bismuth) to radio-opacify the plastics could serve as a marker of surface disruption. Bismuth particles were released by exposure of polyethylene catheters, whereas a layer of fluorine prevented the escape of bismuth from PTFE.

Care is needed in selecting an indwelling endourologic prosthesis if ESWL may follow. Silicone or PTFE prostheses may be recommended, but the latter is more widely applicable. If polyvinyl chloride is necessary, a formulation lacking additives should be used.

▶ Clinical experiences have shown that shock waves do not fracture or fragment nephrostomy tubes or ureteral catheters in patients. This study shows that shock waves do cause minor disruption of all plastic surfaces, more so with some compounds than with others. The silicone and PTFE catheters sustained the least damage. The authors correctly warn against the possible release of inorganic elements used for opacification (e.g., barium and bismuth).—J.Y. Gillenwater, M.D.

Evaluation of Renal Damage in Extracorporeal Lithotripsy by Shock Waves
F.J. Ruiz Marcellán and L. Ibarz Servio (Centro Sanitario de Litiasis Renal, Instituto Dexeus, Barcelona)
Eur. Urol. 12:73–75, March–April 1986   17–10

Enzymatic analyses were done before and after extracorporeal lithotripsy by shock waves for caliceal and renal pelvic stones. Variations of N-acetyl glucosaminidase (NAG) and lactate dehydrogenase (LDH) levels were determined in blood and urine specimens obtained from 44 patients aged 20–67 years to learn whether liberation of lysosomal enzymes was activated by renal tubular affection.

A significant increase in serum and urine LDH levels was observed after treatment as compared with before treatment. The NAG values in blood also increased significantly. In urine, the pretreatment NAG level was not significantly different from the posttreatment value. Whereas the serum results indicated a marked increase in both enzymes, the values were still within normal limits. The data suggest the presence of renal microdamage with the clinical significance of transitory hematuria. No correlation between the number of waves and enzymatic increase was established at the doses required for stone fragmentation. Preventive therapy for the kidney is recommended using a protective agent that exhibits extracellular osmotic effects (e.g., mannitol) to avoid edema and vascular spasms.

▶ The authors postulate that changes in the enzymes NAG and LDH assess renal tubular damage from shock waves. Presumed, but unproved, was the assumption that no enzyme release would occur from other organs in the blast path, e.g., the liver and skeletal muscle. Post lithotripsy, significant elevations were noted in the serum and urinary LDH levels and in serum NAG activity. I am not certain what the small changes mean.—J.Y. Gillenwater, M.D.

Ultrasound Stone Localisation for Extracorporeal Shock Wave Lithotripsy
X. Martin, J.L. Mestas, D. Cathignol, J. Margonari, and J.M. Dubernard (Hôpital Edouard Herriot, Lyon, France)
Br. J. Urol. 58:349–352, August 1986   17–11

For treatment of renal stones, an extracorporeal shock wave lithotriptor using an ultrasound scan head pantograph location system was used. The shock wave ellipsoid reflector position was adjusted to the stone with a computer-assisted positioning device. Human urinary stones of 8–20 mm were implanted in the renal pelvis of seven dogs. Plain radiographs of the renal area were taken every 300–400 shots to monitor stone disintegration and to establish treatment success. Stone fragmentation occurred in all cases, the fragments being less than 3 mm in size. Disintegration was accomplished by administering 700–2,000 shock waves (mean 1,500). Autopsy disclosed renal hematoma in one instance. Kidney exposure to 2,500 shock waves resulted in no abnormalities.

Subsequently, 45 patients were treated for 25 stones in the renal pelvis (8–29 mm in size) and 21 caliceal stones (3–15 mm). Radiopaque as well as poorly opaque or radiolucent stones were treated. Between 800 and 3,000 shock waves were applied (mean 1,900). Radiographs performed after the procedure showed good fragmentation in 38 patients (85%).

Incomplete fragmentation (particle size larger than 3 mm) was observed in four instances. In two patients with stones initially larger than 2 cm, a second shock wave treatment was carried out. Four patients received additional endoscopic treatment. In four cases (8%), the stones appeared unchanged after shock wave therapy and further shock wave treatment was considered. Stone hardness may have contributed to these failures.

Although ultrasound is an effective method for localizing stones, it is less effective in assessing the degree of stone destruction. Plain radiographs taken with portable apparatus appeared to offer the best way of evaluating the degree of stone disintegration. Ultrasound localization and the ellipsoid positioning device avoided the need for expensive fluoroscopic equipment and a hydraulic patient positioning system. Radiolucent, poorly opaque, and even nonopaque stones can be treated with this prototype. Shock waves generated by an underwater spark gap discharge are effective in fragmenting stones and do not harm soft tissue.

▶ This is the first report of a new lithotripter made in France. Shock waves are generated by two electrodes in a hemiellipsoid placed in a water container. Stone localization is by ultrasound. The authors' assessment is that the degree of fragmentation is difficult to determine with the ultrasound. Portable x-ray studies were used to evaluate the degree of disintegration. Adequate fragmentation was seen in 85% of the patients.—J.Y. Gillenwater, M.D.

Extracorporeal Stone Disintegration Using Chemical Explosive Pellets as an Energy Source of Underwater Shock Waves
Masa-Aki Kuwahara, Koichi Kambe, Seiichi Kurosu, Seiichi Orikasa, and Kazuyoshi Takayama (Tohoku Univ., Sendai, Japan)
J. Urol. 135:814–817, April 1986   17–12

The use of chemical explosives to create a controlled microexplosion is an approved therapy for the disintegration of bladder stones. The explosive lead azide was used to disintegrate renal stones in dogs. Adult dogs underwent half ligation to create partial ureteral obstruction. The dilated renal pelvis of each animal was then implanted with a human or artificial calculus. After 3 weeks, the anesthetized animal was exposed to a range of 10–100 focused underwater microexplosions. Ten-mg lead azide pellets were used to create the explosion, which was monitored by holographic interferometry and focused with an ellipsoidal reflector.

The model and human calculi were successfully disintegrated. The largest fragments were 27 cu mm for the human calculi, and the size of the fragments tended to be dependent on the number of explosions. Despite a minor bleeding lesion of the pelvic mucosa in one animal and of the lower lung in another, all organs appeared normal. The focus of the explosion could be confined to an area 10 mm in diameter, and the pressure could be regulated easily by the amount of explosive used. Moreover, damage to the kidney and other organs was slight. It appears, therefore, that extracorporeal microexplosive lithotripsy may be useful in human patients.

▶ This is the first article on another method of lithotripsy. In this case, shock waves are created by exploding lead azide. Patients have now also been successfully treated. Three methods of delivering the shock waves are used. First, an external explosion is created and the shock waves are focused by a pseudoellipsoidal reflector in a water bath. Second, a hole is bored in the stone and the explosion is created in the stone. Third, the explosion is created in a small metal capsule next to a ureteral calculi. The explosion causes a metal pin to strike and fragment the calculi. Interestingly, the explosive has to be stored several blocks from the hospital in a gunsmith's safe.—J.Y. Gillenwater, M.D.

Fragmentation of Gallstones by Extracorporeal Shock Waves

Tilman Sauerbruch, Michael Delius, Gustav Paumgartner, Joseph Holl, Othmar Wess, Werner Weber, Wolfgang Hepp, and Walter Brendel (Univ. of Munich)
N. Engl. J. Med. 314:818–822, March 27, 1986   17–13

Although cholecystectomy has become the standard treatment for symptomatic cholelithiasis, nonsurgical approaches have been pursued with enthusiasm. Nevertheless, the results of medical management of gallstones have been disappointing High-energy shock waves generated extracorporeally have been used successfully for nonsurgical fragmentation of kidney stones. Recent experiments on the effects of extracorporeal shockwaves on human gallstones implanted in the gallbladders of dogs indicated that the stones could be disintegrated by shock waves without serious side effects. Nine patients with functioning gallbladders containing one to three symptomatic, radiolucent stones no larger than 25 mm in diameter and five patients with common duct stones that were not removable endoscopically were treated by extracorporeally generated shock waves during general anesthesia. The patients with gallbladder stones received adjuvant treatment with a combination of ursodeoxycholic acid and chenodeoxycholic acid.

All gallbladder stones were disintegrated into sludge or fragments with diameters of no more than 8 mm. In six of the nine patients the fragments disappeared completely within 1–25 weeks. No adverse effects were detected during follow-ups of 10–34 weeks, except for transient biliary pain in two patients, with mild pancreatitis in one. In four of the five patients with common duct stones, shock wave treatment produced stone disintegration and permitted successful endoscopic extraction or spontaneous passage of fragments.

Gallstones may be treated successfully and without serious adverse effects by extracorporeally generated shock waves in selected patients. This new approach may resolve life-threatening conditions in selected patients with common duct stones unamenable to other nonsurgical approaches. However, it must be emphasized that, according to present criteria for patient selection, only about 5% to 10% of all patients with gallbladder or common bile duct stones referred to the authors appear to be suitable candidates for extracorporeal shock wave treatment.

▶ Gallstones can be fragmented by shock waves. The problems are localization of nonopaque stones and passage of the fragment burden with possible complications of cholecystitis, biliary obstruction, cholangitis, or pancreatitis. Stone localization is achieved with ultrasound. The patient machines do away with the water bath, substituting a plastic water-filled container around the ellipsoid. Recently, ten tests sites were selected for the Food and Drug Administration's studies of the new Dornier Gallstone Lithotripter.—J.Y. Gillenwater, M.D.

Long-Term Follow-up of Extracorporeal Shock Wave Lithotripsy Patients
Daniel M. Newman, John W. Scott, and James E. Lingeman (Indianapolis, Ind.)
J. Urol. 137 (Pt. 2): 141A, 1987   17–14

Three months post treatment, 1,910 patients were evaluated. Of these, 653 had a 1-year follow-up, and 135 had a 2-year follow-up. Analysis of the number of stones treated revealed that the stone-free state decreased as the number of stones treated increased. Evaluation of solitary stones by size indicated a decreasing success rate based on stone size, with an increase in the significant residual fragment rate when stones were larger than 2 cm in size. Patients with pelvic stones had a greater stone-free state than did those with caliceal stones; the success rate in those with ureteral stones was about the same as that in patients with pelvic stones. The stone-free state after treatment of stones in patients with normal anatomy was 71%, compared with 64% for those with obstructed collecting systems. In a small series of patients with severe hydronephrosis, only 33% had a stone-free state after treatment. Those with medullary sponge kidneys and poor function had decreased stone-free states also. Patients with horseshoe

TABLE 1.—Three-Month Follow-Up ESWL: Number of Stones Treated

Number	Total	Stone–Free	Residual Fragments
1	1145	892 (78%)	253 (22%) Insig. 15% Sig. 7%
2	318	189 (59%)	129 (41%)
3	188	82 (44%)	106 (56%)
4	259	81 (31%)	178 (69%)
Overall	1910	1244 (65%)	666 (35%)

Insignificant: 4 mm or less in size; sterile urine; not struvite; asymptomatic.
Significant: more than 4 mm in size; infected urine; struvite; symptomatic.
[Courtesy of Newman, D.M., et al.: J. Urol. 137 (Pt. 2): 141A, 1987. © by Williams & Wilkins, 1987.]

TABLE 2.—Three-Month Follow-Up ESWL: Solitary Stone By Size

Size (cm)	Total	Stone–Free	Insig. Residual Fragments	Sig. Residual Fragments
0.1 – 1.0	809	655 (81%)	110 (14%)	44 (5%)
1.1 – 2.0	272	195 (72%)	53 (20%)	24 (8%)
2.1 – 3.0	56	37 (66%)	8 (14%)	11 (20%)
3.1	8	5 (62%)	2 (25%)	1 (13%)

[Courtesy of Newman, D.M., et al.: J. Urol. 137 (Pt. 2): 141A, 1987. © by Williams & Wilkins, 1987.]

TABLE 3.—Three-Month Follow-Up ESWL: Solitary Stone By Treatment Location

Location	Total	Stone–Free	Insig. Residual Fragments	Sig. Residual Fragments
Pelvis	585	493 (84%)	58 (10%)	34 (6%)
Calyx	466	325 (70%)	99 (21%)	42 (9%)
Ureter	26	22 (84%)	2 (8%)	2 (8%)

[Courtesy of Newman, D.M., et al.: J. Urol. 137 (Pt. 2): 141A, 1987. © by Williams & Wilkins, 1987.]

kidneys had a 50% stone-free state after tretment. Results at 3 months post treatment are shown in Tables 1, 2, and 3.

For those patients who at 3 months were stone free, new stone growth was 8.4% at 1 year and 10.6% at 2 years. If the patient had a fragment at 3 months' follow-up, the fragment growth rate was 21.6% at 1 year and 21.7% at 2 years. Patients who had single stones treated and were stone free at 3 months had a recurrence rate of 5.5%, whereas those with multiple stones who were stone free at 3 months had a recurrence rate of

16.7%. Of 227 renal units with residual fragments at 3 months, 43% had no demonstrable change at 1 year. Also, 20% became stone free at 1 year, and 15% had fewer fragments at 1 year; 21.6% had stone growth at 1 year. For those patients with residual fragments that were unchanged at 3 months and at 1 year, analysis at 2 years revealed 56% with no change, 13% were stone-free, and 9% had fewer fragments; 21.7% had stone growth in 23 kidneys followed for 2 years.

▶ Daniel Newman, John Scott, and Jim Lingeman of Indianapolis, Indiana, kindly supplied me with the long-term follow-up of the ESWL patients they have treated. The data were presented at the 1987 AUA meeting.—J.Y. Gillenwater, M.D.

The following review article is recommended to the reader:

Riehle, R.A., Jr., Naslund, E.B., Fair, W.R., et al.: Impact of shockwave lithotripsy on upper urinary tract calculi. *Urology* 28:261, 1986.

18 Cystic Disease

▶ The comments for this chapter were written by Dr. Marguerite Lippert, Assistant Professor of Urology, University of Virginia School of Medicine.—J.Y. Gillenwater, M.D.

The Natural History of Simple Renal Cysts: A Preliminary Study
Daniel Dalton, Harvey Neiman, and John T. Grayhack (Northwestern Univ.)
J. Urol. 135:905–908, May 1986   18–1

Cystic renal disease is a complex composed of several different groups of cystic lesions. Simple cortical cysts comprise a distinct, recognizable clinical entity. The bulk of the literature regarding simple renal cysts has concentrated on their differentiation from and coexistence with neoplastic renal masses, and renal ultrasonography has become a reliable first-line diagnostic tool to differentiate cystic from solid renal masses. Patients with simple renal cysts are often followed periodically with ultrasonography in the event that a coexistent solid (neoplastic) mass might become evident. However, to date the natural history of simple renal cysts has not been described. Findings were reviewed in 59 patients with simple renal cystic disease followed periodically with ultrasonography.

The ultrasonic examination was performed with commercially available static gray scale and real-time B-mode ultrasonoscopes with either a 3.5-MHz or 5.0-MHz transducer. Examinations during the early years of this review were performed primarily with the patient in the prone and lateral decubitus positions. More recently, supine and oblique scans have been preferred. All ultrasonic examinations evaluated both kidneys, except in patients who had undergone nephrectomy.

The results indicated that simple cysts tend to progress in number than than size. Further, three patients had independent solid or complex lesions. The only patient explored had an adenocarcinoma of the kidney. Periodic reevaluation of patients with an ultrasonic diagnosis of simple renal cyst should be considered seriously.

▶ This paper uniquely examines the natural history of renal cysts by sequentially evaluating the same patients with ultrasonography. Although, 27% of the cysts had an increase in diameter, because all of the increases were no more than 2 cm and only a cyst diameter of 3 cm was believed to be significant, no significant increase in cyst size was established. Further, as another cyst developed in 29% of all patients the author concludes that simple cysts tend to progress in number rather than in size. However, the observation period was only 2–3 years in another series, when decades of years of patients' ages were compared, CT studies revealed that as the patients' ages increased, both the number of cysts per patient and diameter of cyst increased (Laucks, S.P., Jr., and McLachlan, M.S.: *Br. J. Radiol.* 54:12, 1981). However, this method compares different patients.—M.C. Lippert, M.D.

The following review article is recommended to the reader.

Parivar, F., Bradbrook, R.A.: Interstitial cystitis. *Br. J. Urol.*, 58:239, 1986.

19 Renal Infection

▶ The comments for this chapter were written by Dr. Jackson E. Fowler, Jr., Clarence C. Saelhof Professor of Urology, University of Illinois College of Medicine, Chief of the Division of Urology at University of Illinois Hospital.—J.Y. Gillenwater, M.D.

Host-Parasite Relationships in Acute Pyelonephritis
James A. Roberts, George M. Suarez, Bernice Kaack, Gerald J. Domingue, and Stefan B. Svenson (Tulane Univ., Delta Regional Primate Res. Ctr., Covington, La., and Natl. Bacteriological Lab., Stockholm)
Am. J. Kidney Dis. 8:139–145, September 1986   19–1

Colonization of the urinary tract by pathogens results from bacterial adherence to mucosal cell membranes. Hydrophobic interactions and/or more specific ligand-receptor interaction between the bacteria and epithelial surfaces, most frequently caused by bacterial fimbriae of bacterial cell walls, are thought to be responsible for adherence. To determine the importance of host and bacterial factors in the host-parasitic interaction that leads to acute pyelonephritis, 15 patients, including 7 children and 8 adults with nonobstructive pyelonephritis, were observed during a 1-year prospective study. Studies on bacterial adherence to uroepithelial cells were conducted using fluorescein-labeled type I and P-fimbriated reference strains of *Escherichia coli* and fluorescence-activated cell sorting (FACS) analysis.

In all cases, P-fimbriated *E. coli* was the causative urinary pathogen. The identical serotype of P-fimbriated *E. coli* was isolated from the vaginal introitus of 60% of the patients and from the fecal flora in 86%. Analysis by fluorescence-activated cell sorting showed receptor receptivity for both type I fimbriated *E. coli* and P-fimbriated *E. coli*. The latter adhered significantly better to urothelial cells than did type I fimbriae. In addition, more P-fimbriated *E. coli* adhered to the patients' cells. The only host anatomical abnormality was moderate vesicoureteral reflux in 20% of the patients; this resolved with long-term antimicrobial treatment. These data indicate that both colonization with P-fimbriated *E. coli* and urothelial cell-receptor availability are important in the pathogenesis of pyelonephritis.

▶ Using fluorescence-activated cell sorting methodologies, this study confirms previous observations that bacterial adherence to uroepithelial cells is greater among patients susceptible to bacteriuria than among patients resistant to bacteriuria, and that P-fimbriated *E. coli* adhere more avidly to uroepithelial cells than do type I fimbriated *E. coli.*—J.E. Fowler, Jr., M.D.

The following review article is recommended to the reader:

Klein F.: Emphysematous pyelonephritis: Diagnosis and treatment. *South. Med. J.* 79:41, 1986.

20 Hydronephrosis

Effect of Thromboxane Inhibition on Renal Blood Flow in Dogs With Complete Unilateral Ureteral Obstruction
Marcus H. Loo, Donald N. Marion, E. Darracott Vaughan, Jr., Diane Felsen, and Craig T. Albanese (New York Hosp.-Cornell Med. Ctr., New York)
J. Urol. 136:1343–1347, December 1986   20–1

Renal prostaglandins may mediate some of the hemodynamic changes that follow ureteral obstruction, e.g., the transient increase in ipsilateral renal blood flow and the subsequent progressive decline in flow. The effects of inhibiting renal thromboxane on renal blood flow and ureteral pressure were assessed in awake dogs during 18 hours of complete unilateral ureteral obstruction, using the thromboxane synthetase inhibitor OKY-046. Urinary thromboxane B_2 excretion was used as a marker for inhibition of thromboxane synthesis. Urinary prostaglandin E_2 excretion also was estimated.

Infusion of OKY-046 did not alter the triphasic relationship between ipsilateral renal blood flow and ureteral pressure previously observed after unilateral ureteral obstruction. Ipsilateral urinary thromboxane B_2 excretion was inhibited by more than 90%, and ipsilateral prostaglandin E_2 excretion did not decrease consistently. Contralateral urinary prostaglandin E_2 excretion fell significantly below baseline after release of the obstruction.

Ipsilateral renal blood flow did not improve in this model of unilateral ureteral obstruction despite substantial inhibition of ipsilateral urinary thromboxane inhibition. Further studies with a newly synthesized thromboxane receptor blocker may help to elucidate the role of thromboxane A_2 in the pathophysiology of the renal hemodynamic changes associated with chronic unilateral ureteral obstruction.

► Complete unilateral ureteral obstruction causes an initial ipsilateral increase in renal blood flow thought to be prostaglandin mediated. The mechanism of the decrease in ipsilateral renal blood flow after 12 hours of complete unilateral ureteral obstruction is controversial. This study shows that the thromboxane (a vasoconstrictor) synthetase inhibitor OKY-046 does not prevent the afferent vasoconstriction associated with complete ureteral obstruction.—J.Y. Gillenwater, M.D.

Evaluation of Hydronephrosis in Pregnancy Using Ultrasound and Renography
Roland Müller-Suur and Olof Tyden (Univ. of Uppsala, Sweden)
Scand. J. Urol. Nephrol. 19:267–273, 1985   20–2

Normal variations in renal pelvic diameter were assessed sonographically under varying states of diuresis in 20 nonpregnant women and in 31 asymptomatic pregnant women. Both ultrasonography and ^{131}I-hippuran renography were performed on the same day in 35 pregnant women with suspected ureteral obstruction who had flank pain for 1–4 days unaffected by posture. Furosemide was administered intravenously in conjunction with renography.

Renal pelvic diameters in nonpregnant women ranged from 3 mm to 9 mm on the right side and from 2 mm to 6 mm on the left. In the asymptomatic pregnant women, renal pelvic diameters in the first, second, and third trimesters were 5 mm, 10 mm, and 12 mm, respectively, on the right side, and 3 mm, 4 mm, and 5 mm on the left. An increased renal pelvic diameter was confirmed in all but 4 of the 35 symptomatic women. Diuretic renography indicated acute ureteral obstruction in 6 of 27 women with right-sided pain and in 3 of 8 with left-sided pain. Renal function was impaired in six of the nine affected patients. Function sometimes returned to normal after surgical intervention.

Both ultrasound study of the renal pelvis and renography can demonstrate hydronephrosis during pregnancy. Because of the lower radiation dose, renography is recommended in place of urography in pregnant women with flank pain who have an enlarged renal pelvic diameter on ultrasound study. Obstruction to ureteral flow may be associated with impaired renal function on the affected side.

▶ Although hydronephrosis associated with pregnancy is well recognized, the etiology is still debatable. Because of the risks of radiation, studies of renal anatomy and ureteral function have not been adequately evaluated. This study shows that by using ultrasonography and renograms with ^{131}I-hippuran and furosemide diuresis both anatomy and function can be evaluated. I agree with the authors that ultrasonography should be done first. Unless significant dilation is seen, renography is not indicated.—J.Y. Gillenwater, M.D.

21 Renal Transplantation

▶ The comments for this chapter were written by Dr. Arthur I. Sagalowsky, Associate Professor of Urology at University of Texas Southwestern Medical School, and Surgical Director of Renal Transplant at Parkland Memorial Hospital, Dallas.—J.Y. Gillenwater, M.D.

Diagnosis of Tubular Injury in Renal Transplant Patients by a Urinary Assay for a Proximal Tubular Antigen, the Adenosine-Deaminase-Binding Protein
N.E. Tolkoff-Rubin, A.B. Cosimi, F.L. Delmonico, P.S. Russell, R.E. Thompson, D.J. Piper, W.P. Hansen, N.H. Bander, C.L. Finstad, C. Cordon-Cardo, L.H. Klotz, L.J. Old, and R.H. Rubin (Massachusetts Gen. Hosp. and Harvard Univ., Boston, the Cambridge Res. Lab., Cambridge, Mass., and Memorial-Sloan Kettering Cancer Ctr., New York)
Transplantation 41:593–597, May 1986   21–1

Specific and sensitive noninvasive means are needed for diagnosing impending allograft rejection. Two murine monoclonal antibodies that detect epitopes of adenosine-deaminase-binding protein (ABP), a proximal tubular cell glycoprotein antigen, were incorporated into a sandwich enzyme immunoassay for urinary ABP. Urinary ABP is found on the brush border of the proximal tubular epithelial cells. The test is a good marker for proximal tubular injury, and it has reliably distinguished between glomerular and tubular injury in patients with native kidney disease.

Serial urine samples were obtained from 34 renal transplant recipients during a 6-month period after transplantation. The urinary ABP level consistently fell to below 0.35 absorbance unit (AU) in the first postoperative week in 11 patients without either acute allograft rejection or cyclosporine A toxicity. All 29 episodes of acute rejection in 23 patients were associated with urinary ABP levels exceeding 0.6 AU starting 1–7 days before rejection was clinically diagnosed. Declining urinary ABP levels accompanied reversal of acute rejection on treatment with OKT3 or antithymocyte globulin in patients who remained free of further rejection. High ABP levels also accompanied cyclosporine A toxicity, and levels returned to normal after the dose of cyclosporine was reduced. Patients with chronic allograft rejection and no more than minimal tubulointerstitial inflammation had urinary ABP values of less than 0.35 AU.

Serial measurements of urinary ABP are useful in the management of renal transplant recipients having graft rejection or cyclosporine A toxicity. It is hoped that other urinary monoclonal antibody-based assays of renal injury will be developed.

▶ The authors report on the use of a monoclonal antibody that binds to ABP,

125

which is a glycoprotein antigen on the proximal renal tubule. The assay is specific for tubular as opposed to glomerular renal injury, but it cannot distinguish the specific cause of the tubular injury. An increasing urinary level of the marker protein correlated with acute rejection and cyclosporine nephrotoxicity. Because of the prevalence of some degree of tubular injury in most cadaver renal transplants, measurement of a baseline sample of marker urinary protein is necessary for proper interpretation of serial measurements.—A.I. Sagalowsky, M.D.

Is Chronic Renal Transplant Rejection a Non-Immunological Phenomenon?

J. Feehally, K.P.G. Harris, S.E. Bennett, and J. Walls (Leicester Gen. Hosp., England)
Lancet 2:486–488, Aug. 30, 1986   21–2

Immunologic factors have been emphasized in acute renal transplant rejection, but the progressive course of chronic renal graft failure may be independent of immune mechanism, rather analogous to the declining renal function seen in chronic renal failure. Renal impairment in chronic graft failure often is associated with proteinuria, fluid retention, and hypertension. Chronic vascular rejection is considered to be immune mediated, although evidence of antibody mediation is only indirect. The usual management is to maximize immunosuppression and use measures applicable to all chronic renal failure. These include optimal control of blood pressure, serum phosphate level, and fluid status.

There is substantial evidence that, in human beings, progression of chronic renal failure may be slowed by dietary protein manipulation. Protein restriction to 0.6 gm/kg of ideal body weight daily is recommended in chronic renal failure when the serum creatinine level exceeds 500 μmole/L. Five consecutive patients with progressive renal transplant failure and a serum creatinine level of more than 500 μmole/L were managed in this way. All of them had recent biopsy evidence of chronic rejection. The slope of the linear regression relating the reciprocal serum creatinine level to time decreased during dietary management. Body weight was stable after the first 2 months of protein restriction.

Chronic renal transplant failure seems to be closely analogous to chronic renal failure in native kidneys, and the resultant decline in renal function is similarly amenable to manipulation by dietary protein restriction. This is a safe, inexpensive, and well-tolerated approach that holds value for prolonging renal transplant function. Protein restriction is associated with impaired immunity, but only if severe.

▶ The authors point out the clinical parallels between abnormalities identified in both chronic renal transplant rejection and progressive chronic renal insufficiency including proteinuria, hypertension, fluid overload, and phosphorus abnormalities. It is known that dietary protein restriction will prolong the terminal decline in chronic renal insufficiency that results in end-stage renal disease. The authors applied similar protein restriction to renal transplant recipients diagnosed as having chronic rejection. A similar prolongation of residual renal function was observed. This experience suggests a relatively easy adjunct in the management of such patients. However, these findings do not address the issue of whether or not declining renal function in the phase called "chronic rejection" results from an ongoing immunologic process.—A.I. Sagalowsky, M.D.

Cyclosporin-A Nephrotoxicity and Acute Cellular Rejection in Renal Transplant Recipients: Correlation Between Radionuclide and Histologic Findings

E. Edmund Kim, George Pjura, Patricia Lowry, Regina Verani, Carl Sandler, Stuart Flechner, and Barry Kahan (Univ. of Texas at Houston)
Radiology 159:443–446, May 1986   21–3

Serial nuclide studies were performed in 25 patients with clinical findings of either cyclosporine-related nephrotoxicity or acute cellular rejection after renal allografting. All patients were receiving cyclosporine A and prednisone, and all had a rise in serum creatinine level of at least 25% above baseline, with a definitive response to treatment. Fifteen patients had a final diagnosis of cyclosporine nephrotoxicity, whereas ten had acute cellular rejection that responded to steroid pulse therapy. Dynamic nuclide studies were done with ^{99m}Tc-diethylenetriamine pentaacetic acid (DTPA) and ^{131}I-hippuran.

There were no distinctive light microscopic or ultrastructural features of cyclosporine nephrotoxicity. A correct diagnosis was made in 80% of these patients and in the same proportion with acute cellular rejection. Seven patients with cyclosporine nephrotoxicity showed definite improvement in tubular function after dose reduction. Six patients with acute cellular rejection definitely improved after antirejection therapy.

Serial nuclide studies with both ^{99m}Tc-DTPA and ^{131}I-hippuran are useful in the management of renal transplant recipients by providing early distinction between acute cellular rejection and cyclosporine-related nephrotoxicity. A correct diagnosis was made in 80% of the present patients.

▶ Imaging of renal function by radionuclide scans is a relatively sensitive and specific means of detecting decreases in renal function caused by both acute rejection and cyclosporine nephrotoxicity. Decreased renal blood flow and decreased excretion are well described features of acute cellular rejection. Preservation of renal perfusion and a marked decrease in excretion on radionuclide scan during episodes of cyclosporine nephrotoxicity also have been observed by ourselves and others. This is an interesting finding in view of the fact that, in vitro, one can show that cyclosporine induces marked arteriolar constriction even with doses in the therapeutic range and that nephrotoxicity is believed to result, in part at least, from this phenomenon apart from any direct effects of the drug on the renal tubule.—A.I. Sagalowsky, M.D.

Severe Nephrotoxicity Caused by the Combined Use of Gentamicin and Cyclosporine in Renal Allograft Recipients

Ariën Termeer, Andries J. Hoitsma, and Robert A.P. Koene (St. Radboud Hosp., Nijmegen, The Netherlands)
Transplantation 42:220–221, August 1986   21–4

After renal transplantation, patients are at increased risk of infection because of the immunosuppressive drugs used to prevent rejection. Several reports have documented the beneficial effect of intraoperative antibiotic prophylaxis on wound and other infections. However, certain medications are potentially nephrotoxic, especially when used in combination with cyclosporine. For example, the combination of cyclosporine and gentamicin, used prophylactically or therapeutically, may lead to severe nephrotoxicity. This was observed in three patients who received the antibiotic later after transplantation.

Case 1.—Boy, 7 years, received immunosuppression with cyclosporine and low-dose prednisone after transplantation. He experienced acute rejection twice, but 2 months after transplantation stable renal function was reached. At that time he received cyclosporine, 7.5 mg/kg daily; treatment with gentamicin intravenously was started because of a urinary tract infection with *Pseudomonas aeruginosa*. After receiving two doses of gentamicin, the patient became anuric on the first day of treatment. When gentamicin therapy was discontinued, diuresis gradually returned. Subsequently, the urinary tract infection was treated with ceftazidime without further incident.

Case 2.—Girl, 10 years, received prophylactic gentamicin before cystoscopy 7 days after renal transplantation. The cyclosporine dose at that time was 17.5 mg/kg daily. After a single dose of 35 mg of gentamicin, urinary output decreased by more than 50% for 4 days.

Case 3.—Man, 40, took 13.5 mg of cyclosporine per kg daily 1 month after transplantation. Because of a flucloxacillin-resistant high fever, he was given a 7 day-course of gentamicin. The urinary output decreased markedly from the third day of antibiotic treatment. After discontinuation of gentamicin therapy, diuresis gradually increased.

In addition to these three patients, two additional patients were seen who sustained a substantial loss of renal function after a single dose of gentamicin. The combination of cyclosporine with gentamicin can be hazardous, not only perioperatively but also later in the course after renal transplantation. It is conceivable because both drugs are notoriously nephrotoxic. The authors recommend combining cyclosporine with ceftazidime when antibiotic therapy is necessary in renal transplant recipients.

▶ The routine use of perioperative broad-spectrum antibiotics has been associated with a decreased incidence of wound infections in renal transplantation. It should come as no surprise that exposure to several different nephrotoxic agents (e.g., aminoglycosides and cyclosporine) may have an additive detrimental effect on the kidney. Because of the recent development of effective antipseudomonal nonaminoglycoside agents, many renal transplant programs will be altering their standard antibiotic regimen.—A.I. Sagalowsky, M.D.

Functional Preservation of the Mammalian Kidney: VII. Autologous Transplantation of Dog Kidneys After Treatment With Dimethylsulfoxide (2.8 and 4.2 *M*)
Armand M. Karow, Jr., Malcolm McDonald, Tracy Dendle, and Raghunatha Rao (Med. College of Georgia, Augusta)
Transplantation 41:669–674, June 1986   21–5

Screening studies using a rabbit divided kidney model have indicated that the cryoprotectant dimethylsulfoxide (Me_2SO) is more effective and less toxic to renal tissues than either ethylene glycol or glycerol. The utility of this model in predicting preservational efficacy was confirmed in canine kidneys by autologous transplantation. Kidneys were perfused in vitro with Me_2SO in either a K-Mg-rich vehicle or a K-glucose-rich vehicle. The Me_2SO concentration in the vehicle was increased to 2.9 *M* or 4.2 *M* over a period of 28–35 minutes, kept constant for 5–10 minutes, and then decreased in about 1 hour. Kidneys were perfused at 25 C.

A beneficial interaction of the vehicle with Me_2SO was observed in this study, and the efficacy of perfusion at 25 C was confirmed. The optimal concentration of Me_2SO appeared to be 2.8 *M*. The best results were obtained using the K-glucose-rich vehicle. The dividied kidney model is an accurate means of predicting kidney preservation when tested with the autotransplanted canine kidney. The K-glucose-rich vehicle appears to give the best results when its strongly favorable parenchymal effect and marginally unfavorable vascular effect are both taken into account.

▶ The present study explores the use of dimethylsulfoxide as a cryoprotectant for long-term renal preservation in a canine model. In the past, hypothermia to slow cellular metabolism has been the most effective means to minimize the energy requirements of organs during preservation. The present study and much ongoing work also address the provision of energy substrate in the form of glucose or adenine nucleotides in the preservation solution. Further refinement of preservation techniques may allow for longer periods of organ storage, which would permit increased organ sharing, better tissue matches, and "semielective" scheduling of surgery.—A.I. Sagalowsky, M.D.

Kidney Transplantation From Unrelated Living Donors: Time to Reclaim a Discarded Opportunity
Andrew S. Levey, Susan Hou, and Harry L. Bush, Jr., (New England Med. Ctr., Boston, and Michael Reese Hosp. and Med. Ctr., Chicago)
N. Engl. J. Med. 314:914–916, Apr. 3, 1986   21–6

Before dialysis therapy was available routinely in the United States, both related and unrelated living donors were accepted for renal transplantation. With the increased availability of dialysis, transplantation from poorly matched living donors was discouraged because it was thought that a cadaveric kidney provides equal benefit to the recipient without risk to a living donor. Although the results of transplantation have improved dra-

---

<table>
<tr><td colspan="6" align="center">DIALYSIS AND TRANSPLANTATION IN THE UNITED STATES, 1980 TO 1984</td></tr>
<tr><td>YEAR</td><td>NEW DIALYSIS PATIENTS DURING YEAR</td><td>TRANSPLANTATIONS FROM LIVING RELATED DONORS DURING YEAR</td><td>CADAVERIC TRANSPLANTATIONS DURING YEAR</td><td>PATIENTS ON DIALYSIS AT YEAR END</td><td>PATIENTS AWAITING TRANSPLANTS AT YEAR END</td></tr>
<tr><td>1980</td><td>19,687</td><td>1275</td><td>3422</td><td>52,364</td><td>5072</td></tr>
<tr><td>1981</td><td>21,367</td><td>1458</td><td>3427</td><td>58,924</td><td>5773</td></tr>
<tr><td>1982</td><td>22,797</td><td>1677</td><td>3681</td><td>65,765</td><td>6720</td></tr>
<tr><td>1983</td><td>24,218</td><td>1796</td><td>4333</td><td>71,961</td><td>7137</td></tr>
<tr><td>1984</td><td>27,113</td><td>1704</td><td>5264</td><td>78,479</td><td>8562</td></tr>
</table>

*Source of data is the End-Stage Renal Disease Network Coordinating Council.
(Courtesy of Levey, A.S., et al.: N. Engl. J. Med. 314:914–916, Apr. 3, 1986. Reprinted by permission of The New England Journal of Medicine.)

---

matically, living persons who are not related to the recipient are still rejected as potential kidney donors. It is now time to reevaluate the ethical and medical justifications for this policy.

Because of advances in immunologic management, there has been spectacular improvement in the outcome of cadaveric kidney transplantation from unrelated donors. However, the supply of cadaveric kidneys is not adequate to meet the demand and, at present, the rate of kidney transplantation lags far behind the incidence of end-stage renal disease (table). In theory, the success of transplantation from living unrelated donors should be equal or superior to the success of cadaveric transplantation. The potential advantages from living unrelated donors may lead to superior graft function and survival. In fact, preliminary studies have revealed that the results of these procedures are excellent whether or not donor-specific transfusions are used. Furthermore, the risks of nephrectomy to the donor are minimal. Death during the operation is rare, and 2% to 3% of donors experience major but temporary morbidity. There are considerable benefits to the organ donor, with many donors reporting increased self-esteem and sense of worth.

Transplantation from an unrelated living donor is indicated for patients for whom neither a living related donor nor a cadaveric donor is available. In addition, this approach may also be considered as an alternative to cadaveric transplantation for selected patients in whom a planned transplant operation would provide an advantage, i.e., those who would benefit from donor-specific transfusions or other pretransplantation immunosuppression, those who require pretransplantation bilateral nephrectomies, and those who choose to avoid the long wait for a cadaveric organ. Further study of the results of transplantation from unrelated living donors is needed to guide future practice.

▶ This is a very timely and thought-provoking article that can be approached on a number of different levels. Philosophically, if it is moral and ethical to use living related donors, one can make a sound argument that a properly motivated and informed living unrelated donor is equally acceptable. Certainly, ethical standards for proper screening of such prospective donors should ensure that fully informed consent, lack of any form of coercion, or suggestion of monetary gain to the donor are the conditions that must be met. These standards do not differ from what has been applied to prospective living related donors for many years. From a practical standpoint with regard to supply and demand, the topic is also timely. The authors cite distressingly low but valid statistics on individual and family willingness to donate and the actual yield from potential available cadaveric donors. However, more recent evidence suggests more families may be willing to donate than previously thought if they are simply advised of the need and possibility for organ donation. An organized, comprehensive program of generalized public education regarding organ and tissue donation and transplantation is urgently needed.—A.I. Sagalowsky, M.D.

Long-Term Blood Pressure and Renal Function in Kidney Donors
Tore Talseth, Per Fauchald, Sverre Skrede, Ole Djøseland, Knut J. Berg, Jean Stenstrm, Arne Heilo, Erling K. Brodwall, and Audun Flatmark (The Natl. Hosp., Oslo)
Kidney Int. 29:1072–1076, May 1986   21–7

Hemodynamically mediated injury to the hyperperfused nephrons that remain is evident after subtotal resection of a renal mass in the rat, but uninephrectomy has not been shown to produce such injury in healthy man. The renal functional status of 74 family members who donated kidneys between 1969 and 1974 was reviewed. The 35 men and 33 women followed had median ages of 46 years at donation and 56 years at follow-up. Thirty-two healthy persons served as controls.

Morbidity in the donor group included lower urinary tract infections in three, chronic glomerulonephritis in two, and acute pyelonephritis and renal stone formation in one patient each. Ten donors were hypertensive, but only three of them were totally normotensive preoperatively. Abnormal urinary protein excretion usually was attributable to intercurrent disease. The creatinine clearance (C_{cr}) averaged 78% of the preoperative value; it was less than 50% in eight donors. The compensatory increase correlated inversely with both age and blood pressure. No consistent abnormalities of tubular function were documented. The only consistent abnormality found when 32 donors were matched with the healthy controls was increased urinary albumin excretion.

These findings, like those of other studies of kidney donors, do not preclude the continued active recruitment of living donors. Strict criteria, however, are needed in screening potential donors for elevated blood pressure. Longer-term observations are needed to assess adequately the prevalence and extent of hypertension in kidney donors.

► The laboratory observation that subtotal nephrectomy in the rat is followed by a hyperfiltration injury to the remaining nephron mass resulting in proteinuria, hypertension, and progressive renal damage has caused many transplant centers retrospectively to evaluate the long-term results in renal donors. The current study is consistent with all reports to date. Namely, there is significantly elevated urinary protein excretion that is of uncertain clinical import with follow-ups of between 5 years and, in some cases, 20 years. Prior donors have a slight increase in blood pressure but have no higher incidence of true hypertension than an age-matched population followed over the same period of time. The world-wide experience today with long-term follow-up of renal donors for up to 20 years continues to support the safety of this procedure.—A.I. Sagalowsky, M.D.

Long-Term Renal Function in Kidney Donors: A Comparison of Donors and Their Siblings
Susan L. Williams, Jacqueline Oler, and Diane K. Jorkasky (Univ. of Pennsylvania and Drexel Univ., Philadelphia)
Ann. Intern. Med. 105:1–8, July 1986   21–8

That renal disorders and hypertension are often found in family clusters is recognized. However, these hereditary and familial factors have not been taken into account in studies of long-term renal function in kidney donors. A comparison was made of renal function and blood pressure in donors who underwent nephrectomy at least 10 years previously and in their siblings who did not have nephrectomies. The transplantation records at the Hospital of the University of Pennsylvania yielded a final total of 38 kidney donors who entered the study. Seventeen of their siblings also participated. Another 38 unrelated individuals matched with donors for age, sex, and race served as population controls to determine the prevalence of hypertension. Of the 38 donors, 20 had donated a kidney to a brother or sister, and the rest had donated to a child.

The 24-hour urinary protein excretion was increased by about 100 mg in all donors after nephrectomy, with men having greater increases than women and 12 of the 38 donors excreting more than 150 mg/24 hours. However, no significant correlation was found in the years since nephrectomy, degree of proteinuria, and blood pressure. Serum creatinine concentrations were 20% higher in donors than in their siblings, and creatinine clearance was 20% lower in donors than in their siblings. Unilateral nephrectomy, although associated with mild proteinuria of unknown clinical significance, does not appear to affect renal function adversely in the kidney donor.

▶ Yet another carefully controlled long-term study reveals that renal donors have an increase in proteinuria, a slight increase in serum creatinine activity, and a decrease in creatinine clearance, but no increased incidence of hypertension or clinically manifest renal disease.—A.I. Sagalowsky, M.D.

Long-Term Consequences of Renal Donation in Humans
I. Fehrman, U. Widstam, and G. Lundgren (Huddinge Univ., Sweden)
Transplant. Proc. 28:102–105, February 1986   21–9

The living donor transplant is widely considered optimal for use in patients with terminal uremia, but the possibly adverse long-term effects of renal donation remain uncertain. Of 67 patients who served as kidney donors in 1964–1974, 62 were available for assessment. Twenty-one females and 13 males (mean age, 58 years) were examined a mean of 12 years after donation.

Six donors were hypertensive, and two others had borderline hypertension. Five donors reported recurrent urinary tract infections, and five had asymptomatic bacteriuria at follow-up. The serum creatinine level rose significantly immediately after donation but fell subsequently in all patients but one. The glomerular filtration rate, measured by the ^{51}Cr-edetate method, usually was about 2SD lower than reference values for age-matched controls. Eight patients had macroproteinuria and nine had microproteinuria. Four of the nine patients with abnormal excretion of β_2-microglobulin had repeated urinary tract infections. Only 4 of 34 donors had significantly increased excretion of red blood cells in the urine, and 3 excreted significant numbers of leukocytes.

Most renal donors in this study were in good health 10–20 years after donation. About one third of the group had hypertension, urinary tract infections, or asymptomatic bacteriuria with probable involvement of the renal parenchyma. Kidney function nevertheless was adequate in all of them. Regular follow-up should be offered to renal donors to treat possible hypertension or urinary tract infection in a timely manner.

▶ In addition to the usually measured parameters of proteinuria, serum creatinine, renal clearance, and hypertension, this study looked at the incidence of urinary tract infection, and both symptomatic and asymptomatic bacteriuria in prior donors. It is difficult to impune historically distant donor nephrectomy to lower urinary tract infection, and the major thrust of this study reaffirms the safety of living-related renal donation.—A.I. Sagalowsky, M.D.

Comparison of Renal Transplantation and Dialysis in Rehabilitation of Diabetic End-Stage Renal Disease Patients
Raja B. Khauli, Donald G. Vidt, Andrew C. Novick, Magnus Magnusson, Donald R. Steinmuller, Emil Paganini, Caroline Buszta, Martin Schreiber, and Satoru Nakamoto (Cleveland Clinic Found.)
Urology 27:521–525, June 1986   21–10

Chronic hemodialysis, peritoneal dialysis, and renal transplantation are three treatments for patients with end-stage renal disease (ESRD) resulting from diabetic nephropathy. Past work has shown that long-term survival is better in those patients undergoing transplantation. A retrospective study was conducted to determine whether other factors (e.g., level of rehabilitation, stabilization of extrarenal diabetic complications, and quality of life) are also improved with transplantation compared with dialysis.

Data on 100 patients with ESRD secondary to insulin-dependent diabetes were reviewed. The mean duration of diabetes was 20 years. Forty-eight patients underwent renal transplantation. Of 52 patients managed by chronic dialysis, 29 received hemodialysis, 18 were managed with peritoneal dialysis, and 5 used both methods. The incidence of myocardial infarction was lowest among transplant patients, their selection being dependent on an absence of heart disease. In both groups, there was the same 10% rate of peripheral vascular disease requiring limb or digit amputation. Progression of retinopathy occurred in 45% of those on dialysis and in 11% of those who received transplants. Progression of neuropathy was not significantly different among groups. As for rehabilitation, 55% of those with transplants and 26% of those on dialysis are employed.

Rehabilitation and stabilization of retinopathy and neuropathy are greater among transplant patients compared with those undergoing hemodialysis. However, patients having peritoneal dialysis had stabilization of retinopathy equal to that in the transplant group and less severe progression of neuropathy compared with both transplant and hemodialysis patients. Because survival and rehabilitation are better among patients undergoing kidney transplantation, it is the optimum therapy for ESRD secondary to insulin-dependent diabetes.

▶ Several studies have established that the greatest long-term survival of patients with diabetes and renal failure is obtained by successful renal transplantation. The overall degree of rehabilitation in diabetics with renal failure or, conversely, prevention of the diabetic sequelae of retinopathy, neuropathy, and peripheral vascular disease, are less well documented. The authors point out an important preselection bias in the current series favoring transplantation for patients with milder degrees of myocardial disease. The higher incidence of long-term myocardial infarction in patients remaining on dialysis comes as no surprise. Interestingly, the incidence of limb amputation for peripheral vascular disease was identical in transplant recipients and in those not having transplants. Progression of other diabetic sequelae may be slower in patients given transplants.—A.I. Sagalowsky, M.D.

Cancers of the Anogenital Region in Renal Transplant Recipients: Analysis of 65 Cases
Israel Penn (Univ. of Cincinnati)
Cancer 58:611–616, Aug. 1, 1986   21–11

Some renal transplant recipients have an increased incidence of certain cancers. When findings in these patients are compared with those in age-matched controls, skin cancers are found to be increased by up to 21-fold, lip cancers by 29-fold, non-Hodgkin's lymphomas by up to 49-fold, in situ carcinomas of the uterine cervix by 14-fold, and Kaposi's sarcomas by up to 500-fold. The occurrence of cancers of the anogenital region was described in renal transplant recipients in 1979. The anogenital area includes the anus, perianal skin, and adjacent external genitalia: the labia majora and minora, mons pubis, and vaginal introitus in the female, and the penis and scrotum in the male.

A markedly increased incidence of anogenital cancers was noted recently in renal transplant recipients, including a 100-fold increase in the incidence of carcinomas of the vulva and anus compared with findings in the general population. Anogenital carcinomas occurred in 65 of 2,150 renal transplant recipients who presented with 2,298 different types of malignancy. Two thirds of these patients were females. In general, they were much younger than persons with similar tumors in the population at large. At the time of diagnosis, the average age of females was 37 years (range, 20–64) and of males, 45 years (range, 34–62). The neoplasms occurred late after transplantation, i.e., an average of 88 months (range, 9–215 months) compared with an average of 56 months (1–225.5) for all other posttransplant malignancies. The lesions involved the vulva, penis, scrotum, anus, or perianal area. Two patients also had involvement of the urethral meatus. In several women there was a "field effect" with multiple tumors of the squamous epithelium of the anogenital area, vagina, or uterine cervix. The lesions ranged from in situ carcinomas (in one third of the patients) to lesions invading adjacent organs and lymph node metastases. The treatment varied from local excision to radical vulvectomy, abdominoperineal resection, or penile resection, sometimes combined with excision of the inguinal lymph nodes. In several patients there was a previous history of condyloma acuminatum or herpes genitalis, which suggested a possible viral etiology of these tumors.

Prevention and early treatment of suspected precursor lesions is important. Although the cause of these cancers is not known, the two important factors are thought to be immunosuppression and oncogenic viruses.

▶ An increased incidence of malignancy is one of the well-recognized consequences of long-term immunosuppression. Tumors of the skin and mucous membranes and of the hematopoietic system have been described most often in the renal transplant patient population. The current study documents an increase of 100-fold in the incidence of cancers of the anogenital region in renal transplant recipients and provides guidelines for the prospective surveillance and treatment of these patients.—A.I. Sagalowsky, M.D.

Long-Term Results of Dialysis and Transplantation in Patients With End-Stage Renal Failure From Hypernephroma
Jeffrey Mandel and Carl M. Kjellstrand (Univ. of Minnesota)
Nephron 44:111–114, October 1986   21–12

Hypernephroma, an unusual cause of end-stage renal failure, occurs in only 0.1% to 1% of patients treated by dialysis or transplantation. Patients with end-stage renal failure secondary to renal malignancy who received dialysis for 1–2 years until receiving a transplant had good survival and rarely had recurrence of malignant disease. However, the patients who received transplants after a waiting time of less than a year had a high incidence of recurrence (48%) of malignancy with poor survival. It is not known whether the poor survival of those who waited for a shorter period resulted from flare-up of malignancy secondary to immunosuppression used in transplantation or from a more aggressive tumor. Studies were made in 13 patients undergoing chronic dialysis because of nephrectomy for hypernephroma to evaluate the influence of immunosuppression on recurrence.

Eight patients received dialysis only; six of these died, four of metastatic disease. Death occurred in less than 8 months in three patients with metastatic disease. Five of the patients also received transplants; three of these patients died, one of metastatic disease. There were no differences in age and sex between those with early metastatic disease and those without, but stage III–IV disease and time less than 5 years between first and second nephrectomy were more commonly observed in those with early metastatic disease. A 7-month waiting time on dialysis is sufficient to avoid transplantion in those with early recurrence. Patients with stage III–IV disease and early reappearance of tumor in the second kidney are best treated with conservative management rather than a second total nephrectomy.

▶ In evaluating papers such as this one must recall that the chronic dialysis patient is inherently immunosuppressed as part of the clinical picture of renal failure. In addressing the best form of initial therapy for patients with bilateral tumors or tumors in a solitary kidney, the morbidity and mortality rates attendant to dialysis must be weighed against the risk of local tumor recurrence or, rather, persistence in renal-sparing procedures. In patients already rendered anephric because of nephrectomy for renal cell carcinoma, the risk of any tumor relapse—or the timing of such relapse in the transplanted vs. the dialyzed patient—is little understood.—A.I. Sagalowsky, M.D.

22 Hypertension and Vascular Disease

▶ The comments for this chapter were written by Dr. E. Darracott Vaughan, Jr., James J. Colt Professor of Urology, Cornell University Medical Center, Attending Urologist in Chief at New York Hospital.—J.Y. Gillenwater, M.D.

The Captopril Test for Identifying Renovascular Disease in Hypertensive Patients
Franco B. Muller, Jean E. Sealey, David B. Case, Steven A. Atlas, Thomas G. Pickering, Mark S. Pecker, Jacek J. Preibisz, and John H. Laragh (New York Hosp.-Cornell Med. Ctr.)
Am. J. Med. 80:633–644, April 1986   22–1

The relationships between plasma and renal vein renin values in essential hypertension and in unilateral and bilateral renovascular disease have been defined, and plasma renin assays have become more reliable. A simple screening test was developed by defining the criteria for plasma renin or blood pressure response, or both, to captopril to differentiate essential and renovascular hypertension.

A retrospective review was made of data on 317 outpatients given a single oral dose of captopril as part of an evaluation for hypertension. Subsequently, 71 patients were excluded from the study on clinical grounds. Of the other 246, 171 were studied while receiving no antihypertensive medication. The other 75 received a variety of antihypertensive drugs. The patients were further subdivided according to renal function. Plasma renin activity was measured 60 minutes after captopril administration by standard methods.

Of 200 hypertensive patients without evidence of renal dysfunction, all 56 who had renovascular disease were correctly identified by their renin secretory responses to captopril administration. False positive results were found in only 2 of 112 patients with essential hypertension and in 6 with secondary hypertension. The captopril test appears to be a useful screening tool in identification of patients with unilateral or bilateral renovascular disease. The test is much simpler, less expensive, more specific, and less invasive than older screening procedures such as intravenous pyelography, arteriography, nuclear and radionuclide scanning, and the saralasin test.

▶ We continue to believe that this test is the most accurate means to identify patients with renovascular hypertension (see table). However, since publica-

PREDICTIVE VALUE OF SCREENING TESTS FOR RENOVASCULAR HYPERTENSION*

	IVP	DIVA	PRA	SINGLE–DOSE CAPTOPRIL
Sensitivity (%)	75	88	80	100
Specificity (%)	86	89	84	95
False positive (%)	14	11	16	5
False negative (%)	25	12	20	0
Predictive value (%)				
Prevalence				
2	9.9	14.6	9.3	29
5	22.1	30.5	20.8	51.3
10	37.5	48.1	35.7	69
Exclusion value (%)				
Prevalence				
2	99.4	99.7	99.5	100
5	98.5	99.3	98.8	100
10	96.7	98.5	97.4	100

*Calculations:
Predictive value
$$= \frac{\text{sensitivity} \times \text{prevalence}}{(\text{sensitivity} \times \text{prevalence}) + \text{false positive rate} \times (100 - \text{prevalence})} \times 100$$
Exclusion value
$$= \frac{\text{specificity} \times (100 - \text{prevalence})}{\text{specificity} \times (100 - \text{prevalence}) + \text{false negative rate} \times \text{prevalence}} \times 100$$
Abbreviations: IVP, intravenous pyelogram; DIVA, digital angiography; PRA, plasma renin activity.
Data derived from various sources.
[From Gillenwater, J.Y., et al. (eds.): *Adult and Pediatric Urology.* Chicago, Year Book Medical Publishers, Inc., 1987, p. 759.]

tion of this report there have been occasional false negative results with the captopril tests. Accordingly, if a high index of suspicion for renovascular hypertension exists and blood pressure is refractory to antihypertensive treatment, renal vein renin studies should be obtained for the sake of completeness despite a negative result.—E.D. Vaughan, Jr., M.D.

Prevention of Venous Thrombosis and Pulmonary Embolism
Consensus Development Panel, Office of Medical Applications of Research, NIH, Bethesda)
JAMA 256:744–749, Aug. 8, 1986   22–2

Deep venous thrombosis and pulmonary embolism constitute major health problems in the United States. Prevention may prove beneficial in some patients at high risk for the development of venous thromboembolism. The National Heart, Lung, and Blood Institute and the National Institutes of Health Office of Medical Applications of Research convened a Consensus Development Conference on Prevention of Venous Thrombosis and Pulmonary Embolism to define the patients at risk for deep venous thrombosis and the various prophylactic regimens for it.

Deep venous thrombosis and pulmonary embolism are major causes of morbidity in many common medical and surgical procedures. The incidence of deep vein thrombosis in patients aged 40 years and older undergoing general surgical procedures is 25% by fibrinogen scanning and 19% by venography. Advancing age and malignancy are also associated with higher risks of deep vein thrombosis and pulmonary embolism. The incidence of deep venous thrombosis in urologic surgery is also 25%, and ranges from 40% in transvesical prostatectomy to 10% in transurethral surgery. Urologic patients often have a higher risk than other surgical patients because of increasing age. Other patients at high risk for deep vein thrombosis include orthopedic patients undergoing elective surgery on the lower extremity, particularly the hip and knee; gynecologic patients more than 40 years of age with added risk factors, e.g., prior deep vein thrombosis and pulmonary embolism, varicose veins, infection, estrogen therapy, obesity, and prolonged surgery; neurosurgical patients; and patients with multisystemic trauma. Patients with heart failure, acute myocardial infarction, or pulmonary infection are also at risk for deep vein thrombosis.

A prophylactic regimen should be used extensively in these patients and should include treatment with low-dose heparin, adjusted-dose heparin, dextran, and warfarin. Low-dose warfarin, external pneumatic compression, and gradient elastic stockings, alone or in combination with heparin or heparin/dihydroergotamine, are also effective in decreasing the occurrence of deep venous thrombosis. Aspirin has not been beneficial. Although none of these prophylactic regimens is ideal, most are relatively simple to use, complications are generally few, and the need for laboratory monitoring is minimal. Prophylactic therapy should be tailored according to the patient's disease and degree of risk.

▶ The data given for urology in this article are derived from the book *Postoperative Thromboembolism* by David Bergquist (Sandoz, 1983), p. 14, table 5. However, the reader should be aware that the percentages given are based on the ^{125}I-fibrinogen test. Because this test is a scientific tool and is not used to diagnose thrombosis for treatment purposes, the clinical relevance of the finding remains unclear. Moreover, the efficacy of low-dose heparin prophylaxis is less apparent than the panel findings suggest (see Bergquist). I do not think many follow the panel's recommendation to use low-dose heparin prophylaxis in urology patients over the age of 40.—E.D. Vaughan, Jr., M.D.

Continuous Intravenous Heparin Compared With Intermittent Subcutaneous Heparin in the Initial Treatment of Proximal-Vein Thrombosis

Russell D. Hull, Gary E. Raskob, Jack Hirsh, Richard M. Jay, Jacques R. Leclerc, William H. Geerts, David Rosenbloom, David L. Sackett, Christine Anderson, Linda Harrison, and Michael Gent (Chedoke-McMaster Hosps., Hamilton, Ont.)

N. Engl. J. Med. 314:1109–1114, Oct. 30, 1986   22–3

Heparin is the initial treatment for acute venous thrombosis. A randomized, double-blind trial was performed to compare intravenous with intermittent subcutaneous heparin administration in the initial treatment of 115 patients with acute proximal deep vein thrombosis.

Intermittent subcutaneous heparin therapy proved to be inferior in this trial in the prevention of venous thromboembolism. It induced a below-target anticoagulant response in most patients, and there was a 19.3% frequency of recurrent venous thromboembolism. Continuous venous heparin administration induced a therapeutic anticoagulant response in most patients. The frequency of recurrent venous thromboembolism was 5.2%, significantly less than that in the subcutaneous group. The recurrences developed in those patients in whom therapeutic concentrations of anticoagulant were not achieved.

The intravenous administration of heparin is the treatment of choice for proximal venous thrombosis. The study suggests a relationship between the effectiveness of heparin therapy and the levels of anticoagulation achieved. This may explain the failure of the subcutaneous regimen.

▶ This article may possibly explain some of the confusion that exists concerning the use of subcutaneous heparin as prophylaxis against postoperative venous thrombosis.—E.D. Vaughan, Jr., M.D.

23 Ureter

Therapeutic Ureteral Occlusion in Advanced Pelvic Malignant Tumors
Anne-Charlotte Kinn, Hans Ohlsén, Eva Brehmer-Andersson, and Jan Brundin
(Karolinska Hosp., Southern Hosp., and Danderyd Hosp., Stockholm)
J. Urol. 135:29–32, January 1986   23–1

A vesicovaginal fistula often leads to total urinary incontinence, which is treated by nephrostomy. Hygiene is often difficult when an advanced tumor has led to necrosis that prevents all of the urine from draining through the catheters. Supplementary occlusion of the ureters with hydrogel plugs was studied in 15 patients who had undergone nephrostomy. The 12 women and 3 men (average age, 61 years) had received radiotherapy and, in some cases, surgery for malignant tumors. Several weeks before insertion of the plugs, the patients had undergone nephrostomy. Initially, polidocanol, a sclerosing agent, was injected into the ureters through a catheter to induce a fibrotic stricture and to keep plugs in situ. The 1-cm hydrogel plugs were then inserted.

Urinary leakage ceased in 11 patients, was significantly diminished in 2, and appeared unchanged in 2. The most serious complication, plug migration to the renal pelvis in several patients, might have been the cause of pyelonephritis in one case. The long-term risk of tissue damage is not known. Ureteral occlusion with a hydrogel plus and polidocanol is recommended to control urine leakage in patients whose life expectancy is short.

▶ The authors describe a useful technique. Obstruction of the ureter with simple balloons does not always work. Debrun and associates (*Neuroradiology* 9:267, 1975) described another useful technique, i.e., combining a detachable balloon, a catalyst, and silicone rubber.—S.S. Howards, M.D.

Urine-Compatible Polymer for Long-Term Ureteral Stenting
John F. Cardella, Wilfrido R. Castaneda-Zuniga, David W. Hunter, John C. Hulbert, and Kurt Amplatz (Univ. of Minnesota)
Radiology 161:313–318, November 1986   23–2

Internal double-J ureteral stents were made from C-Flex, a urine-compatible polymer, and evaluated in 28 patients having 35 stents placed in 1984–1985. These patients, 16 women and 12 men, had a mean age of 57 years, and most had neoplastic obstructions from a primary or metastatic tumor. A posteriorly directed middlepole or upper pole calix is preferred for entry into the collecting system. Ureteral dilatation was achieved with balloon catheters or Teflon coaxial cancer dilators, and a small pigtail nephrostomy catheter was left in the renal pelvis for up to 48 hours after stent placement.

The overall mean stent follow-up was 5 months. All ureteral obstructions were crossed successfully, 62% of them at the first session. Eight stents remained patent until the patient died, and four others remained patent until they were removed electively from patients with benign disease. The longest time of stent service was 16 months. Seven stents became occluded, three by clots in early cases when the stent was placed in a grossly hemorrhagic collecting system. Physical testing of the C-Flex tubing suggested that exposure to human urine improved the tensile strength of the tubing but also increased its hardness and stiffness and, therefore, its brittleness.

High stent patency rates may be achieved by increasing urine flow through a greater oral intake, by using oral antibiotics prophylactically, and by avoiding stent placement into an infected or grossly bloody collecting system. Prophylaxis is usually with trimethoprim-sulfamethoxazole.

▶ Periodic stent replacement in patients with "permanent" double-J catheters presents an important clinical problem. A material that would prolong the patency of these stents would be a most welcome addition to our armamentarium. Unfortunately, the C-flex stents tested by the authors do not appear to be significantly better than other available products.—S.S. Howards, M.D.

Percutaneous Surgery for Ureteropelvic Junction Obstruction (Endopyelotomy): Technique and Early Results

Gopal Badlani, Majid Eshghi, and Arthur D. Smith (Long Island Jewish-Hillside Med. Ctr., New Hyde Park)
J. Urol. 135:26–28, January 1986   23–3

In 1943, Davis described enlargement of the ureteral caliber by postoperative stenting in the treatment of ureteropelvic junction obstruction. Endopyelotomy provides the advantages of this procedure without an open operation and without damage to the periureteric blood supply.

TECHNIQUE.—A percutaneous nephrostomy is established through a central calix and a guidewire is passed down the ureter. A nephroscope is inserted if necessary, or a guidewire may be passed up the ureter. Alternately, the nephrostomy may be made and the guidewire passed retrograde. A cold knife direct-vision endopyelotome then is passed through a working sheath, and the ureteral wall is incised on the side toward the kidney until the periureteric fat is visible. The ureteropelvic junction is then intubated with a universal ureteral stent, and a nephrostomy tube is inserted.

Thirty-one patients aged 7–79 years who underwent endopyelotomy were followed for up to 2 years. Initial patients had renal stones and moderate to severe ureteropelvic junction obstruction, whereas later patients were treated for obstruction secondary to pyelolithotomy, failed pyeloplasty, or isolated ureteropelvic junction obstruction. No immediate complications occurred. Nephrostograms obtained 6 weeks postoperatively showed an adequate ureteropelvic junction in 27 patients. All of these patients were asymptomatic during follow-up. Four patients required open surgery to correct a nonpatent ureteropelvic junction. The causes of failure included ureteral deviation with adhesions, a massively redundant renal pelvis, and long stricture.

Endopyelotomy is associated with much less morbidity than open surgery and it is a cost-effective procedure. The ureteral blood supply remains intact. A redundant renal pelvis is not corrected by endopyelotomy. Slight constrictions are amenable to treatment by percutaneous balloon dilation and stenting.

▶ Percutaneous treatment of ureteropelvic junction obstruction is a useful technique with a role in the management of certain patients. We have used dilation without incision to treat failed pyeloplasty with good success, as have others. Results are less good for late surgical failures and radiation strictures. Whether percutaneous ureteral incision, as described above, will be more successful remains to be seen. The experience with urethral strictures is that internal urethrotomy is probably a bit better that urethral dilation but is hardly a panacea.

The series by Badlani and associates is difficult to interpret. One suspects that many of the patients did not require treatment in the first place. We have seen 5,000 stone patients in the last 3 years, none of whom needed a pyeloplasty, although some of the initial x-ray findings suggested that there might be a degree of ureteropelvic junction obstruction. At this point we would be reluctant to take a child with a fresh ureteropelvic junction obstruction who required treatment and subject him to this form of therapy for several reasons: It is unproven; if it failed, the child would have a prolonged course and be subjected to two anesthetics; and surgical treatment is relatively simple.—S.S. Howards, M.D.

24 Voiding Function

▶ The comments for this chapter were written by Dr. Alan J. Wein, Professor and Chairman of the Division of Urology at University of Pennsylvania School of Medicine, and Chief of Urology at the Hospital of University of Pennsylvania.—J.Y. Gillenwater, M.D.

Some Clinical Aspects of Uroflowmetry in Elderly Males: A Population Survey
Klaus M.E. Jensen, Jørgen B. Jørgensen, Peter Mogensen, and Niels E. Bille-Brahe (Bispebjerg Hosp., Copenhagen)
Scand. J. Urol. Nephrol. 20:93–99, 1986   24–1

In the present study a random sample of 200 men aged 50 years and older was selected to investigate various aspects of spontaneous uroflowmetry and to estimate the frequency of prostatism and lower urinary tract dysfunction symptoms. However, for various reasons, the final group consisted of 121 persons (60.5%) from which nine were excluded because of circumstances potentially influencing lower urinary tract function. The age range of these 112 individuals was 50–92 years (median age, 64.5 years).

After interviews in the outpatient clinic, uroflowmetry was performed. Experience of voiding problems was recorded, as well as physician consultation. Prostatism was defined as subjective voiding problems. Symptom analysis was based on complaints of decreased stream, hesitancy, intermittency, and terminal dribbling, and the irritative complaints of urge, nocturia, and diuria. Also included was the presence of dysuria and hematuria.

Voiding problems unrelated to dysuria and hematuria were reported by 19 persons. This resulted in a prevalence of prostatism of 17% (95% confidence limits 11% to 26%), whereas 88% (95% confidence limits 83% to 95%) had voiding symptoms of varying degrees. In the group with prostatism, 74% (95% confidence limits 48% to 91%) considered irritation, especially urge, to be the worst single symptom, although obstructive symptoms were equally common.

Only few associations between single symptoms of prostatism and uroflow variables were revealed. Analysis for correlation between symptom scores and uroflowmetry variables demonstrated significant correlations regarding total and obstructive symptom scores on the one hand and maximum and average flow rates on the other. No correlations were found when the irritative score was examined.

Because the correlations were modest and a sizable amount of overlap of uroflow variables in persons with and without prostatism were proved, the diagnostic specificity and sensitivity of maximum flow rate, as well as other uroflow variables, were low in the screening for prostatism. Decreased stream was not associated with any of the uroflow variables. Uroflowmetry therefore hardly appeared to confirm a clinical impression when prostatism is considered.

▶ There are many studies that have tried to look into the deceptively simple-sounding question of whether one can diagnose prostatism in a given individual on the basis of flow rates alone. The conclusion that these authors reach about this problem is a negative one. There is, however, another way of looking at the question. Uroflowmetry is but one part of an overall urodynamic evaluation that itself is only one part of the overall neurourologic evaluation. Uroflowmetry concerns not only flow rates, but an evaluation of flow pattern, and includes residual urine volume determination. Uroflowmetery is not a complicated or invasive study.

The authors seem to approach urinary flow rates as diagnostic indices, as if the study were somewhat simliar in scope to a study such as cardiac catheterization. In a given afternoon, most male patients over 60 in my practice have a symptom score, using the authors' symptom score table, of around 8. The individuals in the authors' series with "prostatism" had an average symptom score of 9, whereas their patients with "no prostatism" had an average symptoms score of 3.

The most important question here, and one that the authors do not address, is whether or not patients whom they label as "having prostatism" should have treatment for bladder outlet obstruction. In their original article, the authors state that "prostatic hyperplasia, however, is a benign lesion and obviously the logical scale to measure successful treatment is the degree of symptom reduction as judged by the patient." The implication of this statement is that whatever measures are used to judge whether or not a patient has "prostatism" should be correlated with the results of treatment to relieve "prostatism." In other words, the real question is, are there any symptoms or signs (such as uroflowmetry variables) that are correlated with more satisfactory symptom reduction following treatment of what has been diagnosed as bladder outlet obstruction? More importantly, are there any symptoms or signs that might prompt one to expect a less satisfactory result, and prompt a more extensive evaluation to see whether bladder outlet obstruction really exists?

There is another very valuable potential advantage to flowmetry and that is being able to compare postoperative to preoperative values in a patient who has in fact not experienced satisfactory symptom resolution after prostatectomy. This can and does serve, on occasion, as valuable information for both physician and patient as to whether outlet obstruction has in fact been relieved. In my opinion, few studies in urologic practice are as easy to do as uroflowmetry, and few studies yield such valuable diagnostic information in proportion to the amount of effort they require. One additional suggestion that might be helpful to improve the information attained is to carry out two uroflow events during whatever testing sequence the patient is to undergo and to take "the best" of the two as more representative of a given patient's average effort. We have found that, in some patients, flow events at the beginning and end of a given diagnostic sequence are not similar, and "the best" generally cor-

relates with what the patients tell you is their usual typical flow sequence.—
A.J. Wein, M.D.

The following review article is recommended to the reader:

McGuire, E.J.: The innervation and function of the lower urinary tract. *J. Neurosurg.* 65:278, 1986.

25 Voiding Dysfunction

▶ The comments for this chapter were written by Dr. Alan J. Wein, Professor and Chairman of the Division of Urology at University of Pennsylvania School of Medicine, and Chief of Urology at the Hospital of University of Pennsylvania.—J.Y. Gillenwater, M.D.

Initial Bladder Management in Spinal Cord Injury: Does It Make a Difference?

L.K. Lloyd, K.V. Kuhlemeier, P.R. Fine, and S.L. Stover (Univ. of Alabama at Birmingham)
J. Urol. 135:523–527, March 1986
25–1

Various forms of initial urologic management were reviewed in 204 patients aged 13–80 years with acute spinal cord injuries. Twenty-one patients (group A) were undergoing intermittent catheterization within 36 hours of injury and continued it until there was consistently acceptable reflex voiding. Twenty-one others (group B) received a suprapubic trocar within 36 hours of injury. Indwelling catheters were in place for 3 days or longer (mean, 36 days) before intermittent catheterization in 106 patients (group C). Twenty-three patients (group D) underwent indwelling urethral catheter drainage throughout hospitalization. Thirty-three patients (group E) were started on intermittent catheterization at a community hospital shortly after injury.

More than half of the patients undergoing early intermittent catheterization or trocar drainage were being treated by condom drainage at the first annual follow-up (Table 1), as were patients managed with a urethral

TABLE 1.—Urologic Management Method 1 Year After Injury for Five Original Groups

Urological Management Method	Group					Totals
	A	B	C	D	E	
Foley catheter	3	1	9	20	4	37
Condom	12	17	61	0	13	103
Credé's maneuver	1	0	11	0	5	17
Normal	3	2	12	1	4	22
Intermittent catheterization	1	1	12	1	6	21
Ileal conduit	0	0	0	0	1	1
Suprapubic drainage	0	0	1	0	0	1
Diapers	0	0	0	1	0	1
Totals	20*	21	106	23	33	203*

*One patient died within 1 year after injury.
Courtesy of Lloyd, L.K., et al.: J. Urol. 135:523–527, March 1986. © Williams & Wilkins, 1986.)

TABLE 2.—Ratio of Patients With at Least One Episode of Chills and Fever Between Injury and Discharge From Hospital, and Between Discharge and 1 Year After Injury

Interval	Group				
	A No./Total (%)	B No./Total (%)	C No./Total (%)	D No./Total (%)	E No./Total (%)
Injury to hospital discharge	4/21 (19.1)	4/21 (19.1)	9/104 (8.6)	4/23 (17.4)	2/33 (6.1)
Discharge to 1 yr. after injury	4/17 (23.5)	8/18 (44.4)	26/97 (26.8)	8/16 (50.0)	6/22 (27.3)

(Courtesy of Lloyd, L.K., et al.: J. Urol. 135:523–527, March 1986. © Williams & Wilkins, 1986.)

catheter in the early stages. Chills and fever were comparably frequent in all groups (Table 2). Renal plasma flow at discharge was lowest in group D, but most patients in this group were females. Group rates of pyelocaliectasis did not differ significantly. No patient had moderate or severe ureterectasis at discharge, but four group C kidneys were so affected at 1 year. Vesicoureteral reflux was infrequent, and the overall incidence of complications was low. Ten operations for outlet obstruction were necessary.

Urethral catheter drainage is an acceptable short-term aproach to cord-injured patients. Intermittent catheterization may be instituted if an established program is available. Suprapubic trocar cystostomy might be best for a patient not entering rehabilitation, or if a delay of 3 months or longer is expected. Long-term urethral catheter drainage is associated with an increased risk of urinary tract complications, especially stone formation.

▶ The authors' conclusions are entirely consistent with their data. It should be remembered that, at the time intermittent catheterization was first described as a method of initial bladder care for patients with acute spinal cord trauma, the high incidence of urologic complications generally was attributed to indwelling catheterization. Since that time there have been many advances in the management of patients with an indwelling urethral catheter, but, at that time, intermittent catheterization certainly circumvented many of these considerations and still remains the benchmark by which other forms of acute management must be measured.

The authors' data indicate that, as long as close follow-up is instituted, it makes little difference whether the lower urinary tract in acute spinal cord injury patients is managed initially by intermittent catheterization, suprapubic trochar, or an indwelling urethral catheter. Whether these conclusions are universally applicable to all spinal cord injury patients in all locales remains to be seen. Temporary and closely attended indwelling tube drainage, careful further evaluation, and patient compliance and follow-up seem to be absolute requirements to support the contention that the method of initial bladder management is relatively unimportant. The reader should note that, though there was no statistically significant difference in the incidence of chills and fever in the various groups (Table 2), the incidence does appear numerically greater in the groups with suprapubic drainge (B) and with an indwelling catheter (D).—A.J. Wein, M.D.

Functional Effects of In Vitro Obstruction on the Rabbit Urinary Bladder
Robert M. Levin, William Memberg, Michael R. Ruggieri, and Alan J. Wein (Univ. of Pennsylvania and Philadelphia VA Med. Ctr.)
J. Urol. 135:847–851, April 1986   25–2

Bladder outlet obstruction, a common pathophysiologic state, has been studied extensively. The long-term compensation by the bladder with muscular hypertrophy and hyperplasia are wellknown. Experiments were undertaken to study the short-term effects of partial obstruction of the bladder in normal white New Zealand rabbits. Bladders were excised and placed on electrode-tipped catheters in a bath, and bladder pressure and volume were monitored constantly. The outlet port was clamped to simulate obstruction.

The location of the obstruction along the urethra had little effect; to empty, the obstructed bladder had to generate a pressure more than double that of a normal bladder. The obstructed bladder emptied 3.5 to 5 times slower than normal, depending on the volume; however, it did completely empty eventually. Control bladders could empty repeatedly during a 3-hour period, whereas obstructed bladders fatigued significantly.

The initial overdistention in response to partial bladder obstruction appears to be related to reduced bladder function. The large increase in pressure needed to empty the bladder may account for the hypertrophy and hyperplasia that develop later.

▶ Experimentally, the use of the whole bladder model has resulted in the demonstration that rapid and significant functional alterations occur in response to partial bladder outlet obstruction. These studies indicate that the obstructed bladder requires increased pressure to empty and, though it can empty completely, the rate of emptying is significantly reduced and the time required to empty is significantly increased. The normal bladder is relatively resistant to fatigue, whereas the obstructed bladder fatigues rapidly with repetitive stimulation. All of these factors seem to participate in the initial overdistention seen shortly after partial obstruction. After this initial insult, compensation is relatively rapidly achieved by bladder muscle hypertrophy and hyperplasia.

One wonders what the end point of reversibility is, and why some obstructed bladders "decompensate" and others do not. Are the degree of obstruction and/or the rate at which it develops important in determining reversibility? Further answers to questions such as this might help us to determine whether, in a given patient, outlet reduction is necessary or elective.—A.J. Wein, M.D.

Oxybutynin Versus Propantheline in Patients With Multiple Sclerosis and Detrusor Hyperreflexia

Jerzy B. Gajewski and Said A. Awad (Dalhousie Univ., Halifax)
J. Urol. 135:966–968, May 1986   25–3

Urinary symptoms occur in at least half of the patients with multiple sclerosis, with detrusor hyperreflexia being the most common single urodynamic finding. Although several therapeutic agents have been used to treat this problem, the results have not always been well documented. The effectiveness of oxybutynin and propantheline was compared in multiple sclerosis patients with detrusor hyperreflexia. Oxybutynin is a tertiary amine having distinct anticholinergic activity as well as a direct smooth muscle relaxant and analgesic effect. Propantheline is a synthetic quaternary ammonium analogue of atropine that exerts its effect by competitive cholinergic blockade at the neuromuscular junction and the ganglion level.

The study population consisted of 34 patients with multiple sclerosis, all of whom had urinary symptoms. Nineteen patients received oxybutynin (5 mg orally three times daily) and 15 received propantheline (15 mg orally

TABLE 1.—CLINICAL RESPONSE

	Oxybutynin No. (%)	Propantheline No. (%)
Over-all No. pts.	15	11
Clinical response:		
Good	10 (67)	4 (36)
Fair	2 (13)	1 (9)
Poor	3 (20)	6 (55)

(Courtesy of Gajewski, J.B., and Awad, S.A.: J. Urol. 135:966–968, May 1986. © by Williams & Wilkins, 1986.)

TABLE 2.—CHANGES IN CYSTOMETROGRAPHY FOLLOWING TREATMENT

	Oxybutynin (12 pts.)		Propantheline (6 pts.)	
	Before	After	Before	After
Maximum cystometic capacity (ml.)	138.3 ± 64	282.5 ± 117.9*	163.3 ± 77.6	198.3 ± 129†
Height of the contraction (cm. water)	50.3 ± 42	36.7 ± 24†	44.7 ± 33	44.1 ± 33†

*Statistical significance ($P < .05$).
†No statistical difference ($P > .05$).
‡Values are given as mean ± standard deviation.
(Courtesy of Gajewski, J.B., and Awad, S.A.: J Urol. 135:966–968, May 1986. © by Williams & Wilkins, 1986.)

three times daily); the duration of treatment was for 6–8 weeks. Urodynamic examination, consisting of cystometrography and electromyography, was performed in all patients before treatment. Both groups of patients had comparable neurologic, urologic, and urodynamic status before treatment. In four patients (21%) treated with oxybutynin and in four (27%) treated with propantheline, side effects were so severe that the treatment had to be stopped. The symptomatic response to oxybutynin was good in ten patients (67%), fair in two (13%), and poor in three (20%). Propantheline produced good results in four patients (36%), fair results in one (9%), and poor results in six (55%) (Table 1). The mean increase in maximum cystometric capacity on cystometrography was substantially larger in the oxybutynin group than in the propantheline group (144 ± 115 vs. 35 ± 101) (Table 2). Oxybutynin is more effective than propantheline in the treatment of detrusor hyperreflexia in patients with multiple sclerosis.

► The authors report that, in their experience, using a randomized but unblinded treatment sequence, 5 mg of oxybutynin three times daily, produced better clinical and urodynamic results than propantheline, 15 mg. three times daily, in patients with detrusor hyperactivity secondary to multiple sclerosis. There is no question that oxybutynin is an excellent drug, and it has certainly found a place in the urologic armamentarium of those who treat detrusor hyperactivity. However, the real question is whether there is a dose of Pro Banthine, as Blaivas' findings would suggest (*J. Urol.* 124:259, 1980), that will produce a similarly good result, as the authors report with oxybutynin, with no more side effects. This question becomes important only if there is a significant difference in price between the two agents within a given area.

Propantheline bromide is strictly an antimuscarinic agent. Oxybutynin chloride also has significant antimuscarinic properties, but it is classified as an antispasmodic or musculotropic relaxant, this designation implying that a major portion of its action is exerted "distal to" the muscarinic receptor (perhaps by affecting calcium translocation). It is also classified as having local analgesic properties. The fact that it has significant anticholinergic properties is well documented by its almost exclusively anticholinergic side effects. To this commentor, the significant point is this: If the actions of oxybutynin chloride on the lower urinary tract are primarily antimuscarinic (anticholinergic at the level of the bladder smooth muscle membrane), one "should" be able to achieve the same beneficial effects on detrusor hyperactivity with some dose of propantheline, a dose that produces a similar pharmacokinetic availability of antimuscarinic action. If the clinical effect of oxybutynin (not in vitro but in vivo) is, in a major fashion, unrelated to antimuscarinic properties, and especially if it also possesses clinically relevant anticholinergic effects on the bladder, then it may well be a "more effective" drug by anyone's standards. Additionally, if the musculotropic relaxant properties of oxybutynin far outweigh the antimuscarinic ones, there certainly exists a rationale for combining it with an antimuscarinic agent such as propantheline to achieve somewhat of an additive effect in selected patients.—A.J. Wein, M.D.

Effect of Vesical Outlet Obstruction on Detrusor Contractility and Passive Properties in Rabbits

Gamal M. Ghoniem, Claude H. Regnier, Piero Biancani, Lewis Johnson, and Jacques G. Susset (Roger Williams Gen. Hosp., VA Med. Ctr., and Rhode Island Hosp., Providence)

J. Urol. 135:1284–1289, June 1986   25–4

The detrusor significantly changes its structure and mechanical properties in response to obstruction of the vesical outlet. Experiments indicate that chronic obstruction leads to muscle cell hypertrophy and hyperplasia. The location and extent of changes in detrusor contractility and passive properties, and the relationship between the degree of obstruction and morphological changes, were examined.

Sixteen male white New Zealand rabbits were divided into groups to determine the optimal parameters of electrical stimulation to effect bladder contraction and the parameters of in vitro vesical contractions in normal, moderately, and severely obstructed animals. Outlet obstruction was incurred by implantation of a polyethlene tube around the bladder neck for 3 months. The excised bladders were measured for their response to electrical stimulation and their force-length characteristics, and then were analyzed histologically.

In all animals, the base of the detrusor was rigid, whereas the upper body was more contractile. There was a significant decrease in maximum active stress in the detrusors of the obstructed rabbits. Histology confirmed that hypertrophy was the major response of the detrusor to moderate obstruction, whereas hyperplasia predominated when severe obstruction was present. The length at which maximum contractility occurred was greatest in the moderately obstructed bladder and least in the severely obstructed bladder, with the normal detrusor in between.

The detrusor's response is proportional to the degree of outlet obstruction and is dependent on the bladder zone. Further studies are needed to characterize various types of and responses to obstruction to improve management of patients with bladder outlet obstruction.

▶ From the basic science literature that concerns bladder contractility, we rapidly learn that one experimental model is not comparable to another, and that different authors, although they may use the same terms, mean different things and seek answers to different questions. These authors have been interested in the biomechanical aspects of bladder contractility for some time and have made significant contributions on this subject. They report here that hypertrophy, with a lesser amount of collagen deposition, is the predominant response to moderate obstruction, whereas hyperplasia, with more collagen deposition, is the predominant response to severe outlet obstruction. They correlate this finding with data regarding passive force, indicating that a higher degree of stretch is needed in a moderately obstructed group than in a severely obstructed group.

Collagen deposition is yet another variable that must be considered in evaluating detrusor response to obstruction and its reversibility. Although these authors did not consider reversibility, perhaps the degree of "collagenosis," itself perhaps dependent on the rate of development and degree of obstruction, is a significant factor in determining the optimal time for relief of bladder outlet obstruction insofar as resolution of urodynamic parameters and symptoms are concerned.—A.J. Wein, M.D.

Late Urodynamic Findings After Surgery for Cauda Equina Syndrome Caused by a Prolapsed Lumbar Intervertebral Disk
Pekka Hellström, Pekka Kortelainen, and Matti Kontturi (Oulu Univ. Central Hosp., Finland)
J. Urol. 135:308–312, February 1986   25–5

After surgery to treat prolapsed lumbar intervertebral disks, most patients have changes in clinical or cystometric findings. Modern urodynamic methods have not been used extensively to evaluate such patients. Therefore, urodynamic measurements of bladder function were made in 20 patients with the cauda equina syndrome who had undergone surgery to treat prolapsed lumbar intervertebral disks within the previous 2 or 3 years. Urodynamic evaluation consisted of measurement of residual urine, water cystometry, pressure-flow electromyography, the ice water test, urethral pressure profilometry, and infusion sphincterometry.

Urodynamic findings were normal in four patients, no detrusor contraction was detected in three, two used the detrusor and straining during voiding, and three had unstable detrusors detected by cystometry. The five remaining patients had increased bladder capacity or decreased maximum flow rate. Neurologic findings were normal in two patients. All patients with decentralized detrusors had abnormal perianal sensations, although three still had detrusor contraction. Several months to years were needed for regeneration of the autonomic nerves supplying the bladder and genitals.

All patients with cauda equina syndrome need urodynamic testing, as bladder function can be seriously impaired even without symptoms. Early treatment is necessary to prevent irreversible sphincter paralysis. Patients with vesical dysfunction or urodynamic abnormalities must be followed for many years to prevent upper urinary tract damage.

▶ Most disk protrusions compress the spinal roots in the L4–5 or L5–S1 interspaces. When voiding dysfunction occurs, the most consistent urodynamic finding is detrusor areflexia. The striated sphincter may be normal or show evidence of denervation. Patients with voiding dysfunction generally present with the onset of difficulty in voiding, straining, or urinary retention. Laminectomy may not improve bladder function, and whether or not it does may be related, as these authors suggest, to the rapidity of surgical intervention after symptoms develop.

When one encounters a patient with voiding dysfunction some time after disk surgery, it is important to ascertain whether the dysfunction is the same as what existed before surgery or whether it is different. It is important to remember that the dysfunction may be a result of irreversible changes caused by the original pathology, uncorrected changes because of poor surgical technique, changes caused by the corrective surgery, or another pathologic factor that has developed since the surgery and may or may not be superimposed on some voiding dysfunction related to the disk itself or the surgery designed to correct it.

Individuals who have seemingly persistent "detrusor areflexia" after disk injury and laminectomy surgery must be watched carefully for the development of decreased compliance, which most likely represents a bladder response to decentralization. Intermittent catheterization is doubtless an excellent method of treatment for these individuals, but this may need to be coupled with anticholinergic and/or musculotropic relaxant therapy to decrease intravesical pressure during storage.—A.J. Wein, M.D.

The following review article is recommended to the reader:

Hinman, F., Jr.: Nonneurogenic neurogenic bladder (Hinman syndrome)—15 years later. *J. Urol.* 136:769, 1986.

26 Bladder Cancer

Bladder Carcinoma in Patients 40 Years Old or Less
J.M. Fitzpatrick and M. Reda (Meath Hosp., Dublin)
J. Urol. 135:53–55, January 1986   26–1

Although bladder carcinoma usually occurs in older persons, it is found occasionally in young individuals. Whether carcinoma in younger patients is less aggressive is the subject of much speculation. A retrospective study was conducted to determine the effect of age on malignant potential of bladder carcinoma.

Forty males and 10 females with transitional cell carcinoma of the bladder were grouped by age. Twenty-four were aged 30 years or younger and 26 were aged 31–40 years; about 64% of both groups smoked approximately a pack of cigarettes a day. All patients were treated by transurethral resection of the tumor or by biopsy and diathermy. Follow-up continued for 5 years in 10 patients, 5–10 years in 16, and more than 10 years in 24. In the younger group, 2 patients (8%) had recurrences, whereas the older group had 14 patients (54%) with recurrences.

The prognosis for bladder carcinoma among persons aged 30–40 years is no different from that in the older population. The prognosis for the group younger than age 30 years was more favorable; however, these patients should still be followed carefully.

▶ This is a nice epidemiologic study showing that low-grade and low-stage bladder cancer in patients younger than 30 years of age had a favorable prognosis. However, these patients will be "at risk" for a very long time, and longer follow-up is needed to determine in how many, if any, the disease progresses to invasive bladder cancer. I think that such patients younger than 30 years of age still require periodic urine paps every 3 months and cystoscopy every 6 months.—J.Y. Gillenwater, M.D.

The Treated Histories of Patients With Ta Grade 1 Transitional-Cell Carcinoma of the Bladder
George R. Prout, Jr., Barbara Bassil, and Pamela Griffin (Massachusetts Gen. Hosp., Boston)
Arch. Surg. 121:1463–1468, December 1986   26–2

Superficial transitional cell carcinomas are recognized as an exceedingly heterogeneous group of neoplasms. The spectrum of neoplasia spans a broad range of grossly and microscopically different morphological tumor types. In most reports, these tumors are clustered and then distinguished according to grade, stage, and response to therapy. A review was made of longitudinal, prospectively collected data concerning 160 patients with grade 1 transitional cell carcinoma. The study was carried out because the treated histories of these patients suggested that grade 1 transitional cell carcinoma may not be a true malignant neoplasm.

The mean follow-up period was 57 months. There were 92 new patients; 68 others had a history of transitional cell carcinoma. Fifty-three (33%) of these 160 patients never had another transitional cell carcinoma. However, 68 (43%) of the remaining 107 patients had recurrent Ta grade 1 transitional cell carcinoma. In 32 patients (20%), the disease progressed in grade and in 7 (4%) invasive transitional cell carcinoma developed; 5 patients underwent cystectomy, and 1 patient died of transitional cell carcinoma. High-risk factors included positive results of cytologic studies after therapy and three or more recurrences. Although multiple therapies were used, it was impossible to determine if anything other than transurethral resection changed the course in these patients. Patients with low-risk factors and Ta grade 1 tumors might be followed up with quarterly cytologic examination and cystoscopy once or twice a year unless a change in symptoms occurs.

▶ In this study patients with Ta grade 1 transitional cell carcinoma of the bladder had a 67% recurrence rate in an average 5-year follow-up. This is similar to the Mayo Clinic's 15-year follow-up study reported by Greene et al. (*J. Urol.* 110:205, 1973) with a 73% recurrence rate. Invasive bladder cancer developed in 10% of the patients, leading to death. This study by Prout et al. defines high-risk factors as multiple recurrences and positive cytologic findings during follow-up. These data support the use of periodic urine cytology and cystoscopy in these patients.—J.Y. Gillenwater, M.D.

Coincident Vesical Transitional Cell Carcinoma and Prostatic Carcinoma: Clinical Features and Treatment
P.A. Androulakakis, H.M. Schneider, G.H. Jacobi, and R. Hohenfellner (Univ. of Mainz, West Germany)
Br. J. Urol. 58:153–156, April 1986   26–3

Bladder urothelial carcinoma and prostatic carcinomas, when occurring together in a patient, are termed "double carcinoma." The treatment of this rare condition is not well documented. A retrospective study was conducted to determine the incidence of double carcinoma, the problems associated with management of both tumors, and the best treatment.

Twenty-two patients with bladder urothelial carcinoma and prostatic carcinoma underwent various treatments with follow-ups lasting for an average of 5 years. Nineteen patients underwent primary local resection, five received radiotherapy, three had primary endocrine treatment, and two underwent radical surgery. Transurethral resection was the most effective treatment for noninfiltrating bladder tumors, whereas radical cystoprostatectomy was the best treatment for deeply infiltrating bladder cancer. Localized intraprostatic tumors responded well to external radiotherapy, and transurethral resection of the prostate was sufficient for incidental prostate carcinoma.

Double carcinoma occurred in 1.5% of patients in whom bladder or prostate tumors were diagnosed. Histology is the first step to rule out the presence of transitional cell carcinoma, which must be treated aggressively. The pathologic stage of the bladder tumor is the best prognostic factor, and treatment is most effective when the two tumors are recognized simultaneously. Infiltrating bladder carcinoma must be treated aggressively, cystoprostatectomy being the most successful method. If radical surgery is contraindicated, radiotherapy is the next choice. Advanced prostatic cancer with noninfiltrating bladder tumors responds to transurethral bladder surgery and hormone therapy.

▶ The simultaneous occurrence and diagnosis of bladder transitional cell carcinoma and prostatic adenocarcinoma were reported in 1.5% of the patients with prostate and bladder cancers. The authors conclude that the prognosis depends on the stage and grade of each tumor, and that their coexistence does not worsen the prognosis.—J.Y. Gillenwater, M.D.

Transurethral Ultrasonography in Bladder Cancer
Martin I. Resnick and Elroy D. Kursh (Case Western Reserve Univ., Cleveland)
J. Urol. 135:253–255, February 1986   26–4

Certain patients with bladder cancer are understaged. The usefulness of transurethral ultrasonography was assessed in 62 patients having bladder tumors initially diagnosed by intravenous pyelography and/or cystoscopy. Initial transurethral biopsy was followed by more extensive resection, or segmental resection or cystectomy in patients with more invasive or diffuse tumor. Two transurethral probes are available, one for general use and one for retrograde imaging of the area around the bladder neck. Superficial bladder tumors are seen as echogenic masses projecting into the bladder lumen (Fig 26–1). Infiltrative tumors tend to have a broader base. Tumors extending through the bladder wall can be identified by the presence of an extravesical mass.

A clear distinction between stages A and B1, or stages B1 and B2, sometimes was difficult to make. The study was, however, generally helpful in determining the degree of tumor invasion of the bladder wall and planning appropriate treatment. Ultrasonography also was useful in monitoring the adequacy of transurethral resection. Markedly increased echogenicity was noted along the bladder wall just below the area of resection. Ultrasound study did not help to image residual tumor, but it did demonstrate the depth of resection into the bladder wall.

Transurethral ultrasonography is helpful in staging bladder tumors and also in monitoring the depth of transurethral resection. The method also may prove applicable to the assessment of gynecologic lesions, large bowel tumors, and malignancies of neural or bony origin. Ultrasonography has not proved useful in assessing the pelvic nodes for metastatic involvement.

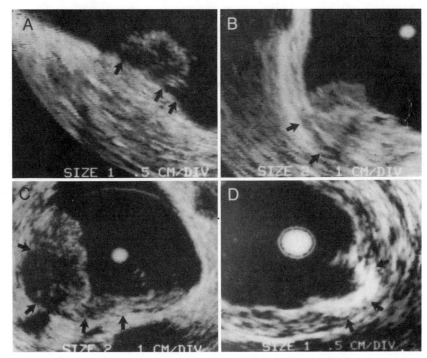

Fig 26–1.—A, transurethral scan of pathologically confirmed stage A bladder tumor. Bladder wall *(arrows)* is well preserved. **B,** transurethral scan of invasive (stage B2) bladder tumor. *Arrows* define limits of tumor. **C,** transurethral scan of stage C bladder tumor *(arrows)* demonstrates complete invasion and infiltration of bladder wall. **D,** transurethral scan obtained following resection of superficial (stage A) bladder tumor. Note increased echogenicity *(arrows)* associated at area of resection. (Courtesy of Resnick, M.I., and Kursh, E.D.: J. Urol. 135:253–255, February 1986. © by Williams & Wilkins, 1986.)

▶ Urologists need to become more familiar with ultrasonography. In the German hospitals I visited, an ultrasound machine is located on each hospital floor and abdominal ultrasonography is performed as a routine part of the physical examination. This article shows that transurethral vesical ultrasonography is useful in staging bladder cancer, but not in evaluating the presence of nodal metastases. Transvaginal ultrasound is also being used to evaluate pelvic organs including the bladder.—J.Y. Gillenwater, M.D.

Long-Term Effect of Intravesical Bacillus Calmette-Guerin on Flat Carcinoma In Situ of the Bladder

Harry W. Herr, Carl M. Pinsky, Willet F. Whitmore, Jr., Pramod C. Sogani, Herbert F. Oettgen, and Myron R. Melamed (Memorial Sloan-Kettering Cancer Ctr., New York)

J. Urol. 135:265–267, February 1986   26–5

Evaluation was made of the long-term therapeutic effect of intravesically administered bacillus Calmette-Guerin (BCG) on flat carcinoma in situ of the bladder. Between March 1978 and July 1981, 47 patients with diffuse, often symptomatic, carcinoma in situ were treated with intravesical BCG and followed every 3–4 months with cystoendoscopy, biopsy, and urine cytology for 3–6 years. All patients had prior or concurrent superficial papillary tumors that were controlled initially by transurethral resection and fulguration 2–3 weeks prior to BCG treatment. Results in patients given BCG were compared with those in patients having only transurethral resection.

Of the 47 patients, 23 received BCG intravesically and percutaneously. Treatment with BCG intravesically alone was initiated in 24 patients with carcinoma in situ. Bacillus Calmette-Guerin was given intravesically (Pasteur strain, 120 mg in 50 ml saline retained for 2 hours) and intradermally (Tice strain, 5×10^7 viable units by multiple time technique) once a week for 6 weeks. Side effects were generally mild, transient, and not dose limiting. Dysuria was the most common complication.

Of the 47 patients, 32 (68%) remained free of disease at 6 years, 15 (65%) after receiving BCG via combined routes for a median duration of 51 months (range, 37–75 months); 17 patients (71%) were disease free after receiving intravesical BCG alone for a median of 45 months (range, 36–53 months). In the randomized study, 4 of 23 patients (17%) required cystectomy because of local progression of disease, as did 17 of 26 controls (65%) who were randomized to transurethral resection and fulguration only. Cystectomy was performed within 3–27 months after BCG treatment. In three patients, tumor was localized to the prostate gland; none was found within the bladder.

Bacillus Calmette-Guerin significantly reduced the number of patients needing cystectomy as well as the time to cystectomy. The interval to alternative therapy in the BCG-treated patients was prolonged. Prior exposure to intravesical chemotherapy did not affect the overall response to BCG. Bacillus Calmette-Guerin is capable of producing long-term remissions of diffuse carcinoma of the bladder in a significant number of high-risk patients. The results confirm that the combination of transurethral resection and BCG is more effective than the former alone.

▶ Patients in this study had three forms of therapy: (1) transurethral resection (TUR) alone, (2) TUR plus BCG, intravesically and intradermally, and (3) TUR plus BCG, intravesically. This study showed that in patients with carcinoma in situ of the bladder, TUR alone was not as effective as TUR plus BCG intravesically. Intravesically administered BCG was as effective as BCG intravesically and intradermally. A one-time, 6-week course was effective for up to 6 years.—J.Y. Gillenwater, M.D.

Prognostic Value of Purified Protein Derivative Skin Test and Granuloma Formation in Patients Treated With Intravesical Bacillus Calmette-Guerin

David R. Kelley, Eric O. Haaff, Michael Becich, Janice Lage, Walter C. Bauer, Steven M. Dresner, William J. Catalona, and Timothy L. Ratliff (Washington Univ. and Jewish Hosp., St. Louis)

J. Urol. 135:268–271, February 1986   26–6

The intravesical administration of bacillus Calmette-Guerin (BCG) appears to be the most effective adjuvant approach in treatment of superficial bladder cancer. The prognostic value of an immunologic response to BCG intravesically was evaluated in 62 patients with superficial transitional cell carcinoma of the bladder who received this treatment once a week for 6 weeks. Purified protein derivative (PPD) skin tests were performed before and after therapy. Cold cup bladder biopsy specimens were examined in a blind retrospective fashion for the presence of granulomas 6 weeks after completion of therapy.

A significant correlation was observed between tumor-free status and the presence of either a positive response to the PPD test or granuloma formation in the bladder. Nineteen of 25 patients (77%) whose PPD test converted from negative to positive remained free of tumor, compared with 11 of 32 (34%) whose PPD test remained negative at follow-up evaluation. Similarly, 28 of 37 patients (77%) who had a granulomatous response remained free of tumor compared with 8 of 25 patients (32%) without a granulomatous response. Similar correlative trends were observed for each parameter in a subgroup analysis of patients treated for carcinoma in situ, residual tumor, or prophylaxis. However, neither parameter alone or in combination provided a highly accurate predictive index of therapeutic response in individual patients. False positive or false negative rates, ranging from 23% to 24% and 32% to 39%, respectively, were observed.

These results suggest a link between immunologic responsiveness and BCG-mediated antitumor response. Neither PPD nor a granulomatous response, although suggestive of therapeutic efficacy, exhibits sufficient immunologic specificity for use as a prognostic indicator in individual patients.

▶ There seems to be little question that intravesically administered BCG is effective in a large percentage of patients in preventing recurrent superficial bladder cancer. These studies show that patients whose PPD test converts from negative to positive and who have a granulomatous response have fewer recurrences of superficial bladder cancer. The mechanism of action of BCG in preventing bladder cancer is not known. These studies suggest an immunologic response. However, BCG has to be in contact with the mucosal surface, as suggested by its lack of effect on the ureter and urethra, which would imply that a systemic immunologic response is not the only mechanism at work.— J.Y. Gillenwater, M.D.

Two Courses of Intravesical Bacillus Calmette-Guerin for Transitional Cell Carcinoma of the Bladder
Eric O. Haaff, Steven M. Dresner, Timothy L. Ratliff, and William J. Catalona (Washington Univ. and Jewish Hosp., St. Louis)
J. Urol. 136:820–824, October 1986   26–7

Intravesically administered bacillus Calmette-Guerin (BCG) immunotherapy is becoming the adjunctive treatment of choice for patients with recurrent superficial transitional cell carcinoma of the bladder, but about 20% of patients fail to respond to the initial BCG treatment regimen. In an effort to determine the appropriate therapy for these patients, response rates were evaluated in 61 patients treated with a single 6-week course of BCG intravesically (120 mg, Pasteur strain); included were 25 patients who failed to respond to the initial course and were treated with a second 6-week course. No intradermal injections of BCG were given. Follow-up consisted of urinary cytology and bladder biopsy every 3 months.

Of 19 patients with carcinoma in situ, 8 (42%) responded to the initial BCG course and remained free of tumor for a mean of 15.1 months; 5 of 9 (56%) became tumor free after the second course. The overall cumulative response rate was 68% at a mean follow-up of 13.5 months. Of 13 patients treated for residual papillary tumors, 6 (46%) responded to the initial course and 3 of 7 (43%) responded to the second course. The overall response rate was 69% with a mean follow-up of 14.8 months. Of the patients treated for prophylaxis against tumor recurrence, 20 of 29 (69%) and 6 of 9 (67%) were free of tumor after the initial and second BCG courses, respectively, for an overall response rate of 90% at a mean follow-up of 12.8 months. The combined response rate free of tumor for all patients, inclusive of the two courses, was 79%. Response rates for the first and second 6-week treatment courses were identical at 56%, indicating that a single 6-week course of BCG intravesically alone was not optimally effective for all patients. In both treatment courses, patients whose purified protein derivative skin test converted from negative to positive were more likely to respond to BCG therapy than were those whose tests remained negative. Side effects were common but well tolerated in both treatment courses and consisted of dysuria/frequency, hematuria, and a flu-like syndrome. However, toxicity was more severe with prolonged treatment. A second 6-week course of BCG immunotherapy is warranted for patients who fail to respond to the initial treatment course.

▶ In this study, a single 6-week course of BCG intravesically resulted in a response rate of 56% in patients with carcinoma in situ of the bladder and 43% in those with residual papillary tumors. An additional 56% responded to a second 6-week course of BCG intravesically. These results are at variance with Harry Herr's at Memorial Hospital, which suggest that a single course is sufficient. I have been using a 6-week course and then instilling through the cystoscope one ampule of BCG with each follow-up cystoscopy. The obvious problem with this is that patients may be receiving unnecessary therapy.—J.Y. Gillenwater, M.D.

Monitoring Intravesical Bacillus Calmette-Guerin Treatment of Superficial Bladder Carcinoma by Serial Flow Cytometry

Robert A. Badalament, Helen Gay, Willet F. Whitmore, Jr., Harry W. Herr, William R. Fair, Herbert F. Oettgen, and Myron R. Melamed (Memorial Sloan-Kettering Cancer Ctr., New York)

Cancer 58:2751–2757, Dec. 15, 1986   26–8

It is now well established that the automated flow cytometry (FCM) can be used to identify and characterize superficial bladder carcinoma. Investigators have proposed that FCM might be of value in predicting response to bacillus Calmette-Guerin (BCG) intravesically in treatment of superficial bladder cancer. In a preliminary report, FCM of bladder irrigations done weekly during therapy and 6 weeks after treatment could differentiate responder from nonresponder. A comparison was made of FCM and cytology in 29 patients with superficial bladder carcinoma who were receiving intravesical treatment with BCG and were followed for 1 year or longer with simultaneous FCM, cytology and cystoscopic examinations at 3-month intervals.

Automated flow cytometry and cytology were in agreement in 57 of 103 examinations, with both FCM and cytology being positive in 38 instances and carcinoma confirmed by biopsy specimens in 35 (92.1%). In 16 instances, results of FCM and cytology were negative, but carcinoma was observed in a biopsy specimen in 5 instances (31.3%). Three examinations were suspicious by both techniques. The 46 determinations with discordant FCM and cytology were further divided into pathologically confirmed recurrences (25 patients) and no evidence of pathologic or cystoscopic disease (21). In the 25 patients with recurrence, FCM was positive in 18 (72.0%), suspicious in 3 (12.0%), and negative in 4 (16.0%), whereas cytology was positive in 3 (12.0%), suspicious in 9 (36.0%), and negative in 13 (52.0%). Most patients had a severe BCG-induced inflammatory response that caused an elevation of the hyperdiploid population. This was thought to be secondary to epithelial regeneration and proliferation. In the 21 patients without detectable recurrence, hyperploidy led to a relatively high proportion of positive (15) and suspicious (4) results by FCM, but only 8 had distinct aneuploid populations. This latter group, at least, is probably harboring occult carcinoma. Conventional cytology in the group with nonrecurrence was positive in 1 (4.8%), suspicious in 7 (33.3%), and negative in 13 (61.0%). When tumor was confirmed by biopsy examination, the false negative rate for FCM was 19.7% and that for cytology, 40.9%.

Automated flow cytometry appears to be more sensitive but less specific than conventional cytology, having a lower false negative but a higher false positive rate. Although serial FCM provides an objective quantitative measure of aneuploid stemlines and hyperdiploid populations in bladder irrigation specimens and can be helpful in following the effect of BCG intravesically in superficial bladder carcinoma, it should still be used with conventional cytology. The greatest difficulty with FCM at present, as with conventional cytology, is when substantial inflammation is present. The present results were obtained under the most stringent conditions and represent the minimum level of accuracy. Potential improvements in the technique with the addition of immunologic or other markers hold hope of further increasing the accuracy of FCM.

▶ Automated flow cytometry in this study is based on DNA measurements to recognize cell populations with aneuploid DNA and hyperdiploid DNA as characteristic of carcinoma. In this study, FCM was more sensitive but less specific than conventional cytology. More studies are needed to compare these two techniques.—J.Y. Gillenwater, M.D.

Complications of Bacillus Calmette-Guerin Immunotherapy in 1,278 Patients With Bladder Cancer
Donald L. Lamm, Valerie D. Stogdill, Brian J. Stogdill, and Ray G. Crispen (West Virginia Univ., Morgantown)
J. Urol. 135:272–274, February 1986   26–9

Data on 1,278 patients were reviewed to determine complications associated with bacillus Calmette-Guerin (BCG) therapy. Included were 195 patients seen by the authors, 134 reported in the literature, and 949 studied by various other physicians. The most commonly used substrains of BCG were Armand Frappier, followed by Tice and Connaught. The latter caused the fewest reported complications of any of these three substrains. Less commonly used strains included Paris Pasteur, Glaxo, and Moreau.

Cystitis occurred in 91% of the patients, usually with frequency and dysuria. Symptoms commonly began after two or three instillations and lasted for about 2 days. Chronic administration increased the duration and severity of cystitis. The complications identified included fever of more than 103 F in 50 patients (3.9%), granulomatous prostatitis in 17 (1.3%), BCG pneumonitis or hepatitis in 12 (0.9%), arthritis and arthralgia in 6 (0.5%), hematuria necessitating catheterization or transfusion in 6 (0.5%), skin rash in 5 (0.4%), skin abscess in 5 (0.4%), ureteral obstruction in four (0.3%), epididymo-orchitis in 2 (0.2%), bladder contracture in 2 (0.2%), hypotension in 1 (0.1%), and cytopenia in 1 (0.1%).

If patients experience severe or prolonged symptoms, treatment with 300 mg of isoniazid daily, diphenhydramine, and acetaminophen or ibuprofen is recommended. Treatment is continued during the course of symptom manifestation and reinstituted and continued for 3 days prophylactically the morning of subsequent BCG instillations. Isoniazid prophylaxis can also prevent constitutional symptoms and complications. Patients with life-threatening systemic BCG infection or anaphylaxis should be given 500 mg of cycloserine twice a day for 3 days in addition to combination antituberculous therapy, because the rapid action of this medication can be life-saving.

Bacillus Calmette-Guerin should never be injected directly into the skin because skin abscess formation, necrosis, and ulceration can result. Intravesically administered BCG generally appeared to be well tolerated in more than 95% of patients treated. Although deaths have been recorded after BCG treatment of numerous malignancies, none is known to have occurred in bladder cancer patients.

▶ This is a good review of the complications associated with the intravesical instillation of BCG, showing that there are relatively few serious side effects. Adverse side effects increase with the prolonged and frequent administration

166 / Urology

of BCG. I think before the use of simultaneous prophylactic isoniazid becomes routine, controlled studies must be done to prove that this approach does not prevent or modify the antitumor effects of BCG.—J.Y. Gillenwater, M.D.

Transpubic Cystectomy and Ileocecal Bladder Replacement After Preoperative Radiotherapy for Bladder Cancer
Kenneth Steven, Peter Klarskov, Henrik Jakobsen, H. Bay-Nielsen, and Finn Rasmussen (Univ. of Copenhagen)
J. Urol. 135:470–475, March 1986   26–10

Radical cystectomy requires urinary diversion and usually leads to erectile impotence. Urinary cystectomy is most often performed via an external conduit with an ileal stoma. To increase the quality of life after radical cystectomy, the operation was modified by leaving the apical prostatic capsule. This technique facilitates anastomosis of an isolated segment of intestine to the urethra and makes it possible to create an internal urinary diversion and retain normal micturition. Because it also avoids injury to the autonomic innervation of the corpora cavernosa, it preserves erectile potency. From February 1983 to January 1985, 15 consecutive patients with invasive bladder cancer underwent transpubic radical cystectomy with ileocolic bladder replacement.

The operation, modified radical cystectomy, left the apical prostatic capsule to facilitate anastomosis of the isolated ileocecal segment to the urethra and preserve erectile potency. The transpubic approach was used to increase exposure and facilitate dissection and anastomosis (Fig 26–2).

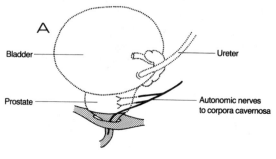
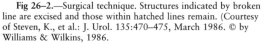
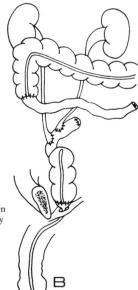

Fig 26–2.—Surgical technique. Structures indicated by broken line are excised and those within hatched lines remain. (Courtesy of Steven, K., et al.: J. Urol. 135:470–475, March 1986. © by Williams & Wilkins, 1986.

Fifteen patients with stages T1 to T4 bladder tumors underwent the operation, 13 after preoperative radiotherapy with 4,000 rad and 2 for salvage cystectomy after 6,000 rad.

One patient died postoperatively. The remaining 14 patients underwent urodynamic evaluation 3–6 months postoperatively. The maximum urine flow rates were almost normal, and none of the patients had significant residual urine. Although daytime urinary continence was satisfactory in 13 patients, 1 was moderately incontinent. However, all of the patients were incontinent at night, probably because of peristaltic contractions in the intestinal bladder and relaxation of the pelvic floor muscles. Preoperatively, eight patients experienced erections and seven had intercourse. Postoperatively, erectile potency was preserved in four patients, three of whom had sexual function. No orthopedic disability occurred postoperatively. The median follow-up was 20 months (range, 3–30 months). One year postoperatively, six of nine patients had sterile urine. The described technique avoids the need for a urinary stoma, obtains satisfactory voiding and urinary continence in almost all instances, and preserves sexual function in some patients.

▶ Urinary continence is important to all patients. Intestinal bladder replacement in continuity with the urethra is preferable to catheterization through a continent stoma. These patients were salvage cystectomies after radiation failure, which was a significant factor in causing the major and minor complications. Potency was preserved in 50%, which is not as high as the 85% rate reported by Walsh and Mostwin (*Br. J. Urol.* 56:694, 1984). The 100% rate of nocturnal incontinence was attributed to relaxation of pelvic floor muscles during sleep and continued peristaltic activity of the intestines. The long-term effect of reflux will have to be monitored.—J.Y. Gillenwater, M.D.

Selective Urethrectomy Following Cystoprostatectomy For Bladder Cancer

David P. Hickey, Mark S. Soloway, and William M. Murphy (Univ. of Tennessee, Baptist Mem. Hosp. and VA Hosp., Memphis)
J. Urol. 136:828–830, October 1986   26–11

The optimal management of the retained male urethra after cystectomy for bladder carcinoma remains controversial. Some investigators advocate prophylactic urethrectomy because of the poor prognosis associated with symptomatic urethral carcinoma. In 1976–1985, 75 cystoprostatectomies for bladder cancer were performed. Three underwent simultaneous urethrectomy because of tumor in the prostatic urethra, whereas the remaining 72 were monitored rigorously with urethral wash cytology studies every 6 months.

Of the 72 men followed for 6 months to 9 years after cystectomy, 7 (10%) had positive cytology findings after 2–40 months (mean, 11 months). In all seven, carcinoma in situ was found in subsequent urethral resections. To date, six are free of disease and one died 18 months after urethrectomy without evidence of tumor. There were no false positive findings in urethral wash cytology studies and no patient had local recurrence in the absence of a positive cytology result.

Simultaneous urethrectomy and cystectomy are indicated in the presence of tumor or carcinoma in situ in the urethra. Performing prophylactic urethrectomy in most patients with bladder cancer is unnecessary for a disease that has a 1 in 10 chance of urethral recurrence and would preclude future attempts at innovative urinary diversion techniques should they become necessary.

▶ In the future, many patients will request preservation of the urethra to allow bladder substitution with continent diversion and voiding through the urethra. I favor not doing a urethrectomy unless there is evidence of cancer or carcinoma in situ in the urethra. This study documents that urethral cytology evaluation is adequate to diagnose urethral recurrences.—J.Y. Gillenwater, M.D.

Intra-Arterial Infusion Chemotherapy in Combination With Angiotensin II for Advanced Bladder Cancer
Naoki Mitsuhata, Masaomi Seki, Yosuke Matsumura, and Hiroyuki Ohmori (Kure Mutual Aid Hosp., Kure, and Univ. of Okayama, Japan)
J. Urol. 138:580–585, September 1986   26–12

Twenty patients (16 men) aged 41–87 years with advanced bladder cancer were treated with intra-arterial infusion of angiotensin II in conjunction with cis-platinum administration. Twelve patients had clinical stage T3 disease, and 8, T4 disease. Seven patients had previously received systemic chemotherapy or radiotherapy. Patients were given cis-platinum infused in a dose of 50–80 mq/sq m via the internal iliac artery; they also received doxorubicin or the new anthracycline, tetrahydropyranyl-doxorubicin. Angiotensin II was infused at a rate of 1.5–2.0 μg/minute for 20 minutes on both sides. Patients were hydrated and underwent furosemide-induced diuresis. Two patients also received systemic chemotherapy, and two, radiotherapy.

A complete response was obtained in nine patients and a partial response in eight. Eight patients with a complete response had clinical stage T3 disease; grade IV disease was documented histologically in four of these. Marked tumor destruction without viable cells was observed histologically in 6 patients, and no tumor was seen in 4 of 15 who were evaluable. Arterial ^{81m}Kr infusion showed selective enhancement of regional flow in the tumor area after infusion of angiotensin II.

Intra-arterial infusion chemotherapy combined with angiotensin infusion is an effective regional treatment of bladder cancer that persists regionally. It also may be used to control intrapelvic disease in patients with advanced bladder cancer and distant metastases. Early regional control of cerebral, pulmonary, or hepatic metastases may be obtained. Pain from bone metastases may be controlled, as may intractable bleeding.

Intra-Arterial Chemotherapy as an Adjuvant to Surgery in Transitional Cell Carcinoma of the Bladder
Thomas J. Maatman, James E. Montie, Ronald M. Bukowski, Barbara Risius, and Michael Geisinger (Cleveland Clinic Found.)
J. Urol. 135:256–260, February 1986   26–13

The treatment of patients with locally advanced invasive bladder cancer remains unsatisfactory. A regimen using regional chemotherapy with intra-arterial cis-platinum alone, or combined with intra-arterial doxorubicin and cyclosphosphamide intravenously (intra-arterial CISCA) was developed as an adjuvant to radical cystectomy and urinary diversion in patients with transitional cell carcinoma of the bladder. The preliminary results of phases I and II of this treatment regimen in 25 patients were reviewed.

Intra-arterial chemotherapy was administered through a percutaneous catheter placed in the hypogastric artery. A total of 17 patients received intra-arterial CISCA, which consisted of 40–75 mg of cis-platinum per sq m intra-arterially for 30 minutes (17 patients), 30–40 mg of doxorubicin per sq m intra-arterially for 60 minutes (11 patients) or 12 hours (6 patients), and 400–500 mg of cyclophosphamide per sq m intravenously. Eight patients received 70–100 mg of cis-platinum per sq m intra-arterially for 30 minutes. Courses were repeated at 4-week intervals.

Patients treated with CISCA intra-arterially received 41 courses (median, 2 per patient). Clinical staging was T3aNxMo in six patients, T3bNx-2Mo in eight, and T4a-bNxMx-1 in three. Patients treated with intra-arterial cis-platinum alone received a total of 17 courses (median, 2 per patient). Clinical staging was T3aNxMx in two patients, T3bNxMx in four, and T4a-bNxMo-x in two. Overall, the clinical response was assessed in 24 patients: Six had a complete clinical response with disappearance of measurable disease preoperatively, 12 had a partial response with a decrease of more than 50% in size of mass with no new lesions identified, and 7 had no response. Sixteen patients underwent total cystectomy and urinary diversion with pathologic staging as follows: ToNoMo in three, T1NoMo in one, T3aNoMo in five, T3bNo-2Mo in six, and T4NoMo in one. Survival in patients treated with intra-arterial CISCA ranged from 2 to 30+ months (median, 12 months), and for those treated with intra-arterial cis-platinum alone, from 1 to 24+ months (median, 3.5 months). No death was attributed to intra-arterial chemotherapy. Myelosuppression and hematologic toxicity were minimal even in patients who had radiotherapy. The significant toxic effects noted included buttock pain, skin erythema, ulceration, and plexopathy, and were seen mostly in patients treated with intra-arterial CISCA, with doxorubicin the most likely causative agent. All toxic effects resolved with conservative treatment.

Intra-arterial CISCA and cis-platinum alone can produce a complete pathologic response as well as an objective partial response in patients with locally advanced transitional cell carcinoma of the bladder. Regional intra-arterial chemotherapy is safe and well tolerated by most patients, with moderate but reversible side effects.

▶ The value of intra-arterial chemotherapy in bladder cancer has not been defined. The major problems in B_2-C stages of bladder cancer are that 50% to 60% of patients have distant metastases, which are not cured by local chemotherapy. If local intra-arterial chemotherapy could be demonstrated to provide local control, then bladder preservation could be considered for some patients. There are still too many unanswered questions about this therapy for it to be used except under research protocols designed to better define its value.—J.Y. Gillenwater, M.D.

Treatment of Invasive Bladder Cancer With a Neodymium:YAG Laser
Joseph A. Smith, Jr. (Univ. of Utah)
J. Urol. 135:55–67, January 1986   26–14

Management of muscle-invading bladder tumors often requires radical cystectomy or, occasionally, segmental cystectomy. However, excessive bleeding and perivesical urinary extravasation can be the outcome of full-thickness transurethral resection of large segments of the bladder wall. Neodymium: yttrium/aluminum/garnet (Nd:YAG) laser treatment has minimal vaporizing or ablative tissue effects. Coagulative necrosis with good hemostatic properties develop, and healing occurs with collagen deposition so that the bladder wall maintains its structural integrity. The value of Nd:YAG laser therapy was assessed in 21 patients with muscle-invading bladder cancer who were unsuited for surgery.

Electrocautery resection was done to reduce tumor bulk and permit histologic staging of the disease. Five patients with clinical stage B_1, six with stage B_2, four with stage C, and six with known metastases received Nd:YAG laser energy by transurethral endoscopic application. Four of five patients with stage B_1 and three of six with stage B_2 lesions had normal findings in posttreatment biopsy specimens. Of the four patients with stage C tumors, only one had local tumor control. Of the patients previously known to have metastases, only palliative debulking was accomplished. Sigmoid colon perforation that was possibly treatment-related was the only complication (one patient).

Laser therapy appears to be most useful in patients with stage B_1 tumors and is much less effective in patients with more progressed tumors. The difficulty in correctly staging the tumor and detecting treatment failure makes laser therapy risky. Thus, laser therapy should be restricted to patients who refuse cystectomy or are not candidates for other therapies because of age or poor health.

▶ As the author states, the problem with Nd:YAG laser treatment of bladder cancer is the difficulty in correctly staging the tumor and detecting treatment failure. Adjacent bowel perforation is a risk but did not occur in this series. Four of five patients with B_1 bladder cancer appeared to have tumor eradication.

Further studies are needed to define how this therapy will be used clinically.—
J.Y. Gillenwater, M.D.

The following review articles are recommended to the reader:

Friedell, G.H., Soloway, M.S., Hilgar, A.G., et al.: Summary of workshop on carcinoma in situ of bladder. *J. Urol.* 136:1047, 1986.
Klimberg, I.W., Wajsman, Z.: Treatment for muscle invasive carcinoma of bladder. *J. Urol.* 136:1169, 1986.

27 Urinary Diversion

Accurate Determination of Renal Function in Patients With Intestinal Urinary Diversions
W. Scott McDougal, and Michael O. Koch (Vanderbilt Univ.)
J. Urol. 135:1175–1178, June 1986   27–1

In patients with intestinal segments interposed in the urinary tract, assessment of renal function is needed to determine the correct dose of antibiotics or antimetabolites, the progression of renal insufficiency, and the long-term efficacy of different forms of urinary diversion. However, nondiuretic creatinine or urea clearances and urine concentrating ability are no longer thought to give correct assessment of renal function. A prospective study was undertaken to determine whether urinary clearances of inulin, creatinine, and urea are dependent on urine flow rate, and whether they provide an accurate assessment of renal function.

Twenty-one patients with intestinal segments inserted into the urinary tract and eight normal individuals were tested after fasting overnight. Bolus and constant infusions of inulin were given, and urine and blood samples collected, before and after infusion of furosemide and large volumes of saline. Osmolality, inulin, creatinine, and urea were measured in the urine and serum samples. In the patients with urinary diversion, the glomerular filtration rate (GFR) was measured using technetium-labeled diethylenetriaminepentaacetic acid (DTPA).

In controls, inulin and creatinine clearances were independent of urine flow whereas in the patients with diversion, this independence occurred only at high rates of urine flow. Serum osmolality was similar in both groups, although urine osmolality was lower in patients with diversion. Cockcroft estimation of creatinine clearance significantly underestimated the true GFR in patients with intestinal segments in the urinary tract.

Assessment of renal function in patients with intestinal segments interposed in the urinary tract is most accurate when inulin clearance is determined under diuretic conditions. The GFR can also be estimated from serum and urine creatinine levels when urine output in these patients is 200–300 ml/hour. Under circumstances of diuresis, when intestinal reabsorption is minimized, these values correlate well with the true GFR.

▶ A significant number of patients have intestinal urinary diversions. If they are healthy with relatively normal renal function, precise measurement of their renal function is not of practical importance, although long-term trends in their GFR can be clinically significant. These patients can be followed by serum creatinine determination. However, a corollary of the message in this study is that the determinations should be made under similar conditions of hydration. It has long been known that patients with intestinal diversion reabsorb urea from the intestinal segment and thus have an elevated blood urea nitrogen-to-creatinine ratio. McDougal and Koch provide us with the important information that creatinine is also absorbed in significant amounts.

They also documented that creatinine clearances in these patients underestimate the true GFR unless the patient is very well hydrated. This could be important in patients receiving certain medications, e.g., cis-platinum. Some years ago we demonstrated that in children without urinary diversion the creatinine clearance is dependent on the state of hydration. Thus this effect may be even more pronounced in children with urinary diversions. It is also interesting that there was a very poor correlation between the DTPA-determined GFR and the GFR estimated from inulin clearance. We have always believed that GFRs estimated from nuclear studies had to be interpreted with caution.—S.S. Howards, M.D.

Bladder Reconstruction Following Cystectomy by Uretero-Ileo-Coloureth-rostomy
W. Scott McDougal (Vanderbilt Univ.)
J. Urol. 135:698–701, April 1986   27–2

After excision of the bladder, urine must be diverted to another reservoir, either one that is external or one constructed from the intestines. However, external reservoirs give the patient a changed body image and impede physical activity, and when the intestines are used for a reservoir, pyelonephritis, deterioration of the upper urinary tract, ureteral obstruction, and an increased risk of colon cancer occur. A review was made of the benefits and problems accompanying the use of the right colon as the urine reservoir.

Five patients, four adults with bladder carcinoma and one boy with congenital and iatrogenic injuries, underwent cystectomy and ileo-ascending bowel bladder construction. During surgery, the ileocecal valve was altered to form an antirefluxing valve. A Foley catheter was left in place for 3 weeks postoperatively, after which time the patients began intermittent self-catheterization.

During follow-up, ranging from 9 to 16 months, the anastomoses healed in all of the patients without complications. Within 3 months, all five patients urinated spontaneously, although one required self-catheterization intermittently. One patient who had decreased renal function experienced many episodes of bacteremia. Oral doses of bicarbonate and nicotinic acid were successful in treating abnormal serum bicarbonate and chloride levels. Urine output averaged 2.9 L daily, with an osmolality of 286 milliosmoles per kg.

Uretero-ileo-colourethrostomy is beneficial in patients who have benign or focally malignant bladder disease. Because so little of the bladder need remain, the cancer operation is not compromised. One problem is that the colonic bladder that is created holds only 300–500 ml, thus the patient must void frequently to avoid damaging the upper tract. This procedure was well received by all patients because their body image is normal, short-term renal function is maintained, and metabolic disturbances can be controlled easily.

Bladder Replacement With Use of a Detubularized Right Colonic Segment: Preliminary Report of a New Technique
Benad Goldwasser, and David M. Barrett, and Ralph C. Benson, Jr. (Mayo Clinic and Found.)
Mayo Clin. Proc. 61:615–621, August 1986   27–3

Dissatisfaction with the long-term results of cutaneous urinary diversion prompted development of a relatively simple means of bladder replacement for men having cystoprostatectomy. An internal reservoir is made from reconstructed bowel segments and anastomosed to the urethra, providing continence and transurethral urination. A detubularized right colonic segment was used. The ureters may be reimplanted into the bowel segment by submucosal tunneling, split-cuff nipple reimplantation, or the Camey technique. The bowel segment used for bladder replacement is retroperitonealized, and omentum is brought down, if available, and wrapped around the suture lines of the new bladder.

Three males who underwent bladder replacement after radical cystoprostatectomy for bladder cancer were followed for up to 2 months. All were completely continent at follow-up. Cystometry done 6 weeks postoperatively in one patient showed a "bladder" contraction of 44 cm water at a volume exceeding 300 ml. It is expected that even this high-volume contraction will eventually disappear, as has been observed in detubularized bowel segments used in augmentation cystoplasty.

The early results of this bladder replacement procedure are encouraging. Low-pressure collection and storage of urine are provided, and reflux is prevented. A low-pressure reservoir is created through detubularization of the bowel segment, a large-capacity reservoir, and a new "bladder" of large diameter.

▶ The 1986 YEAR BOOK had a dozen articles on continent diversions. One must distinguish between operations that involve a bladder replacement anastomosed to the urethra (please see Abstracts 27–2, 27–3, and 27–4) and those that involve a continent abdominal stoma (please see Abstracts 27–5 and 27–6). It still is not clear which operations are the best. A few trends are developing: (1) It is clear that some patients are not good candidates for continent diversions and are better off with standard ileal conduits. (2) The Camey procedure is losing popularity because of the problem of nocturnal enuresis, although this can be treated with condom drainage. (3) A large capacity is essential to avoid incontinence, particularly in patients without the normal urethral continence mechanisms. (4) Many, but not all, centers are abandoning the Kock pouch for simpler procedures. At the 1987 meeting of the AAGUS, several speakers emphasized that in selected patients ureterosigmoidostomy is a good option.

The two papers above (Abstracts 27–2 and 27–3) discuss different techniques of using the right colon for bladder replacement. Both methods seem reasonable. McDougal believes detubularization is not necessary if the capacity is adequate, and his results support this contention. We prefer to use the King technique for ileal intussusception, making incisions to allow suturing muscle to muscle. King has reported excellent long-term results with this method. Zinman and others have advocated preservation of the distal prostate to decrease the incontinence rate.—S.S. Howards, M.D.

The Mainz Pouch (Mixed Augmentation Ileum and Cecum) for Bladder Augmentation and Continent Diversion
J.W. Thüroff, P. Alken, H. Riedmiller, U. Engelmann, G.H. Jacobi, and R. Hohenfellner (Johannes Gutenberg Univ., Mainz, West Germany)
J. Urol. 136:17–26, July 1986   27–4

The Mainz pouch bladder augmentation procedure uses cecum, ascending colon, and two ileal loops. The goal is to create a low-pressure reservoir of adequate capacity from the cecum and longitudinally split ileal loops. Antirefluxing ureteral implantation into the cecum or ascending colon is achieved by a submucosal tunneling method. In urinary diversion, continent pouch closure is achieved by isoperistaltic ileoileal intussusception or by implantation of an alloplastic stomal prosthesis. Eleven patients have had Mainz pouch bladder augmentation since 1983, five in conjunction with undiversion. Twelve other patients have had Mainz pouch urinary diversion, the most frequent indication being radical cystoprostatectomy for bladder cancer. The mean patient age was 36 years.

Three patients had major operative complications, but there were no operative deaths. Ten of the 11 patients having augmentation were completely dry day and night at follow-up, with normal intervals of bladder evacuation. Two patients with myelomeningocele were on intermittent catheterization, but the rest voided spontaneously without significant residual urine. Six of the 12 patients with urinary diversion had an ileoileal intussusception valve and were completely continent. Three of four with an alloplastic stomal prosthesis also were completely continent. Two patients in this group are awaiting implantation of a sphincteric prosthesis. The mean follow-up has been 5 months.

This technique appears to meet all requirements for reconstruction of a urinary reservoir. Antirefluxing implantation of the ureters into the pouch permits subtotal cystectomy, and this is especially advantageous in patients with interstitial cystitis and detrusor hyperreflexia. Further applications of the Mainz pouch will allow avoidance of an abdominal stoma.

▶ This report is similar to the paper by the same group reviewed in the 1986 YEAR BOOK (p. 188). The Mainz pouch certainly meets virtually all of the considerations for an ideal continent reservoir. However, it may be that the simple procedures outlined above by the Mayo Clinic group (Abstract 27–3) will prove to be adequate.—S.S. Howards, M.D.

Long-Term Management of Patients Who Have Had Urinary Diversions Into Colon

S.H. Silverman, C.R.J. Woodhouse, J.R. Strachan, J. Cumming, and M.R.B. Keighley (Univ. of Birmingham, and Inst. of Urology and Royal Postgraduate Med. School, London)
Br. J. Urol. 58:634–639, December 1986   27–5

Prior to 1950 and the advent of the ileal conduit, diversion of urine into the colon was widely practiced. Many of these patients have grown up in good health and routinely attend urology clinics. Currently, there are a few circumstances in which ureterosigmoidostomy remains the treatment of choice. Because of this, it is important to know the long-term results of this form of diversion and to have a protocol for the management of problems that may arise.

Thirty-four patients with urinary-colonic diversion were followed for 13–41 years (mean, 20.3 years). The most common long-term complication was hyperchloremic acidosis (50%). The most serious long-term complication was neoplasm at the anastomotic site, with benign lesions occurring in three patients and carcinomas occurring in two. Staining for sialomucins in colonic biopsy specimens adjacent to the anastomoses was positive in 17 of 19 patients. This finding represents a premalignant change. Analysis of fecal flora in 17 patients with diversion and in 27 controls disclosed a significant difference in the carriage rate and viable count of *Peptostreptococcus* species. This species could have a role in the etiology of the neoplasms.

The patients in this group who still have a colonic form of urinary diversion are in general happy with it. The high incidence of hyperchloremic acidosis is of concern, however, and it is recommended that estimation of the plasma bicarbonate and chloride levels be made at least annually. Further, the risk of neoplasia is considerable and constant surveillance by colonoscopy is needed. Although the etiology of the tumors is unknown, the mixed and metabolically highly active fecal flora that are present after urinary diversion may promote nitrosamine production and degradation of bile. Both processes could be important in tumor development.

► Ureterosigmoidostomy (usig) remains a useful form of diversion in selected patients. Indeed, as pointed out above, there is some increase in support for this procedure. The problems, of course, include urinary tract infections, hyperchloremic acidosis, and colonic malignancies. Hyperchloremic acidosis can be treated with bicarbonate to replace bicarbonate losses, and nicotinic acid blocks chloride absorption. The mean duration from diversion to neoplasm has been approximately 25 years. Certainly, all patients who have had usigs for more than 10 years should undergo yearly colonoscopy. If a usig is converted to another form of diversion, the colon at the anastomotic site should be resected because it appears to remain at risk (Spence, H.M., et al.: *Br. J. Urol.* 51:466, 1979). Although Crissey and associates (*Science* 207:1079, 1980) presented experimental data in the rat to suggest that the combination of urine and feces is necessary to form neoplasms, this is not supported by all of the experimental data and there are now at least 12 reports of malignancy in colonic segments used for urinary diversion not in the fecal stream.—S.S. Howards, M.D.

Jejunal Conduit Urinary Diversion
Eric A. Klein, James E. Montie, Drogo K. Montague, Robert Kay, and Ralph A. Straffon (Cleveland Clinic Found.)
J. Urol. 135:244–246, February 1986   27–6

The jejunal conduit for patients needing urinary tract diversion has the advantage of avoiding damaged or diseased ileum or colon and ureters. However, the jejunal conduit syndrome, a characteristic electrolyte imbalance, has led to abandonment of this form of urinary diversion. The jejunal conduit was used in 14 selected high-risk patients to determine how best to decrease the incidence of jejunal conduit syndrome. In these patients irradiation, adenocarcinoma, rectal laceration, previous colostomy, or ligation of the inferior mesenteric artery rendered other intestinal segments unusable. Follow-up lasted for a mean of 34 months.

The most common complications were obstruction of the ureterojejunal anastomosis and enteric fistula, each of which occurred in four patients. Only three patients had jejunal conduit syndrome, the symptoms being mild azotemia, hyponatremia, hypochloremia, hyperkalemia, and acidosis. These patients required hospitalization for intravenous fluid and electrolyte replacement therapy. Subsequently, oral electrolyte therapy was instituted successfully, with no recurrence of electrolyte imbalance or azotemia. Of nine patients with normal renal function after surgery, six continued to have normal function throughout the follow-up period.

When irradiation, surgery, or concurrent disease prevents the use of either ileum or colon, the jejunal conduit is a satisfactory alternative for urinary diversion. The occurrence of jejunal conduit syndrome is lower among patients with normal baseline renal function, and it can be minimized by (1) using the shortest jejunal loop necessary to bridge the gap from the ureters to the skin, thereby decreasing potassium and urea reabsorption and sodium and chloride excretion in the intestine, and (2) instituting prophylactic oral electrolyte replacement therapy.

▶ The authors point out that, in patients who have contraindications to the use of ileum and colon, the jejunum can be used as a conduit. We certainly agree and have on occasion performed jejunal urinary diversion. However, if at all possible we use transverse colon in patients who have had pelvic irradiation because sodium loss can be very significant and annoying to manage. We have seen several patients with jejunal conduits done by nonurologists who were ill for prolonged periods because their sodium loss was not recognized.— S.S. Howards, M.D.

The following review article is recommended to the reader.

Goldwasser, B., Webster, G.D.: Augmentation and substitution enterocystoplasty. J. Urol. 135:215, 1986.

28 Prostate, Benign Prostatic Hyperplasia

Amino-Terminal Sequence of a Large Form of Basic Fibroblast Growth Factor Isolated From Human Benign Prostatic Hyperplastic Tissue
Michael T. Story, Frederick Esch, Shunichi Shimasaki, Joachim Sasse, Stephen C. Jacobs, and Russell K. Lawson (Med. College of Wisconsin, Milwaukee, Salk Inst., LaJolla, and Harvard Univ. and the Children's Hospital, Boston)
Biochem. Biophys. Res. Comm. 142:702–709, Feb. 13, 1987   28–1

Prostatic growth factor was isolated from human benign prostatic hyperplastic (BPH) tissue by homogenization in high ionic strength alkaline buffer containing protease inhibitors and purified by ammonium sulfate, heparin-sepharose chromatography, and cation-exchange chromatography. The growth factor was shown to be structurally related to basic and fibroblast growth factor. Homogenization of the BPH tissue in high ionic strength alkaline buffer containing protease inhibitors resulted in the isolation of a growth factor having a molecular weight of 17,400. When tissue was homogenized in ammonium sulfate of pH 4.5 without protease inhibitors, a smaller, 16,600-dalton growth factor was isolated.

Both growth factors reacted with antisera against synthetic peptides whose sequences responded to the amino-terminal (1–12), internal (33–43), and carboxyl-terminal (135–145) portions of basic fibroblast growth factor (bFGF). This suggested that the smaller growth factor was not a truncated form of bFGF (1–46) and that the larger growth factor may contain additional sequences. Amino terminal sequencing showed the larger growth factor to have the following sequence: Ala-Ala-Gly-Ser-Ile-Thr-Thr-Leu-Pro-Ala-Leu-Pro-Glu-Asp-Gly-Gly-Ser-Gly-Ala-Phe-Pro. The larger growth factor is an 8-amino acid extended form of (1–146) bFGF, and the smaller growth factor is probably a proteolytic cleavage product of the larger growth factor produced during the extraction procedure.

▶ This is the first isolation of a prostatic growth factor thought to be responsible for benign prostatic hyperplasia. The growth factor was similar to basic fibroblast growth factor. We are anxiously awaiting more information about this important discovery.—J.Y. Gillenwater, M.D.

The Role of Transabdominal Ultrasound in the Preoperative Evaluation of Patients With Benign Prostatic Hypertrophy

Claus G. Roehrborn, Herbert K.W. Chinn, Pat F. Fulgham, Kenny L. Simpkins, and Paul C. Peters (Univ. of Texas at Dallas and VA Med. Ctr., Dallas)
J. Urol. 135:1190–1193, June 1986   28–2

Transabdominal sonography is a reasonably accurate means of estimating prostatic size. Fifty-nine consecutive patients with obstructive voiding symptoms underwent transabdominal ultrasound study of the prostate along with excretory urography, urethrocystoscopy, and uroflowmetry. The mean age was 65 years. A real-time sector scanner with a 3.5-MHz transducer was used. Fifty-three patients had transurethral prostatic resection and six had open prostatectomy. Follow-up uroflowmetry was carried out 4 weeks postoperatively.

Specimen weight correlated poorly with the postvoiding residual. The preoperative flow rate index correlated negatively with specimen weight to a significant degree, but improvement in flow could not be related to specimen weight. Flow rate indices rose markedly after surgery. Both rectal examination and cystoscopy tended to overestimate small glands and underestimate large ones. Sonographic estimates were most accurate. Patients with a difference of more than 10 gm between predicted and actual specimen weights consistently had residual tissue demonstrated sonographically 4 weeks postoperatively.

Transabdominal sonography of the prostate is recommended preoperatively because the study is noninvasive and provides an accurate estimate of prostate size. Bladder abnormalities and intravesical growth are detected sonographically. Patients requiring open surgery for relief of bladder neck obstruction can be identified sonographically.

▶ These studies showed that transabdominal ultrasound is accurate in determining the size of the prostate gland. The major clinical importance of this is to provide the surgeon with better information in determining whether to do open as opposed to transurethral surgery. As expected, no significant correlation was found between prostate size, voiding symptoms, and residual urines. Transabdominal ultrasound did not detect the three patients with A2 prostate cancer.—J.Y. Gillenwater, M.D.

The Echogenic Focus in Prostatic Sonograms, With Xeroradiographic and Histopathologic Correlation

Wolfgang F. Dähnert, Ulrike M. Hamper, Patrick C. Walsh, Joseph C. Eggleston, and Roger C. Sanders (Johns Hopkins Univ.)
Radiology 159:95–100, April 1986   28–3

The nature of highly echogenic foci in ultrasound scans of the prostate is controversial. Prostatic ultrasound scans were obtained from 42 patients with adenocarcinoma before and after radical prostatectomy. These were reviewed and correlated with xeroradiographs and pathologic sections of the specimens to identify the source of the strong signal.

The comparisons showed that all echogenic foci, with or without acoustic shadowing, represented prostatic calcifications. They were adjacent to the urethra or at the margins of the "internal gland." Calculi were found surrounded by tumor when there was carcinomatous spread toward the urethra. This was considered to reflect secondary involvement.

Echogenic foci represented calcifications on xeroradiographs in this series. The simultaneous occurrence of prostatic cancer and calculi appears to be coincidental. In the past, calcifications may have been mistaken for neoplastic changes.

▶ This is a nice study that correlates radiologic, histologic, and ultrasonic images of the prostate. The authors showed that the bright echogenic foci were calcifications.—J.Y. Gillenwater, M.D.

Excretory Urography in Patients With Prostatism

Thomas J. Bundrick and P. Gary Katz (McGuire VA Med. Ctr, Richmond, Va.)
AJR 147:957–959, November 1986   28–4

The value of using routine screening excretory urography in patients with prostatism was evaluated prospectively in 180 patients aged 50 years and older (mean age, 65 years). All had signs and symptoms of prostatism or acute urinary retention, findings of benign prostatic hypertrophy on physical examination, and negative urine cultures. Excluded were high-risk patients, e.g., those with hematuria, urinary tract infections, a history of bladder tumors, or significantly elevated serum creatinine levels. Patients who fulfilled these criteria underwent excretory urography followed by cystoscopy. Cystometry and urinary flow rate determinations were also performed on select patients. As long as other criteria were met, those in whom excretory urology showed an abnormality were included.

Upper tract abnormalities were detected in 49 patients (27%) by excretory urography, but most of the findings were insignificant and minor. The excretory urography appearances led to an alteration in clinical management in four patients (2.2%), including three with malignant tumors and one whose renal cyst was aspirated because it was atypical. One patient experienced a severe contrast reaction manifested by laryngeal edema that responded to epinephrine subcutaneously. Despite the attempt to preselect patients without high-risk factors, findings in four resulted in an alteration of patient management. Results in other patients were potentially valuable, e.g., a solitary kidney in one, renal calculi in five, papillary necrosis in one, and chronic pyelonephritis in three. However, none of these findings directly influenced patient management. The discovery of three asymptomatic cancers (1.7%) represented a higher rate than previously reported but this could be explained in part by the prospective nature of the study, which prevented loss of any patients with significant excretory urinary findings. Most patients had no acute urinary retention, unlike findings in many retrospective studies. The inclusion of nephrotomography allowed visualization of more subtle lesions. The upper urinary tract should be assessed in patients under evaluation for prostatism.

▶ Whether or not to do routine excretory urography in patients with prostatism is a complex subject with no easy answer. There is general agreement that, if the patient has hematuria or recurrent urinary tract infections or renal failure, information is needed about the anatomy of the kidney, ureter, and bladder. Also, there is some agreement that it is proper to use ultrasound or excretory urography to evaluate patients with signs and symptoms of prostatism as to whether they have residual urine or hydronephrosis. The unanswered question concerns the patient who needs a prostatectomy and has not had excretory urography. Is it justified, from a cost/benefit ratio, to do excretory urographic screening for significant renal and ureteral pathology or cancer? In a review of other series (Talner, L. B.: *AJR* 147:960, 1986) the prevalence of renal cancer was 15 of 3,828 patients (0.4%). Autopsy series report the prevalence of renal cancer to be 0.18% to 0.3% (Harvey, N.A.: *J. Urol.* 57:669, 1947; Lucke, B. et al.: *Atlas of Tumor Pathology,* Washington, D.C., Armed Forces Inst. of Pathology, 1957; Bell, E. T.: *Renal Diseases,* ed. 2, Philadelphia, Lea and Febiger, 1950). In this study, 2.2% of patients had significant lesions found on a screening excretory urogram with the authors concluding that routine screening of patients with prostatism is warranted. This happens also to be my prejudice, but we will have to have more prospective studies to see if this is correct.—J.Y. Gillenwater, M.D.

Distribution of Current During Transurethral Resection
L. Kay and H. Bay Nielsen (Glostrup County Hosp., Denmark)
Scand. J. Urol. Nephrol. 19:257–259, 1985   28–5

Because the surgeon performing transurethral resection (TUR) may receive an electric shock that causes ocular damage, attempts have been made to develop a resectoscope fitted with an earthing wire from its sheath. The metal sheath of a resectoscope was fitted with an earthing lead and prostatic TUR was carried out using coinducting chlorhexidine-lidocaine gel. The current passing to the cutting loop and returning through the sheath and earthing wire was monitored during the operation. In vitro studies were carried out when considerable current was found to be passing through the earthing wire.

In vivo measurements showed that 45% of the high-frequency current returned to earth via the earthing lead. In vitro tests showed that bleeding had little effect on the amount of current returning through the earthing lead. Current was reduced when an insulated Teflon sheet was used.

Because the current in the resectoscope sheath generates heat that may produce a urethral stricture, it appears best for both the patient and surgeon to use an insulated sheath. Nonconductive lubricating jelly must be applied, and regular checks made, to ensure that the insulation is intact.

▶ This is a good discussion of a subject of importance to all urologists: protection of the surgeon during transurethral resection. Their basic recommendation of the use of an insulated resectoscope and of insulating lubricant is good advice.—J.Y. Gillenwater, M.D.

Bladder Neck Incision or Transurethral Electroresection for the Treatment of Urinary Obstruction Caused by a Small Benign Prostate? A Randomized Urodynamic Study
P. Hellström, O. Lukkarinen, and M. Kontturi (Oulu Univ., Finland)
Scand. J. Urol. Nephrol. 20:187–192, 1986   28–6

A prospective randomized study was carried out that compared bladder neck incision and transurethral resection (TURP) in 24 patients with a prostate estimated ultrasonographically to weigh less than 30 gm. Eleven patients, with a mean age of 63 years, underwent bladder neck incision and 13, with a mean age of 59 years, underwent TURP. All patients had symptoms of infravesical obstruction. Baseline urodynamic findings were comparable in the two groups.

The maximum flow rate increased to a nearly significant degree after bladder neck incision. After TURP the rate rose from 7.5 ml/second to 16.5 ml/second. The measured mean prostatic length decreased after TURP, as did sphincterometric measurements with the bladder empty. Detrusor pressure at maximum flow decreased from 58 cm to 26 cm water. Detrusor pressure at maximum flow was lower after TURP than after bladder neck incision and prostatic length was shorter. Mean operating time was longer in the TURP group. Detrusor instability disappeared in two of four patients after TURP and developed after bladder neck incision in two. Urethrocystoscopy done 6 months after operation showed a mild penile urethral stricture in one patient in the bladder neck incision group. Few significant complications occurred. Eight patients experienced retrograde ejaculation after TURP.

Bladder neck incision can provide subjective results as good as those obtained by TURP in patients with minimal prostatic hypertrophy, but many urodynamic parameters are better after TURP. The long-term effects of bladder neck incision are unknown. The procedure can be recommended for men younger than 60 years who have minimal prostatic hypertrophy and are sexually active. Elderly men are best managed by TURP.

▶ This is a nice prospective, randomized series comparing TURP with bladder neck incisions in a small group of patients. The symptomatic response was comparable. Urodynamically, the TURP group had better results than the bladder neck incision group. None of the bladder neck incision group had retrograde ejaculation, whereas 62% of the TURP group had retrograde ejaculation.

We reported in the 1986 YEAR BOOK OF UROLOGY (p. 201) Orandi's large series of patients who underwent transurethral incision of the prostate. Dr. Orandi believes that transurethral incision works best in small glands. For transurethral incision of the prostate to work there must be some obstruction by some midline tissue.—J.Y. Gillenwater, M.D.

Transurethral Resection of the Prostate With Local Anesthesia in 100 Patients
Binod Sinha, George Haikel, Paul H. Lange, Timothy D. Moon, and Perinchery Narayan (Univ. of Minnesota and VA Med. Ctr., Minneapolis)
J. Urol. 135:719–721, April 1986   28–7

Local anesthesia is feasible for transurethral prostatic resection (TURP) in selected patients. All eligible men seen in a 1-year period underwent resection under local anesthesia, supplemented intravenously when appropriate (Table 1). Patients with normal levels of anxiety and pain tolerance and a prostate estimated at 50 gm or less were accepted into the study. Initially, a local anesthetic was injected transurethrally only; later in the study the perineal route was used as well. Patients usually were premedicated with hydroxyzine and meperidine. Both 0.25% bupivacaine and 1% lidocaine were used for local anesthesia. The lateral prostatic lobes and area of the verumontanum were injected.

TABLE 1.—Anesthesia Data

	Phase 1	Phase 2
Median cc local (range):		
Transurethral	20 (15–35)	10 (5–20)
Perineal	0	20 (10–35)
% intravenous supplement	100	35
Median mg. intravenous supplement (range):		
Diazepam	5.8 (2–13)	3 (2–10)
Fentanyl	2.5 (0–7)	2 (1–5)
% given diazepam plus fentanyl	50	15

(Courtesy of Sinha, B., et al.: J. Urol. 135:719–721, April 1986. © Williams & Wilkins, 1986.)

TABLE 2.—Pain Control

	Phase 1 No. (%)	Phase 2 No. (%)
Pt. estimate:		
Would do it again	35 (87)	59 (98)
No pain	5 (13)	31 (52)
Mild pain	25 (63)	29 (48)
Significant pain	5 (13)	0
Would not do it again	5 (13)	1
Estimate of tolerance by anesthetist or nurse monitor:		
Good–excellent	18 (45)	50 (87)
Fair	11 (28)	8 (13)
Poor	2 (5)	0

(Courtesy of Sinha, B., et al.: J. Urol. 135:719–721, April 1986. © Williams & Wilkins, 1986.)

Forty patients had transurethral injection only, whereas 60 received perineal infiltration as well. No patient had to be converted to general anesthesia. None had significant hypotension, but one patient had mild respiratory distress after receiving excessive intravenous doses of morphine. Intraoperative procedure-related complications were minimal. Five patients had transient hypotension, and three, transient hypertension. Immediate postoperative complications also were infrequent. Pain tolerance was improved by added perineal infiltration. Patients' acceptance of local anesthesia was excellent, particularly when perineal supplementation was used (Table 2).

Transurethral prostatic resection can be done under intravenous-assisted local anesthesia in many cases, and this approach is especially useful in patients at high risk from lower spinal or general anesthesia. The cost of surgery may be reduced and "catheter-free" resection may be feasible. At present, nursing personnel or physician assistants monitor vital signs, and the surgeon makes the decision regarding intravenous supplementation.

▶ This is a significant contribution. We do not have any experience with this technique. I would suggest using only Xylocaine because Marcaine (bupivacaine) has a much less safe tolerance level. With elevated blood levels of bupivacaine, cardiac conduction blockade develops, with cardiac arrest, which can last longer than 24 hours.—J.Y. Gillenwater, M.D.

The following review article is recommended to the reader:

Drach, G.W., Nolan, P.E.: Chronic bacterial prostatitis: Problems in diagnosis and therapy. *Urology* 28 (Suppl. 2):26, 1986.

29 Prostate Cancer

Patterns of Progression in Prostate Cancer
John E. McNeal, David G. Bostwick, Robert A. Kindrachuk, Elise A. Redwine,
Fuad S. Freiha, and Thomas A. Stamey (Stanford Univ.)
Lancet 1:60–63, Jan. 11, 1986   29–1

Prostatic cancer has been considered for a long time to be unpredictable, making valid therapeutic decisions difficult. It is not clear whether certain histologic grades of disease evolve from initially well-differentiated cancers. The hypothesis of tumor progression was examined in 100 prostates with carcinoma obtained at autopsy. Measured tumor volume was related to differentiation, capsular invasion, seminal vesicle involvement, and metastasis. Quantitative measures then were applied to 38 specimens obtained from radical prostatectomies.

Tumor volume was less than 1.4 ml in 80% of the specimens and less than 0.46 ml in 60%. Progressive loss of differentiation accompanied increasing tumor volume. In older patients, increasing volume was associated with an increase in the number of poorly differentiated cancers and fewer better-differentiated tumors. In both the autopsy and surgical series, metastases were associated only with tumors larger than 4 ml in volume, which represented 13% of the autopsy series. Only Gleason grade 4 or 5 tumors had metastasized.

Metastasis of prostatic cancer probably is limited to tumors much larger than 1 ml in volume that have acquired poorly differentiated areas as a result of tumor progression. The prognosis could be improved by identifying subgroups of grade 4 tumors and by estimating cancer volume and the extent of capsule penetration by in vivo imaging.

▶ This is a nice study that helps to define the natural history of prostate cancer. Distant metastasis correlates with grade, volume, and capsular or seminal vesicle penetration.—J.Y. Gillenwater, M.D.

Expression of *ras* Oncogene p21 in Prostate Cancer
Michael V. Viola, Frank Fromowitz, Sheila Oravez, Swati Deb, Gerald Finkel,
Joel Lundy, Patricia Hand, Ann Thor, and Jeffrey Schlom (SUNY at Stony
Brook and Natl. Cancer Inst., Bethesda)
N. Engl. J. Med. 314:133–137, Jan. 16, 1986   29–2

An immunohistochemical assay for *ras* p21 was used to determine the relationships between its expression and the biologic potential of prostate tumors. The antigen was detected by a monoclonal antibody, RAP-5, specific for p21. Normal ducts and acini of prostates did not stain for antigen.

187

Nineteen biopsy specimens of benign prostatic hyperplasia were examined. Whereas glandular or epithelial cells did not stain in any case, neoplastic epithelial cells in some grade 1 and in all higher grade neoplasms expressed detectable p21. Two anaplastic lesions showed heterogeneity of staining. The anti-p21 antibody titers in assays of grade II through grade V carcinomas were significantly higher than in assays of benign or grade I lesions. Anti-p21 antibody titers had a significant positive correlation with tumor grade.

Expression of *ras* p21 antigen correlated significantly with tumor grade, whether tumors were graded according to pattern of gland formation or degree of anaplasia. Therefore, *ras* p21 may represent a new class of exploitable tumor markers.

▶ Oncogenes are normal cell genes that, when activated, express a gene product capable of transforming the cell. The most frequently identified transformation-inducing genes found in human solid tumors are members of the *ras* family of cellular oncogenes. The *ras* oncogene p21 was found to correlate with prostatic cancer tumor grade and was not seen in benign prostatic hyperplasia (BPH). The latter showed no staining for the *ras* oncogene. Simoneau from Houston [*J. Urol.* 137 (Pt. 2):113A, 1987], using the proto-oncogene C-SIS, found increased C-SIS expression in both BPH and cancer, with more expression in the cancer.—J.Y. Gillenwater, M.D.

Latent (pTO) Prostatic Carcinoma: A Retrospective Study of Frequency and Natural History
R. Haapiainen (Univ. Central Hosp., Helsinki)
Ann. Chir. Gynaecol. 75:172–176, 1986   29–3

A comparison was made of the pTO prostatic cancer frequency in two 5-year periods 10 years apart. Data concerning therapeutic modalities for benign prostatic hyperplasia (BPH) and the frequency of pTO carcinomas were also compared with findings from eight other hospitals. The outcome in 34 patients aged 58–81 years (mean, 69 years) with incidentally discovered prostatic carcinoma was analyzed; more had received primary treatment for a small carcinoma focus found after transurethral resection.

The proportion of prostatectomies performed transurethrally was 19% in 1967–1971 and 88% 10 years later. A general progressive trend toward more transurethral resections and incidentally diagnosed prostatic carcinomas was observed. The mean frequency of unsuspected microscopic adenocarcinomas after transurethral resection was 6% during the 5-year period 1977–1981, with an 11% increase during the last year. A diversity of methods in pathologic examination by the various hospitals resulting in only one third to one half of all resected chips being studied. This accounted for pTO carcinoma frequency ranges of 5% to 10%.

Prostatic cancer cases rose to 24% in the second 5-year period from

9% 10 years previously. The only significant change took place in the therapeutic modalities for BPH. Overall, 90% of surgical interventions were done transurethrally and at least 50% of the surgical specimen was examined. Only the macroscopically suspect portion of the specimen had been sent for pathologic study previously when adenomas were enucleated.

All 34 patients studied retrospectively had undergone transurethral resection because of urinary outlet obstruction. At the time of carcinoma diagnosis by microscopy, 53% of the patients had focal and the remainder had diffuse disease. During the follow-up period of 58 months, 24% had disease progression. The progression rate in patients with diffuse involvement was 38% and in those with focal involvement, 11%. To date, one third of the patients studied have died: three of prostatic cancer with distant progression, one of cardiovascular disease, and six of other disorders. From the data analyzed, it appears that a latent tumor will develop in most men who live long enough. This age group is also more at risk of death from other causes.

▶ Of 34 patients with incidental prostate cancer followed for 5 years (53% focal and 47% diffused, 82% well differentiated), 8 (24%) had progression of the disease requiring therapy. Three died of prostatic cancer. Six of the eight patients with progression of the disease had diffuse cancer (more than three chips). The clinical problem is to determine which of these incidentally discovered prostate cancers will progress and metastasize so that the cancer can be treated aggressively initially.—J.Y. Gillenwater, M.D.

Prognosis of Untreated Stage A1 Prostatic Carcinoma: A Study of 94 Cases With Extended Followup
Jonathan I. Epstein, Gerson Paull, Joseph C. Eggleston, and Patrick C. Walsh (Johns Hopkins Univ.)
J. Urol. 136:837–839, October 1986   29–4

The prognosis and management of patients with incidental (stage A) carcinoma of the prostate are controversial matters. It was found in one series that if the tumor involved 5% or less of the tissue and was not of high grade (stage A1), only 2% of the tumors progressed at 4 years. Ninety-four men with stage A1 disease were followed for an extended period to determine whether such patients would still have such a low risk of progression during longer follow-up.

Twenty-six patients died of other causes, without evidence of progression, less than 4 years after diagnosis. Eighteen patients had no evidence of progression 4–8 years after diagnosis. Of the 50 who remained at risk 8 years or longer from the time of diagnosis, 8 (16%) had disease progression. The average interval from diagnosis to progression was 7 years (range, 3.5–8 years), with six of eight patients dying of cancer. Neither volume nor grade predicted progression, because of the eight tumors that progressed, four involved less than 1% of the tissue and six were of low grade. The mean age of the patients who died of unrelated causes less than 4 years after diagnosis was 10 years older than those who remained alive and at risk for at least 4 years after diagnosis, 75 years and 65 years, respectively.

Stage A1 prostatic carcinoma progresses at longer intervals from diagnosis and at lower frequency than do stage A2 tumors. Patients with stage A1 tumors, however, are not entirely free of progression, and because 16% of the men who remained at risk for 8 or more years had disease progression, this factor must be recognized in the management of young men with stage A1 tumors.

► Previous studies (Cantrell, B.B., et al.: *J. Urol.* 125:516, 1981) showed A2 prostatic cancers to have a 33% risk of progression at 4 years, and A1 prostatic cancers had 2% progression at 2 years. This study shows that these same patients have 16% progression by 8 years. Six of the eight with progression died of the disease.

Blute (*J. Urol.* 136:840, 1986) reported the long-term follow-up of young patients with stage A cancer of the prostate. Of the eight with A2 tumors, two had disease progression and one died of the disease. Of the 15 with A1 disease, four had disease progression (three systemically and one locally) 10 years after diagnosis.

Careful surveillance of young patients with stage A1 prostatic cancer is necessary. I think routine follow-up transurethral resection is not justified. In addition to monitoring rectal examinations and measurement of serum acid phosphatase levels, periodic thin-needle biopsies should be done.—J.Y. Gillenwater, M.D.

Transrectal Sonography of Benign and Malignant Prostatic Lesions

Deland D. Burks, Leo F. Drolshagen, Arthur C. Fleischer, Hal T. Liddell, W. Scott McDougal, Edward M. Karl, and A. Everette James, Jr. (Vanderbilt Univ.)
AJR 146:1187–1191, June 1986   29–5

Transrectal prostatic sonography is sensitive to textural changes produced by both benign and malignant disease, but no sonographic features appear to be predictive of cancer. One laboratory, using the real-time linear array probe, reported that thick, brightly echogenic foci and shadowing were highly suggestive of a benign condition. In all, 117 patients with sonographic and pathologic correlation of prostatic lesions were evaluated by linear-array transrectal prostatic sonography; 43 had adenocarcinoma and 74 had benign disease, predominantly benign prostatic hyperplasia.

There was considerable overlap in the sonographic appearances of benign and malignant lesions. Mixed echogenicity was the most common pattern in cancer (65%), but represented only 28% of benign diseases. Hypoechogenicity, a common finding in cancer (58%), was highly suggestive of malignancy when present posterior or posterolateral in the peripheral zone. In addition, thick, brightly echogenic foci with or without shadowing within or adjacent to a lesion did not exclude cancer.

Although certain sonographic features may be suggestive of benign or malignant disease, there are no sonographic features that can reliably predict malignancy of the prostate. Biopsy should be performed on all suspicious palpable lesions of the prostate.

▶ I think the lay press and public expectations have gone ahead of technology. All of the carefully done studies with histologic correlation have shown that transrectal sonography cannot accurately detect prostate cancer nor distinguish benign from malignant disease.—J.Y. Gillenwater, M.D.

Intraductal Dysplasia: A Premalignant Lesion of the Prostate
John E. McNeal and David G. Bostwick (Stanford Univ.)
Hum. Path. 17:64–71, January 1986   29–6

Several noninvasive lesions having certain histologic features of adenocarcinoma have been described in the prostate, but they are not established as biologic precursors of invasive cancer. Foci of cytologic atypia having histologic characteristics of malignancy were sought in the ductal and acinar lining epithelia in 100 serially sectioned prostates with adenocarcinoma and in 100 benign prostates obtained at autopsy. The lesion, termed intraductal dysplasia, was recognized as sharply demarcated clusters of glandular units having deeply stained, variably thickened epithelium. The acini and ducts usually were comparably involved.

Foci of dysplasia were found in 82 prostates with adenocarcinoma and in 43 benign prostates. Dysplasia was both more marked and more extensive in the prostates with carcinoma. Grade 3 dysplasia was identified in one third of this group and in 4% of benign prostates. The frequency of multiple independently invasive carcinomas was increased in prostates containing multiple foci of dysplasia. Multicentric carcinoma was present in 28% of prostates without dysplasia, in 44% of those with one to four foci of dysplasia, and in 58% of those with more than four foci of dysplasia. Half of the prostates with more than four foci of dysplasia contained three or more primary cancers.

Intraductal dysplasia is probably a biologic precursor of invasive prostatic carcinoma. Most prostatic cancers may develop from this type of morphological change. Nearly half of the prostates without carcinoma may contain dysplasia by the sixth decade of life. The pathogenetic events that eventually end in invasive cancer may be present at a much earlier age than previously thought.

▶ Dr. McNeal continues his superb investigative studies into prostatic disease. In this study he identified cytologic atypia in the prostatic ductal and acinar lining epithelia, which he thinks is the antecedent lesion of the majority of prostatic cancers.—J.Y. Gillenwater, M.D.

Measurements of Serum γ-Seminoprotein and Prostate Specific Antigen Evaluated for Monitoring Carcinoma of the Prostate
Jill K. Siddall, Sugandh D. Shetty, and Edward H. Cooper (Univ. of Leeds, England)
Clin. Chem. 32:2040–2043, 1986   29–7

Serum γ-seminoprotein (γ-SM) is a glycoprotein in seminal fluid that appears to be a potential marker of prostatic cancer. Two commercial enzyme immunoassays for γ-SM were used, along with prostate specific antigen (PSA), to assess findings in 20 patients with localized prostatic cancer for a median of 22 months. Both are antigens of prostatic origin that are synthesized independently of prostatic acid phosphatase. Seventy-one other patients with prostatic cancer were studied before treatment, as were 30 healthy males and 25 patients with benign prostatic hyperplasia. A radioimmunoassay was used to estimate the PSA content.

There was a highly significant correlation between γ-SM and PSA values at presentation. All but 3 of 30 patients with metastases had a PSA value of more than 10 ng/ml at presentation, and all but 1 had a γ-SM concentration of more than 10 ng/ml. An abnormal PSA concentration was found in 34% of patients without metastases, and an abnormal amount of γ-SM was found in 38%. The 13 patients followed up who had signs of local spread or bony metastases had median γ-SM, PSA, and prostatic acid phosphatase values of 58 ng/ml, 34 ng/ml, and 2.1 units per liter, respectively. Corresponding values for patients who remained clinically stable were 2.5 ng/ml, 3.9 ng/ml, and 2.3 units per liter.

Estimations of either PSA or γ-SM are able to predict disease progression in prostatic cancer patients with normal prostatic acid phosphatase activity. Further experience is needed to determine which tests are most helpful in the management of patients with prostatic cancer.

▶ In this study two specific antigens were tested to monitor prostatic cancer. One, PSA, is confined to the cytoplasm of the acinar and ductal epithelium of the prostate gland. Immunologic assays have increased the accuracy of estimating the PSA concentration. The second antigen is a glycoprotein (γ-SM) found in seminal fluid. In patients with metastasis, 90% had elevated PSA concentrations and 97% elevated levels of γ-SM. Preliminary studies suggest that patients with disease progression have early elevation of these tumor markers. Further studies are needed.

At the 1987 AUA Annual Meeting, Stamey and Ercole presented papers showing that serum PSA is a more sensitive indicator than serum prostatic acid phosphatase. Teillac found that serum PSA was elevated in 40% of patients with benign prostatic hyperplasia. Oesterling et al. found the half-life of PSA to be 3 days. They concluded that PSA was not a sufficiently reliable marker to predict the final pathologic stage on an individual basis. [See *J. Urol.* 137 (Pt. 2), a special supplement containing the *Proceedings* of the 1987 AVA annual meeting.]—J.Y. Gillenwater, M.D.

The Role of Transrectal Aspiration Biopsy in the Diagnosis of Prostatic Cancer

Gerald W. Chodak, Gary D. Steinberg, Marluce Bibbo, George Wied, Francis S. Straus, II, Nicholas J. Vogelzang, and Harry W. Schoenberg (Univ. of Chicago)
J. Urol. 135:299–302, February 1986   29–8

Although it is possible to detect prostatic cancer by physical examination, the specificity of the examination is only 50%. This means that a biopsy must always be done. In the United States, the major means used to document the presence of this tumor are the transperineal and the transrectal needle core biopsy. In Sweden and Europe, another method used extensively is transrectal thin-needle aspiration biopsy. Although this technique has several reported advantages, it is used only infrequently in the United States. An attempt was made to define an appropriate role for this method in evaluation of men with abnormal findings on prostatic examination.

During an 18-month period, transrectal aspiration thin-needle biopsy was the sole technique used in 75 men, of whom 19 were discovered to have prostatic cancer. Two patients were not treated because a core biopsy performed at another hospital was negative for carcinoma. In 62 others, aspiration and transperineal core biopsies were carried out. The sensitivity of aspiration in the diagnosis of prostatic cancer was 98% (45 of 46 biopsies), compared with only 81% (37 of 46 biopsies) for the core biopsy method. No complications developed after aspiration biopsy.

Transrectal aspiration biopsy is a sensitive, simple-to-perform means of sampling an abnormal prostate. More widespread use of this technique in the United States is recommended.

Fine Needle Aspiration of the Abnormal Prostate: A Cytohistological Correlation

H. Ballentine Carter, Robert A. Riehle, Jr., June H. Koizumi, James Amberson, and E. Darracott Vaughan, Jr. (James Buchanan Brady Found. and the Papanicolaou Cytology Lab., New York)
J. Urol. 135:294–298, February 1986   29–9

Although fine-needle aspiration biopsy of the prostate has been used extensively and successfully in Europe, it is only beginning to be accepted in the United States. Cytologic diagnosis by fine-needle aspiration of the prostate was compared with histologic diagnosis by either perineal needle biopsy or transurethral prostatic resection in 110 patients with abnormal rectal findings suggestive of prostatic cancer. Fine-needle aspiration was followed by perineal needle biopsy in 108 patients.

TECHNIQUE.—Fine-needle aspiration is performed with a flexible 22-gauge disposable, prostatic aspiration needle, needle guide, and aspiration syringe. With a metal steering ring secured on the gloved index finger, the finger is inserted into the rectum and the suspicious area palpated. A fine needle is introduced into the suspected lesion through the steering ring and moved back and forth within the nodule while maintaining negative pressure suction. Suction is released before needle is withdrawn from the prostate to avoid loss of sample and contamination of the sample with rectal mucosa or contents.

Histologic correlation was evident in 85 of 94 (90.4%) prostatic aspiration specimens that could be given a definite cytologic diagnosis. The false negative rate was 2.7% for fine-needle aspiration and 5.3% for perineal needle biopsy. There was histologic confirmation of malignancy in 49 of 57 malignant aspiration specimens. Inadequate cytologic samples were obtained in 3.6% of cases, mainly at the beginning of the study. An accurate correlation between cytologic and histologic grading was demonstrated in 69%. Complications, which occurred in 2.7% of the patients, included hematoma, clot retention, and transient bacteremia.

Fine-needle aspiration of the abnormal prostate is an easily performed, diagnostically reliable outpatient procedure with minimal complications. It accurately reflects histologic grading and has prognostic significance in terms of response to therapy.

▶ We had similar excellent results with transrectal fine-needle aspiration in the diagnosis of prostatic cancer. I use two sterile gloves, placing the Franzen needle guide over the first glove. The second glove is punctured to obtain the specimen, reducing the chance of contamination of the prostate. In this series no incidence of posttreatment prostatitis was encountered. I have usually given 80 mg of gentamicin intramuscularly prior to biopsy. We have had no false positive results. I have performed radical prostatectomies on three patients with negative core biopsy findings but positive results on fine-needle aspiration. All of the surgically removed specimens contained prostatic cancer. This procedure is painless and can be performed on an outpatient basis with a report back in 30 minutes.—J.Y. Gillenwater, M.D.

Ultrasound Versus Digitally Directed Prostatic Needle Biopsy
Hal T. Liddell, W. Scott McDougal, Deland D. Burks, and Arthur C. Fleischer (Vanderbilt Univ.)
J. Urol. 135:716–718, April 1986   29–10

The diagnosis of prostatic malignancy can be made by transperineal needle biopsy; however, there is a 20% to 30% rate of false negative results, probably because of incorrect needle positioning. A study was undertaken to determine whether ultrasound scanning during needle biopsy can increase its accuracy in cancer detection.

Fifty-five patients with prostatic nodules underwent paired transperineal biopsy, the needle directed digitally in one case and by ultrasound in the other. The 5.0-MHz ultrasound probe was inserted into the rectum directly beneath the prostate and rotated, so that freeze-frame images could be obtained of the entire gland. The images were then studied to determine the most appropriate segment of prostate for biopsy. Biopsies were performed with the needle guided by either a palpating finger in the rectum or by ultrasound scan. Digitally directed biopsies were performed in the usual manner. When ultrasound was used, the needle was inserted into the previously determined suspicious areas.

Of the 55 patients, needle biopsy proved the existence of adenocarcinoma in 15. Nodular hyperplasia or prostatitis was the diagnosis in the remainder. The digitally guided needle biopsies uncovered only 9 of the 15 adenocarcinomas, whereas the ultrasound-guided biopsies detected all 15.

Hypoechogenicity is common among cancerous lesions, and posterior-lying hypoechoic lesions are especially suspect for cancer. Ultrasound guidance was uniquely able to guide the needle past the urethra, bladder, and rectum without causing damage. The high rate of diagnostic accuracy with ultrasound-guided biopsy and the simplicity of the technique make it a superior method for detection of prostatic malignancies.

▶ We have no experience using rectal ultrasound to direct perineal needle biopsies. I have been using the transrectal thin-needle biopsy. Thin-needle biopsies have the advantage of sampling a higher proportion of the prostate and should detect more cancer. Our cytologists can now tell if the cancer cells are well or poorly differentiated. Layfield reported an 80% correlation between cytology and Gleason grade in studies at UCLA [*J. Urol.* 136 (Pt. 2): 194A, 1987].—J.Y. Gillenwater, M.D.

The Prognostic Significance of Post-Irradiation Biopsy Results in Patients With Prostatic Cancer
Peter T. Scardino, Jeffrey M. Frankel, Thomas M. Wheeler, Randall B. Meacham, George S. Hoffman, Carie Seale, John H. Wilbanks, James Easley, and C. Eugene Carlton, Jr. (Baylor College of Medicine, The Methodist Hosp., and St. Luke's Episcopal Hosp., Houston)
J. Urol. 135:510–515, March 1986   29–11

Radiotherapy is the most frequent treatment of early-stage prostatic cancer, but its efficacy in eradicating local disease remains uncertain. Combined radioactive gold seed implantation and external irradiation were used in virtually all patients with stage A2, B, or C1 prostatic cancer in 1966–1979. A total of 475 evaluable patients completed treatment and received hormone therapy or chemotherapy before tumor recurrence was documented. Transrectal needle biopsies were done annually for 1–3 years in 124 patients, 6–36 months after completion of radiotherapy. The mean length of follow-up was 64 months.

One fourth of the patients had nodal metastases at pelvic node dissection. Postirradiation biopsy specimens were positive for cancer in 35% of the patients. Positive findings correlated with the initial clinical stage, but not with tumor grade. Significant correlation with the state of the pelvic nodes was observed. Local recurrences and distant disease were much more frequent in patients with positive biopsy findings. Biopsy retained its strong prognostic importance in patients with proved negative nodes. The results of biopsy and digital rectal examination agreed in 78% of cases. Among patients with abnormal prostatic findings, those with negative biopsy results did as poorly as those with positive results, suggesting sampling error.

Treatment failed locally in at least one third of the patients in this series. Postradiation prostatic biopsy can indicate how effective a given radiotherapy regimen is in controlling local disease, but some patients with positive biopsy findings do not have local recurrence, whereas some with negative findings do have.

▶ Until proven otherwise, I think postirradiation biopsy specimens showing cancer have to be considered cancer. It is like "a touch of pregnancy"! Musselman and associates [*J. Urol.* (Pt. 2):114A, 1987] presented a paper showing that there were no differences in the in vitro biologic potential between irradiated and nonirradiated human prostatic tissue. Local recurrence in those with positive biopsy findings in this series was 82% by 10 years, and significantly more distant metastases attest to the malignant potential of these positive biopsy results.—J.Y. Gillenwater, M.D.

First Clinical Experiences on Neodymium-YAG Laser Irradiation of Localized Prostatic Cancer
Hans O. Beisland and Sten Sander (Aker Hosp., Oslo)
Scand. J. Urol. Nephrol. 20:113–117, 1986   29–12

A review was made of clinical experience with neodymium-yttrium/aluminum/garnet (Nd:YAG) laser irradiation in treatment of localized prostatic cancer during a 4-year period (1981–1985). Tumor bulk was removed first by transurethral resection extending to the capsule. The remnants of cancer tissue in the capsule could then be destroyed by irradiation. Inclusion criteria were tumors of stage $T_{1-2}N_xM_o$ as per the tumor-node-metastasis classification. The 63 patients followed for 6–48 months (mean, 22 months) ranged in age from 51 to 86 years (mean, 69 years). The first ten were treated by the transurethral approach only; afterward, the method was improved by insertion of a suprapubic trocar cystoscope that allowed complete access to the prostatic cavity.

There were no perioperative complications. Postoperatively, acute cystitis, acute epididymitis, and spinal headache prolonged the hospital stay in one patient each. Many patients experienced mild micturition discomfort and hematuria during the first weeks.

Fifty-six patients were disease-free. The overall actuarial disease-free survival rate was 98% at 1 year and 80% at 2–4 years. No deaths occurred, but treatment failed in seven patients. Tumors recurred within the prostate in three patients. In one patient, tumor progression was detected with infiltration behind the bladder and right ureter obstruction. These four patients were laser irradiated initially by only the transurethral route. Dissemination of disease occurred in three patients with poorly differentiated cancer.

In 20 patients with no clinical local tumor recurrence, thin-needle biopsies were done because of hard capsule consistency or unclear ultrason-
ographic findings. Malignant cells were found in five, but cancer cells could
not be found in one of these patients 6 months later.

Transurethral resection combined with Nd:YAG laser irradiation of
localized prostatic cancer is a simple procedure with few complications.
It is well tolerated even in high-risk patients. Satisfactory comparison can
be made with radiotherapy and/or interstitial implantation procedures.
Further experience is necessary for a definitive comparison with established
treatment modalities, however.

▶ The authors evaluated local treatment of prostatic cancer by transurethral
resection of the prostatic capsule to remove the bulk of the tissue followed by
Nd:YAG laser irradiation of the remaining tissue. They have shown that the
treatment can be given safely. However, a follow-up of only 22 months is too
short a period to evaluate the response adequately—J.Y. Gillenwater, M.D.

**Adjuvant Radiotherapy Following Radical Prostatectomy: Results and
Complications**
Robert P. Gibbons, B. Sharon Cole, R. Garratt Richardson, Roy J. Correa,
Jr., George E. Brannen, J. Tate Mason, Willis J. Taylor, and Mark D. Hafer-
mann (Mason Clinic, Seattle)
J. Urol. 135:65–68, January 1986   29–13

There is incomplete evidence as to the efficacy of adjuvant radiation
after radical prostatectomy when the disease extends beyond the prostate
gland or surgical excision is incomplete. A study was undertaken to define
more precisely the role of radiotherapy after total prostatectomy.

Forty-five patients with microscopic disease outside the prostatic capsule
were put into two groups, one of which underwent irradiation approximately 6 weeks after radical prostatectomy when the wound was healed.
These patients received a mean of 6,325 rad of treatment. Follow-up
histories were conducted every 6 months and continued for at least 5 years
or until the patient's death.

One of 22 patients (5%) receiving radiotherapy had a palpable local
recurrence of adenocarcinoma, whereas 7 of 23 patients (30%) treated by
surgery alone had local recurrences. Of the eight local recurrences, seven
were fatal. Of 11 patients who died of the disease, 3 had received adjuvant
radiotherapy. Severe complications occurred in 14% of irradiated patients
and in 6% of those undergoing only surgery. The complications associated
with irradiation appeared to result from the use of low-energy beams early
in the study.

Adjuvant radiotherapy can decrease the incidence of prostatic recurrence
in those patients who have clinical stage B prostate cancer, but who have
pathologic stage C cancer after radical perineal prostatectomy. The risks
of radiotherapy, especially in patients whose tumors have begun to spread,
must be weighed carefully.

▶ In this series adjuvant radiotherapy improved local prostatic cancer control. The question is whether the 14% rate of severe local complications of chronic cystitis, proctitis, and fistula formation is too high a price to pay. Three of 22 patients given adjuvant radiotherapy and 8 of 23 without radiotherapy died of disease. Seven of eight patients with local recurrence died of metastatic disease.—J.Y. Gillenwater, M.D.

Management of Localized Prostate Cancer

Malcolm A. Bagshaw (Stanford Univ.)
Hosp. Pract. 21:73–88, Dec. 15, 1986   29–14

External beam irradiation has been used since 1956 to treat some 900 prostatic cancer patients at Stanford. Survival rates as high as 60% have been obtained in certain subgroups of patients, particularly those with the least disease. Definite benefit also is apparent in patients having locally advanced disease. With modern linear accelerators, a greater treatment volume, including primary and secondary node groups, may be treated. At present, an isocentrically localized four-field technique is used. The prostate and pelvic nodes are treated through parallel opposed anterior and posterior fields, and smaller opposed lateral fields also are treated. Medium energies of 4–10 Mv are applied. Typically, a total dose of 7,000

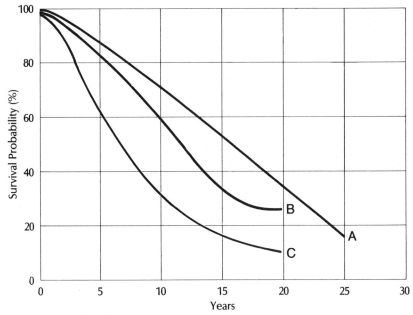

Fig 29–1.—In the Stanford series of approximately 900 prostate cancer patients treated with radiotherapy (1956–1984), actuarial survival was better for those with disease clinically limited to the prostate than for those with extracapsular extension; expected survival for U. S. males of the same age is included for comparison. A, expected age-adjusted survival; B, disease limited to prostate; C, extracapsular extension. (Courtesy of Bagshaw, M.A.: Hosp. Pract. 21:73–88, Dec. 15, 1986.)

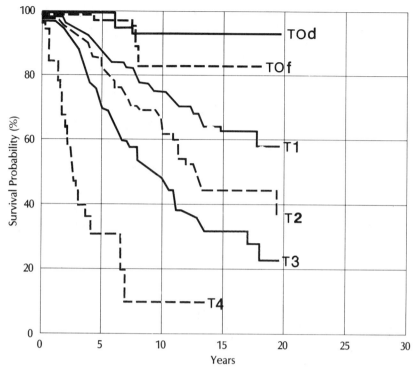

Fig 29–2.—When disease-specific survival in the Stanford series was plotted against Stanford T-stage category, patients who had had the small tumors (TOf and TOd) had the best prognoses after radiotherapy. Probability of survival worsened with increases in tumor size and spread (T1, T2, T3, T4). (Courtesy of Bagshaw, M.A.: Hosp. Pract. 21:73–88, Dec. 15, 1986.)

rad is delivered to the prostate and 5,000 rad to regional nodes during a 7-week period.

Patients with disease limited to the prostate had actuarial survival rates of 81% at 5 years and 35% at 15 years. Lower rates were observed in patients with extracapsular extension (Fig 29–1). Advancing clinical stage also was associated with lower survival rates (Fig 29–2). Radiotherapy led to a 60% actuarial survival rate at 15 years in patients with surgically curable Jewett B_1 disease (Fig 29–3). Patients with clinical stage A_2 disease, who might have been considered suitable for radical prostatectomy, had a disease-specific survival rate at 14 years of about 70%. Radiotherapy may be as effective as prostatectomy in patients with clinical stage A_2 or B disease (Fig 29–4).

Extended-field irradiation appears to be advantageous to some groups of patients with prostatic cancer, although it is not clear that treatment of regional nodes overcomes the adverse effects of adenopathy on patient survival. Long-term survival may be achieved in a significant minority of patients with more advanced primary disease. Several patients having incomplete excision or locally recurrent disease have been salvaged by radiotherapy. Early detection of prostatic cancer remains the critical factor in effective treatment.

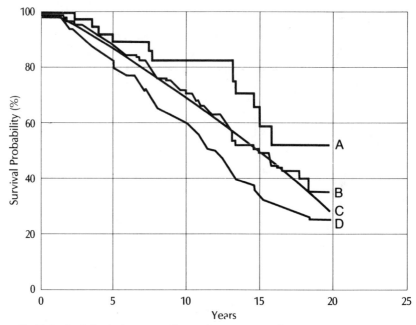

Fig 29–3.—In 40 Stanford patients with 1-cm B_1 tumors surgically curable by Jewett's criteria, radiotherapy resulted in 60% 15-year actuarial survival. In 138 other surgical candidates given radiotherapy for B_1 tumors involving up to half of one lobe, rate was about 50%. Results for both groups were equal to or better than expected survival of healthy men of the same age and superior to actuarial survival in all Stanford patients treated for disease limited to the prostate. A, 1-cm nodule; B, half of one lobe; C, expected age-adjusted survival; D, disease limited to prostate. (Courtesy of Bagshaw, M.A.: Hosp. Pract. 21:73–88, Dec. 15, 1986.)

▶ This is an excellent review by Bagshaw of the Stanford data on the treatment of cancer of the prostate with external beam radiation. The significant data are a 35% *actuarial* survival at 15 years for disease limited to the prostate and 18% for the extracapsular extension group. Their data show no statistically significant evidence that prophylactic lymph node irradiation improves survival. The results in 64 patients showed positive biopsy findings in 39. Only 11 of these 39 patients were alive without evidence of metastases or disease progression (18 died of metastatic prostate cancer). Nineteen of the 25 patients with negative postirradiation biopsy results were alive without evidence of metastases or disease progression.—J.Y. Gillenwater, M.D.

Cardiovascular Side Effects of Diethylstilbestrol, Cyproterone Acetate, Medroxyprogesterone Acetate and Estramustine Phosphate Used for the Treatment of Advanced Prostatic Cancer: Results From European Organization for Research on Treatment of Cancer Trials 30761 and 30762

Herman J. de Voogt, Philip H. Smith, Michele Pavone-Macaluso, Marleen de Pauw, Stefan Suciu, and members of the European Organization for Research on Treatment of Cancer Urological Group (Free Univ., Amsterdam, St.

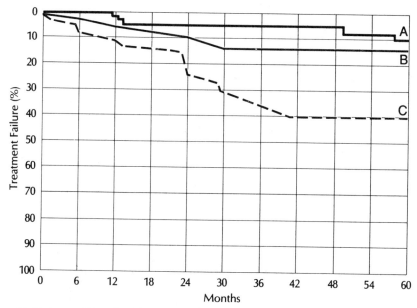

Fig 29–4.—In a VA study of 97 patients with A₂ or B tumors, treatment failure was less frequent after radical prostatectomy than after radiotherapy. In contrast, among 51 comparably staged patients in a Stanford study, radiotherapy was more effective, equaling or perhaps slightly improving on surgery in the VA group. Both studies used time to first evident distant metastasis as their endpoint. **A**, Stanford radiation therapy; **B**, VA radical surgery; **C**, VA radiation therapy.

James's Univ. Hosp., Leeds, England, Univ. of Palermo, Italy, and EORTC Data Ctr., Brussels)
J. Urol. 135:303–307, February 1986   29–15

Randomized trials were begun by the European Organization for Research on Treatment of Cancer urologic group in 1976, one comparing 1 mg of diethylstilbestrol orally, three times daily, with both 250 mg of cyproterone acetate orally daily and 500 mg of medroxyprogesterone acetate intramuscularly three times weekly for 8 weeks, followed by 200 mg orally daily. The other trial compared 3 mg of diethylstilbestrol with estramustine phosphate in an oral dose of 560 mg for 8 weeks, followed by 280 mg daily. Cardiovascular toxicity was evaluated in 239 patients in the first trial and 226 patients in the second.

Fluid retention was the most frequent form of cardiovascular toxicity in both trials. Cardiovascular toxicity as a whole was more frequent with diethylstilbestrol therapy than with either estramustine or medroxyprogesterone (table). It was least frequent with cyproterone acetate therapy. Severe cardiovascular complications occurred most often in the first 6 months of treatment. Risk factors for cardiovascular toxicity included higher age, body weight exceeding 75 kg, and previous cardiovascular disease.

Cyproterone acetate treatment for advanced prostatic cancer was least

SEVERITY OF CARDIOVASCULAR MANIFESTATIONS BY TYPE OF TOXIC SIDE EFFECTS IN TRIALS 30761 AND 30762 IN 465 PATIENTS WITH OR WITHOUT PREVIOUS CARDIOVASCULAR DISEASE BEFORE TREATMENT WAS STARTED

	Trial 30761			Trial 30762	
	Cyproterone Acetate	Medroxyprogesterone Acetate	Diethylstilbestrol	Estramustine Phosphate	Diethylstilbestrol
With previous cardiovascular disease					
No. pts.	30	28	31	34	31
Degree of toxicity (%):					
None	86.7	82.1	54.8	58.8	54.8
Mild	6.7	10.7	35.5	14.7	3.2
Severe	0.0	7.1	6.5	14.7	19.4
Lethal	6.7	0.0	3.2	11.8	22.6
Without previous cardiovascular disease					
No. pts.	54	54	42	81	81
Degree of toxicity (%):					
None	92.6	81.5	73.8	69.0	61.7
Mild	3.7	14.8	19.0	19.8	11.1
Severe	1.9	3.7	4.8	6.2	13.6
Lethal	1.9	0.0	2.4	5.0	13.6

(Courtesy of de Voogt, H.J., et al.: J. Urol. 135:303–307, February 1986. © Williams & Wilkins, 1986.)

often associated with cardiovascular toxicity in these trials. Diethylstilbestrol, in a dose of 3 mg daily, carries a definite risk of cardiovascular toxicity. Estramustine phosphate also is associated with such toxicity. All patients given hormonal therapy should be monitored closely for the first 6 months. The use of diethylstilbestrol probably should be restricted in high-risk patients, e.g., older and obese patients and those with previous cardiovascular disease.

Orchidectomy Versus Estrogen for Prostatic Cancer: Cardiovascular Effects

Peter Henriksson and Olof Edhag (Karolinska Inst., Huddinge, Sweden)
Br. Med. J. 293:413–415, Aug. 16, 1986   29–16

It is not clear that the lower doses of estrogen now used to treat prostatic cancer are associated with an increased risk of cardiovascular morbidity. Morbidity was assessed in prostatic cancer patients treated with current doses of estrogen or orchidectomy. Of 91 patients younger than age 75 years, seen in 1980–1984 with newly diagnosed prostatic cancer, 47 were randomized to receive estrogen and 44 underwent orchidectomy. The former patients received 160 mg of polyestradiol phosphate intramuscularly, monthly, for 3 months, and then 80 mg each month. They also received 1 mg of ethinylestradiol orally daily for 2 weeks, followed by 150 μg daily. The treatment groups were comparable with regard to risk factors for cardiovascular disease.

Thirteen patients experienced major cardiovascular events in the first year after initiation of hormonal therapy. These included three myocardial infarctions and a cerebral infarction. No major cardiovascular events occurred in the orchidectomy group, and the group difference was significant. Only 75% of estrogen-treated patients had escaped major events at the end of the first year of treatment. The mean interval from the start of treatment to a major cardiovascular event in the first year was 5 months.

Cardiovascular morbidity occurs at an increased rate during the first year of estrogen therapy in prostatic cancer patients despite use of a low-dose regimen. Even patients without clinically apparent atherosclerosis may be affected. This cardiovascular morbidity should be considered when deciding whether to use estrogen therapy or orchidectomy in patients with prostatic cancer.

▶ In de Voogt et al.'s study (Abstract 29–15), lethal cardiovascular toxicity at 3 years was 20% with diethylstilbestrol treatment (3 mg/day) and 11% with estramustine phosphate. No significant difference was noted whether or not the patient had previous cardiovascular disease. Cyproterone acetate caused the least cardiovascular toxicity. In the study by Henricksson and Edhag (Abstract 29–16), patients given low-dose estrogen had a major cardiovascular toxicity rate of 25% vs. none in the orchiectomy group. These studies add support to previous investigations showing the cardiovascular toxicity of estrogens and showing that significant cardiovascular toxicity is seen with diethylstilbestrol in doses of 3 mg/day. I favor orchiectomy for hormonal therapy.—J.Y. Gillenwater, M.D.

Testosterone and Gonadoptropin Profiles in Patients on Daily or Monthly LHRH Analogue ICI 118630 (Zoladex) Compared With Orchiectomy

J.B.F. Grant, S.R. Ahmed, S.M. Shalet, C.B. Costello, A. Howell, and N.J. Blacklock (Withington Hosp. and Christie Hosp., Manchester, England)
Br. J. Urol. 58:539–544, October 1986   29–17

The availability of luteinizing hormone/releasing hormone (LHRH) agonist analogues offers a nonoperative approach to treatment of prostatic cancer. Early observations with both daily subcutaneous injections and slow-release depot treatment have been encouraging. Diurnal patterns of gonadotropin and testosterone secretion were studied in 9 patients treated by orchiectomy and in 12 patients given daily subcutaneous injections of the LHRH analogue ICI 118630 (Zoladex) for 6–24 months, usually in a dosage of 250 μg, and 8 patients given at least three depot injections of the 3.6-mg depot preparation of Zoladex. Depot injections were made subcutaneously into the anterior abdominal wall at 28-day intervals.

All patients treated by orchiectomy had testosterone values in the castrate range and significantly elevated basal gonadotropin levels (Fig 29–5). Most testosterone values in patients given daily injections of Zoladex

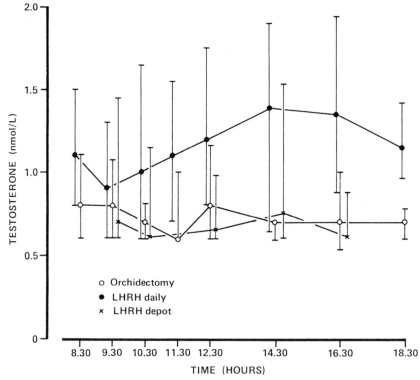

Fig 29–5.—Comparison of testosterone concentrations throughout the day in patients after orchiectomy or during long-term treatment with LHRH analogue administered by daily or monthly injection (median and interquartile ranges). (Courtesy of Grant, J.B.F., et al.: Br. J. Urol. 58:539–544, October 1986.)

were less than 2 nmole/L, but levels were significantly higher than in orchiectomy patients. Patients given depot analogue treatment had a median testosterone level of 0.6 nmole/L, not significantly different from that in the orchiectomy group. Some patients in whom the interval between depot injections was extended to 6 weeks had testosterone levels higher than the castrate range.

Treatment of prostatic cancer with depot LHRH agonist analogue avoids surgery and operative castration. Depot treatment has produced circulating testosterone levels comparable to those achieved by orchiectomy. Long-term studies are needed to determine the effect of analogue therapy on tumor behavior. Depot treatment should be compared with orchiectomy or other treatments that may incorporate drugs to suppress adrenal androgens or antiandrogens.

► Chronic LHRH analogues suppress the pituitary gonadal axis, causing serum testosterone levels to be in the castrate range. The slow-release depot preparation of an LHRH analogue was more convenient and gave lower serum testosterone levels. No toxicity and efficacy data were available in this study.— J.Y. Gillenwater, M.D.

Persistent Blockade of the Pituitary-Gonadal Axis in Patients With Prostatic Carcinoma During Chronic Administration of D-Trp-6-LH-RH

David Gonzalez-Barcena, Patricia Perez-Sanchez, Hector Berea-Dominguez, Alicia Graef-Sanchez, Margarita Bercerril-Morales, Ana Maria Comaru-Schally, and Andrew V. Schally (Instituto Mexicano del Seguro Social, Calzada Vallejo y Jacarandas, Mexico, VA Med. Ctr., New Orleans, and Tulane Univ.)
Prostate 9:207–215, 1986   29–18

Agonistic analogue of luteinizing hormone-releasing hormone (LHRH) comprise an effective treatment for metastatic prostatic cancer. Forty patients with biopsy-proved stage D_2 prostatic adenocarcinoma were treated for up to 30 months with one of these analogues, D-Trp-6-LH-RH. A dose of 1 mg daily was given subcutaneously for 1 week, followed by a daily dose of 100 μg. Thirty patients continued treatment for up to 2 years.

Initial treatment with 1 mg of the analogue led to marked elevations of LH and FSH that lasted for more than 24 hours; a month later, however, baseline gonadotropin levels were below the normal range and did not increase with analogue administration. Plasma testosterone values fell to castration levels during analogue treatment. Acid phosphatase levels, initially elevated in all but four patients, declined progressively after the second week of treatment. In four patients relapse occurred despite persistent pituitary-gonadal blockade.

Long-term treatment with LHRH agonists is preferable to surgical castration or estrogen therapy in men with metastatic prostatic cancer. Chronic treatment with D Trp 6 LH RH effectively blocks the pituitary-gonadal axis, and escape from the effects of blockade may be less frequent than with other analogues.

▶ This study shows that another LHRH analogue in chronic administration is able to suppress serum testosterone levels. An obvious disadvantage is the daily drug injection required. These drugs do not offer any therapeutic advantage over orchiectomy or estrogen therapy.—J.Y. Gillenwater, M.D.

Frozen Section Detection of Lymph Node Metastases in Prostatic Carcinoma: Accuracy in Grossly Uninvolved Pelvic Lymphadenectomy Specimens

Jonathan I. Epstein, Joseph E. Oesterling, Joseph C. Eggleston, and Patrick C. Walsh (Johns Hopkins Univ.)
J. Urol. 136:1234–1237, December 1986   29–19

Even minimal nodal metastases from prostatic carcinoma substantially reduce the likelihood of cure. The accuracy of frozen-section study of apparently uninvolved pelvic lymph nodes was assessed in a series of 310 pelvic lymphadenectomy specimens obtained from 1981 to 1985, just before planned radical prostatectomy. An average of about six lymph nodes per unilateral pelvic node dissection was identified. Superficial and deeper sections were taken from each frozen node. An average of about two nodes were frozen per unilateral dissection.

Forty dissections (13%) yielded metastatic prostatic cancer. Only four patients with positive nodes had elevated serum acid phosphatase levels. Results of frozen-section studies were positive in all six patients having grossly involved lymph nodes. Findings in frozen sections were reported as positive for tumor on at least one side in 68% of the patients with microscopic metastases on permanent sections. Tumor was identified by frozen section on both sides in two of seven patients with confirmed bilateral metastases. False negative findings were obtained in 3.5% of all patients, 27.5% of those with positive nodes, and 32% of those with only microscopic involvement of nodes.

These findings support the routine use of frozen-section study of grossly uninvolved pelvic lymph nodes as a staging procedure preceding radical prostatectomy for prostatic carcinoma. Random frozen-section examination identified about two thirds of the patients with microscopic metastases in the present series.

▶ This is a nice study showing a 27.5% false negative rate by frozen section in those patients with positive nodes on permanent sections. Pelvic node dissections are an excellent way of staging the tumor and obtaining valuable information about prognosis. There is, however, little information to support pelvic node dissection as a curative procedure, because most patients with positive nodes also have other systemic spread of the cancer.—J.Y. Gillenwater, M.D.

(Sexual Function After Radical Prostatectomy)
J. Edson Pontes, R. Huben, and R. Wolf (Cleveland Clinic Found. and Roswell Park Mem. Inst., Buffalo)
Prostate 8:123–126, 1986

29–20

Until recently, erectile impotence was considered an inevitable sequel to radical prostatectomy for cancer, but it now is clear that many patients can retain sexual function if the neurovascular bundle is preserved. Sixty-five patients underwent radical retropubic prostatectomy for clinically localized prostatic carcinoma in 1980–1984. A technique similar to that described by Walsh et al. was used, but it was not until 1983 that the need to preserve the neurovascular bundle was recognized.

Four of the 45 patients interviewed had clinical stage A2 disease, 9 had stage B1 disease, and 32 had stage B2 disease. Many patients had more extensive disease than expected. Twenty-six of the 45 patients were sexually impotent after operation, but 19 others reported erectile potency. The latter were among 35 patients who were potent preoperatively. The outcome could not be related to stage of disease. All patients who failed to respond to irradiation and underwent salvage prostatectomy were impotent postoperatively. Four patients received a semirigid penile prosthesis.

More than half of the patients in this series who were potent before radical prostatectomy had erectile potency postoperatively. Several patients were able to have satisfactory intercourse, and only a few were unable to perform sexually. It seems possible for a significant proportion of patients to retain sexual potency after radical retropubic prostatectomy; however, for many patients sexual potency is secondary in importance to treatment of the disease. At present, an attempt is being made to preserve the neurovascular pedicles in patients with a small tumor volume who wish to preserve sexual function.

▶ Weldon and associates of San Rafael, California, presented their results of nerve-sparing *perineal* prostatectomy at the 1987 AUA Annual Meeting [*J. Urol.* 137 (Pt. 2):225A, 1987]. Fifty-six percent of 16 patients were potent postoperatively.—J.Y. Gillenwater, M.D.

Early Complications of Combined Pelvic Lymphadenectomy and Radical Prostatectomy Versus Lymphadenectomy Alone
Pinhas M. Livine, Robert P. Huben, Richard M. Wolf, and J. Edson Pontes (Roswell Park Mem. Inst., Buffalo)
Prostate 8:313–318, 1986

29–21

Evaluation of the pelvic lymph nodes is critical in staging prostatic carcinoma. Some workers recommend performing pelvic lymphadenectomy as a separate procedure before radical prostatectomy. Fifty-one patients with a mean age of 61 years underwent radical prostatectomy with curative intent in a 4-year period. Twenty-nine patients with a mean age of 63 years had pelvic adenectomy alone for staging of clinically localized prostatic cancer in the same period; three of them had gross node involvement and were excluded. Retropubic radical prostatectomy followed lymphadenectomy.

About 17 lymph nodes were excised in both groups. Twelve patients in the combined surgical group and ten in the lymphadenectomy group had positive nodes. One patient in the combined surgery group died operatively of cardiorespiratory failure. Morbidity rates were 35% in this group and 25% with adenectomy alone. Two iliac vein injuries and one rectal injury occurred in conjunction with combined prostatectomy and lymphadenectomy. There were no ureteral or obturator nerve injuries in either group. In two patients in the lymphadenectomy group lymphoceles developed.

An attempt should be made to evaluate the state of the pelvic lymph nodes nonoperatively in patients with prostatic cancer, but, if this fails, pelvic lymphadenectomy is indicated. Morbidity appears to be low enough to warrant performing lymphadenectomy at the time of radical prostatectomy rather than as a separate procedure.

▶ This paper reports the complications associated with combined radical prostatectomy and pelvic lymphadenectomy and concluded that node dissection does not add significant morbidity. Most authors report complications in about 30% of patients. Lymphedema of the genital region or lower extremities occurs more frequently with extended node dissection or with the addition of radiation therapy. Lymphocele formation is decreased by careful occlusion of the distal lymphatics.—J.Y. Gillenwater, M.D.

The following review articles are recommended to the reader:

Chu, T.M., Murphy, G.P.: What's new in tumor markers for prostate cancer? *Urology* 27:487, 1986.
Fair, W.R.: Perioperative use of carbenicillin in transurethral resection of prostate. *Urology* 28 (Suppl. 2):15, 1986.
Grossman, H.B.: Hormonal therapy of prostatic carcinoma: Is there a rationale for delayed treatment? *Urology* 27:199, 1986.
Huben, R.P., Murphy, G.P.: Prostate cancer: An update. *CA* 33:274, 1986.
Walker, A.R.P.: Prostate cancer—some aspects of epidemiology, risk factors, treatment and survival. *S. Afr. Med. J.* 69:44, 1987.

30 Infertility

Chronic Human Chorionic Gonadotropin Administration in Normal Men: Evidence That Follicle-Stimulating Hormone Is Necessary for the Maintenance of Quantitatively Normal Spermatogenesis in Man
Alvin M. Matsumoto, Anthony E. Karpas and William J. Bremner (VA Med. Ctr., Population CTR. for Research in Reproduction, and Univ. of Washington, Seattle)
J. Clin. Endocrinol. Metab. 62:1184–1192, June 1986   30–1

Eight normal men aged 30–39 years participated in a study for 19–23 months to determine whether normal FSH serum levels are necessary for maintenance of sperm production. After a 3-month control period, a selective deficiency of FSH levels was produced by chronic human chorionic gonadotropin (hCG) administration for 7 months; hCG and testosterone intramuscularly were then given for the next 6 months. Afterward, FSH was replaced in four men by hCG for 3 months. While continuing hCG treatment, they received human FSH, 100 international units (IU), or 75 IU of human menopausal gonadotropin (hMG) daily for 5–8 months.

The mean sperm concentration during the control period was 88 million per ml. Administration of hCG (5,000 IU, intramuscularly, twice daily) resulted in mean sperm suppression in all of the men to 22 million per ml during the final 4 months of treatment. Sperm counts remained suppressed after testosterone was added. Sperm motility and morphology were normal throughout the study in all but one man, who became azoospermic. Serum FSH levels were undetectable during the hCG and hCG plus testosterone periods; the urinary FSH level compared with that in prepubertal children and hypogonadotropic hypogonadal adults. During the second period of hCG administration only, serum FSH levels were not detected and sperm concentrations were suppressed. On adding FSH to hCG, the mean FSH levels increased to 213 ng/ml and the mean sperm concentration rose to 103 million per ml from 34 million per ml during the last 2 months of treatment.

All four men had at least two sperm concentrations within their own control range. Two had mean sperm concentrations during the final 2 months of hCG and FSH treatment that were less than the mean control values. Although FSH replacement was 2–3 months longer in these men, it did not result in sperm concentration increases, making it unlikely that the duration of FSH replacement contributed to failure of the sperm count to normalize. Patients who received human FSH had higher serum FSH levels than those who received human menopausal gonadotropin replacement. In five patients an increase in palpable breast tissue developed during treatment with hCG alone; this remained unchanged or decreased with continued hCG administration.

Prolonged selective FSH deficiency induced by hCG resulted in partial suppression of spermatogenesis, and FSH replacement stimulated sperm production to near control levels. This suggests that the suppressive effects of hCG may result from the low levels of FSH induced by hCG. Normal levels of FSH do not appear to be an absolute requirement for sperm production, but are needed for quantitatively normal sperm production.

▶ There is a consensus that, in man, testosterone and FSH are both necessary to initiate spermatogenesis, but that testosterone alone can maintain it. The data in this paper do not refute the latter point but do document that sperm production is higher with testosterone plus FSH than with testosterone alone. This observation is of both scientific and potential clinical interest. The clinical relevance is that this observation may explain why some men with normal testosterone levels seem to respond with increased sperm production to drugs that elevate the serum FSH level (e.g., clomiphene).—S.S. Howards, M.D.

Pregnancy Following Insemination With Sperm Aspirated Directly From Vas Deferens

Maria Bustillo and Jacob Rajfer (Univ. of California at Los Angeles and Harbor-UCLA Med. Ctr., Torrance, Calif.)

Fertil. Steril. 46:144–146, July 1986

30–2

Current treatment of male infertility resulting from inability to have a seminal emission includes pharmacologic stimulation of the denervated vas deferens or electroejaculation. However, the success rates of obtaining sperm are poor and pregnancy has never been reported. A patient with paraplegia underwent direct aspiration of sperm from the vas deferens in an attempt to establish a pregnancy.

Man, 27, had functional T-12 paraplegia. His wife received clomiphene citrate for more precise ovulation. On her cycle day 17, a day when sonographic and hormonal studies indicated impending ovulation, direct aspiration of sperm was performed on the patient. The right vas deferens was isolated distal to the convolutions and then cut tangentially to expose a half-open lumen. A 3.5 Tom Cat catheter was inserted into the proximal end of the vas and about 0.25 ml of semen was withdrawn. The catheter was flushed with Ham's F-10 medium with 5% human serum albumin to make a total volume of 2.0 ml. The entire volume was used for transcervical intrauterine insemination of the patient's wife. The technique was successful and a healthy infant was born after an uncomplicated gestation.

Direct aspiration of sperm from the vas deferens is simple and does not require an anesthetic. However, certain problems may be encountered. For example, sperm may not be found at the time of aspiration, and complete transection of the vas may occur. The actual success rate, in terms of pregnancies achieved, remains to be determined with similar treatment of additional couples.

▶ This is an important and interesting observation. The aspiration technique along with the electroejaculation work of Bennett (Carol Bennett, M.D., Univ. of Michigan, Ann Arbor) provide new hope for men who are infertile because they cannot ejaculate. This report, of course, describes only one pregnancy. Bennett now has a small but significant experience with a reasonable success rate. Which, if either, of these techniques will ultimately prove practical remains to be seen.—S.S. Howards, M.D.

The Role of the Human Epididymis in Sperm Maturation and Sperm Storage as Reflected in the Consequences of Epididymovasostomy

Robert J. Schoysman and J. Michael Bedford (Univ. of Brussels and Cornell Univ.)
Fertil. Steril. 46:293–299, August 1986   30–3

Relatively little is known about the contribution of the epididymis to sperm maturation. The epididymal milieu provides support for sperm maturation, and androgen and the low temperature of the scrotum allow mature spermatozoa storage in the cauda. Examination of specific sperm parameters known to change during epididymal maturation could indicate segmental limits needed for sperm maturation and which cellular facets require epididymal factors for completion.

Ejaculates were obtained from 117 men who had undergone epididymovasostomy. The exact level of the anastomosis on the epididymis, recorded at surgery as the distance between the proximal border of the caput and the proximal border of the anastomosis site and measured in millimeters, had to be known for the investigation. The patients had 20×10^6/ml or more spermatozoa in a previous ejaculate after unilateral or bilateral anastomosis at a similar site on both epididymides. The anastomosis be-

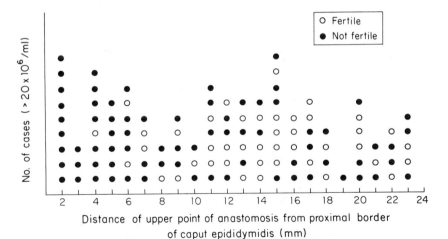

Fig 30–1.—Pregnancies established by epididymovasostomy patients, displayed as a function of the level of anastomosis, measured at the time of surgery. In cases of bilateral anastomosis, the lowest point is indicated. (Courtesy of Schoysman, R.J., et al.: Fertil. Steril. 46:293–299, August 1986. Reproduced with permission of the publisher. The American Fertility Society.)

tween the epididymis and vas deferens was laterolateral, the upper border essentially coinciding with the tubule that had continuous sperm leakage after an incision above the blockage.

The chances for pregnancy are better when the anastomosis is made at the corpus instead of at the caput epididymidis level (Fig 30–1). Pregnancies were occasional when the anastomosis was 8 mm or less from the proximal border of the caput, but common when the anastomosis was more than 10 mm from the proximal border in men with fewer than 20×10^6 spermatozoa in a previous ejaculate. None of the spermatozoa appeared "immature," irrespective of the level of the anastomosis. Spermatozoa from the caput of a normal epididymis failed to bind Fe^{+++} colloid at pH 1.8, in contrast to caudal spermatozoa, yet there was no difference between the binding pattern of cationized Fe^{+++} colloid to spermatozoa surfaces from epididymovasostomy and control samples.

In man, as in animals, the epididymis contributes to the spermatozoa's ability to fertilize. The reason for the importance of making the anastomosis low, near the corpus epididymidis, is not clear; however, the percentage motility could be important. Although the cauda epididymidis may not be of major importance to the delivery of the first ejaculate, it is probably crucial in delivering repeated ejaculates of high fertility in a short time.

▶ I have long awaited the publication of this paper because I quoted these data in the last two editions of Campbell's *Urology*. There are several important points: (1) The overall fertility rate of the 565 of 723 patients available for follow-up was 18%. (2) The motility of ejaculated sperm after an anastomosis in the proximal 9 cm of the epididymis was 0% in 16, less than 10% in 3, and 30% to 60% in 3. (3) The fertility rate associated with proximal anastomosis was poor in spite of the good numbers of spermatozoa in these selected patients. (4) Except for motility and fertility, spermatozoa from proximal anastomoses were mature by the parameters tested. These findings fit with all of the previous animal literature but differ markedly from those noted by Silber, who reported good motility and fertility after proximal anastomoses (*Fertil. Steril.* 34:149, 1980). There is no obvious explanation for this difference. Silber did do a single-tubule anastomosis, but it seems unlikely that this could explain a motility and fertility difference in the presence of large numbers of spermatozoa.—S.S. Howards, M.D.

Percutaneous Sclerotherapy of Varicocele
J. M. Bigot (Hôpital Tenon, Paris)
Ann. Radiol. 29:173–177, 1986

30–4

Of 160 patients who underwent percutaneous sclerotherapy of varicoceles, 86% were referred for subfertility. There were 151 left-side and 69 right-side varicoceles.

TECHNIQUE.—Light premedication and local anesthesia are used. Spermatic phlebography is performed; this includes a higher series centered on the lumbar zone to determine localization of anastomoses and a lower series at the level of the scrotum to assess the volume of the varicocele and venous drainage of the scrotum. Sclerosis is performed with a 3F-coaxial catheter, or a Kunnen 7F catheter for right-side varicoceles, using 2–6 ml of 3% sodium tetradecyl sulfate. At the time of injection, the patient's abdomen is compressed for 10 minutes at the level of the deep fossa of the inguinal canal to prevent reflux of the sclerosing agent toward the scrotum and to reduce flow in the spermatic vein.

Sclerosis was bilateral in 40% of the patients. Sclerotherapy was successful in 142 of 147 patients with a left-side varicocele and in 61 of 69 with a right-side varicocele. Failures in left-side varicoceles were anatomical in four instances, with a valve at the end of the left spermatic vein and anastomoses originating from the hilum of the kidney reinjecting the spermatic venous trunk. Early failures in three patients with right-side varicoceles resulted from unstable catheterizations. Complications were unusual and included venous extravasation or thrombosis of the pampiniform plexus. The recurrence rate was 2%, a figure lower than that associated with surgical ligation (8% to 10%).

Percutaneous sclerotherapy, as an outpatient procedure, is the procedure of choice in the treatment of varicocele. Knowledge of anatomical variants is necessary to ensure successful catheterization. Surgery should be performed only when sclerotherapy fails.

▶ This is another of many reports of successful percutaneous therapy of varicoceles. The method is more popular in Europe than in the United States. There is no doubt that in the hands of a skillful international radiologist the technique works. However, in less experienced hands the failure rate is high and the procedure may take a long time. We manage primary varicoceles surgically but correct recurrent or surgical failures with the percutaneous balloon technique after vasography.—S.S. Howards, M.D.

Comparison of Fecundability With Fresh and Frozen Semen in Therapeutic Donor Insemination

Brenda L. Bordson, Eda Ricci, Richard P. Dickey, Heber Dunaway, Steven N. Taylor, and David N. Curole (The Fertility Inst. of New Orleans)
Fertil. Steril. 46:466–469, September 1986   30–5

Cryopreserved semen has been substituted for fresh semen in therapeutic donor insemination for reasons of availability and convenience, but past studies have indicated reduced pregnancy rates when using frozen semen. The efficacy of fresh and frozen semen was examined by reviewing data obtained in the first 16 months of a therapeutic donor insemination program in which the minimal number of grade 3 active sperm per insemination was 40×10^6. A total of 120 patients began therapeutic donor insemination in 1984–1985. Impaired fertility was diagnosed in 42 women. Inseminations were performed after ovulation was induced or after the natural urinary LH surge, either once or on 2 consecutive days in the periovulatory period.

Of 77 women studied until they conceived or for a total of three insemination cycles, 57% became pregnant. Fecundability was greater for the first three cycles of insemination than for the ensuing three cycles. Fecundability averaged 11.5% with fresh semen and 10.3% with frozen semen, not a significant difference. The number of inseminations per cycle was not a significant factor. Women aged 20–25 years had the highest fecundability rate. The rate for women with impaired fertility was 7%, compared with 15% for those with apparently normal fertility potential.

Pregnancy rates comparable to those obtained with fresh semen may be achieved with frozen samples given well-timed inseminations of at least 40×10^6 grade 3 motile sperm. The use of only frozen sperm in a therapeutic donor insemination program avoids the transmission of human T lymphotropic virus type III. Female factor infertility was the most significant factor determining the success of this procedure.

▶ The finding that frozen semen is as effective as fresh semen is most encouraging and important. It is becoming increasingly difficult to use fresh semen because of concerns regarding the acquired immunodeficiency syndrome. Indeed, many experts recommend that no fresh semen be used. However, we believe that there still is a place for fresh semen if proper caution is exercised. It should be noted that the authors used only donors with excellent-quality prefreeze semen, which showed a post-thaw motility of more than 30% at grade III/IV. There is a very large body of literature that contradicts the authors' findings, documenting a significantly lower fecundity rate with cryopreserved semen.—S.S. Howards, M.D.

Successful Pregnancy in Primary Glomerular Disease
P. Barceló, J. López-Lillo, L. Cabero, and G. Del Río (Universidad Autónoma, Barcelona)
Kidney Int. 30:914–919, December 1986   30–6

The effect of pregnancy on women with primary glomerular disease is controversial. Most studies have included patients with primary and secondary glomerulonephritis and diverse renal disease but follow-up has been too short. Clinical and histologic details are scarce, and the prognosis remains unclear. Some authors discourage pregnancy in these patients because serious deterioration in histologic lesions and renal function is possible; others believe that the renal consequences are insignificant and that pregnancy is not dangerous if hypertension is absent and renal function is normal.

Fetal viability and the consequences of pregnancy were reviewed in 48 women with primary glomerular disease. Before pregnancy, biopsies and routine urine analyses were done. Biopsy specimens underwent light and immunofluorescence microscopy. Histologic types included membrano-proliferative glomerulonephritis in 16, glomerulosclerosis in 13, IgA nephropathy in 10, membranous nephropathy in 7, and focal glomerulonephritis in 2. Five women had moderate renal failure, eight had permanent hypertension, and eight had nephrotic range proteinuria. Neuropathy progression was analyzed by determining the plasma creatinine level, blood pressure, and proteinuria and compared with these findings in nonpregnant women with the same disease after 1 year and 5 years. There was no significant difference between the groups in serum creatinine levels, diastolic pressure, or proteinuria, or in the incidence of nephrotic syndrome, before the study began. Women taking contraceptives were excluded.

Of 66 pregnancies, 51 infants were born at term with normal weight, 7 were preterm, 3 had low birth weight but subsequent normal development, 2 were stillborn, and 3 were aborted spontaneously. Thus fetal viability was 92.4%; preterm deliveries, 10.6%; low birth weight, 4.5%; and perinatal mortality, 31%. A significant linear correlation was found between proteinuria and fetal weight. Proteinuria of less than 1 gm/day was present in five women who had deteriorating renal function before pregnancy. In eight patients with hypertension, 11 pregnancies resulted in four births at term, two preterm, two with low birth weight, one stillbirth, and two spontaneous abortions. Obstetric complaints varied with the presence of risk factors. Serum creatinine, blood pressure, and urinary protein determinations did not show nephropathy progression in most pregnant women. However, renal function declined in two patients, four had a permanent blood pressure increase, and four had increased proteinuria. Renal function continued to worsen in one patient after delivery and reached end-stage failure in 6 months.

Fetal viability in women with primary glomerular disease reached 92%, but decreased in women with glomerulonephritis and hypertension. The incidence of perinatal complications in women with hypertension was 62%, confirming that this is a serious prognostic factor.

▶ This study provides the good news that most women with glomerular disease do well with pregnancy and deliver normal term infants. It does seem clear that women with moderate renal failure and hypertension are at increased risk and should be so advised. There also may be a small but significant risk in patients with membranoproliferative glomerulonephritis and focal glomerulosclerosis. Included in this series were two patients with renal failure, nephrotic syndrome, and hypertension who did have severe deterioration of renal function with pregnancy.—S.S. Howards, M.D.

Diet and Vasectomy: Effects on Atherogenesis in Cynomolgus Macaques
Thomas B. Clarkson, Donna M. Lombardi, Nancy J. Alexander, and Jon C. Lewis (Wake Forest Univ. and Oregon Primate Res. Ctr., Beaverton, Ore.)
Exp. Mol. Pathol. 44:29–49, February 1986   30–7

It was reported previously that more extensive atherosclerosis develops in vasectomized cynomolgus macaques fed diets high in cholesterol content than in sham vasectomized monkeys fed the same diet. These studies were based on the premise that immunologic injury to the arterial wall exacerbates atherosclerosis and because, after vasectomy, antibodies to sperm develop in about 50% of men and most males of other species. The immune response to vasectomy shares many of the characteristics of serum sickness in which foreign antigens have been injected repeatedly. The exacerbation of atherosclerosis among vasectomized monkeys fed atherogenic diets was the result of immunologic endothelial injury. An attempt was made to show that modest hypercholesterolemia injures the endothelium of cynomolgus macaques, and that vasectomy reduces the effect of modest hypercholesterolemia on endothelial cell replication rates and atherogenesis in this model.

The study was performed using adult male feral cynomolgus macaques whose average age was about 9 years. There were three groups: Groups I and II were fed a diet containing the equivalent of 0.19 mg of cholesterol/cal; group III was fed Purina Monkey Chow, which is essentially devoid of cholesterol. Group I monkeys underwent bilateral vasectomy 13 weeks after beginning the diet. On the same schedule, groups II and III monkeys underwent sham vasectomies. Slight hyperlipoproteinemia induced by the moderately atherogenic diet increased endothelial cell replication rates and led to the development of intimal lesions among sham vasectomized monkeys. Unexpectedly, vasectomy led to reduced leukocyte adherence to arterial surfaces and reduced endothelial cell replication rates in response to the moderately atherogenic diet; at most arterial sites, smaller intimal lesions were produced.

With slight hyperlipoproteinemia, vasectomy may result in a small protective effect against atherosclerosis. However, other studies have shown that marked hyperlipoproteinemia in cynomolgus macaques, along with vasectomy, leads to exacerbation of atherogenesis.

▶ In 1978 Alexander and Clarkson published a paper (*Science* 201:538, 1978) suggesting that vasectomy in monkeys might accelerate atherosclerosis. We have now come full circle. At the time of the first report we, among others, warned that the original study was not convincing because it was based on only a few animals given a highly atherogenic diet that were studied at only one point in time and that certain critical backup data were lacking. However, a near-panic occurred, resulting in a special NIH program to study the problem. Fortunately, none of the many very carefully designed studies sponsored by the NIH documented any problem in man (please see 1982 YEAR BOOK, p. 61; 1983 YEAR BOOK, p. 82; 1985 YEAR BOOK, p. 260). Now the authors of the original article offer us further reassuring evidence that, given a mildly atherogenic diet (more comparable to that of the average man), monkeys with a vasectomy may have even less atherosclerosis than nonvasectomized animals.—S.S. Howards, M.D.

The following review articles are recommended to the reader:

Acosta, A.A., Chillik, C.F., Brugo, S., et al.: In vitro fertilization and the male factor. *Urology* 28:1, 1986.

Santoro, N., Filicori, M., Crowley, W.F.: Hypogonadotropic disorders in men and women: Diagnosis and therapy with pulsatile gonadotropin-releasing hormone. *Endocr. Rev.* 7:11, 1986.

Stillman, R.J., Rosenberg, M.J., Sachs, B.P.: Smoking and reproduction. *Fertil. Steril.* 46:545, 1986.

31 Urethra

Perineal Transpubic Repair: A Technique for Treating Post-Traumatic Prostatomembranous Urethral Strictures

George D. Webster and Benad Goldwasser (Duke Univ.)
J. Urol. 135:278–279, February 1986
31–1

Perineal repair of prostatomembranous urethral strictures does not rely on graft take and achieves an accurate suture anastomosis without significantly shortening the penis. Morbidity is considerably less than with the transpubic procedure, but it has been limited to strictures 2 cm or less in length with a healthy distal urethra. Transperineal wedge excision of the pubis permits single-stage perineal repair of strictures up to 5 cm in length.

TECHNIQUE.—The perineum is explored via a midline perineal excision that is bifurcated posteriorly to improve access to the posterior urethra (Fig 31–1). Dissection of the urethral bulb from the midline perineal tendon allows complete mobilization of the posterior urethra. The urethra then is dissected distally and

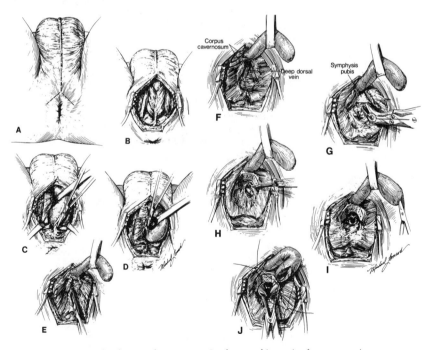

Fig 31–1.—Surgical technique of one-stage perineal transpubic repair of posttraumatic prostatomembranous urethral strictures. (Courtesy of Webster, G. D., and Goldwasser, B.: J. Urol. 135:278–279, February 1986. © by Williams & Wilkins, 1986.)

transected at the distal limit of the stricture. The apical prostatic urethra is spatulated anteriorly, and a wedge is resected from the inferior surface of the pubic symphysis to shorten the distance to the apex of the prostate. The margins of the prostatic urethra are sutured to surrounding tissues, everting its mucosa and, after ventral spatulation of the distal urethral end, an end-to-end bulboprostatic urethral anastomosis is achieved with 3–0 polyglycolic acid sutures. A fenestrated silicone urethral catheter supports the repair. The bulbospongiosus muscle is raised on a posterior vascular pedicle and used to close the dead space where the pubic bone was resected. The perineal tissues are reapproximated before skin closure.

Prostatomembranous urethral strictures up to 5 cm long may be managed by a one-stage perineal end-to-end anastomotic repair. If a stricture 3–5 cm long is present, excision of a wedge of pubic bone via a perineal approach will facilitate the repair. There is no need to ligate the dorsal vein of the penis. This approach has been used to repair four strictures 2–5 cm in length with uniformly good results.

▶ Complete transections of the membranous or proximal bulbous urethra often present challenging problems. There is considerable controversy over initial and definitive therapy. We believe that if careful evaluation reveals complete transection, placement of a suprapubic tube is usually best. Definite repair can also be successful but often the patient's condition, the lack of an experienced surgeon, and difficulty in defining the extent of the injury mitigate against this option. Several authors have recommended endoscopic resection to reestablish continuity after traumatic urethral injury (Gonzalez, R., et al.: *J. Urol.* 130:785, 1983; Marshall, F., personal communication). This may require several procedures and long-term results are not available. We have generally used a perineal approach with a vascularized single-stage repair (Blandy, J.P., Singh, M.: *Br. J. Urol.* 47:83, 1975). One must be prepared to go above if exposure is not adequate. The approach described by Webster and Goldwasser might obviate the need for a second suprapubic incision. We also have been pleased with the results of the Waterhouse technique for difficult cases, particularly second operations.—S.S. Howards, M.D.

The following review article is recommended to the reader:

Blacklock, N.J.: Catheters and urethral strictures. *Br. J. Urol.* 58:475, 1986.

32 Gynecology

Antibiotic Treatment of Pelvic Inflammatory Disease: Trends Among Private Physicians in the United States, 1966 Through 1983
David A. Grimes, Joseph H. Blount, Juanita Patrick, and A. Eugene Washington (Ctrs. for Disease Control, Atlanta)
JAMA 256:3223–3226, Dec. 19, 1986   32–1

Pelvic inflammatory disease remains the most frequent serious infection in women of reproductive age in this country. Nationwide data on patterns of antibiotic therapy in the management of this disease have not been available. An attempt was made to document trends in antibiotic therapy using data from the National Disease and Therapeutic Index survey for 1966–1983. The survey is a stratified national random sample of physicians in fee-for-service, office-based practices, selected each year from more than 200,000 physicians in 19 primary care specialties.

Office-based physicians provided about 1.4 million prescriptions annually for antibiotics to treat pelvic inflammatory disease during the survey period. The proportion of prescriptions by general practitioners declined, whereas that given by obstetricians-gynecologists nearly doubled. Natural penicillins were used less often over the years, whereas the number of aminopenicillin prescriptions more than doubled. Cephalosporins also are used more frequently today. Tetracyclines and aminopenicillins were by far the most frequently prescribed agents in 1980–1983. About one fifth of all antibiotics were prescribed for hospitalized patients. Most patients receive a single antibiotic for pelvic inflammatory disease. Cephalosporin-based combinations were most frequent in recent years.

Pelvic inflammatory disease in the United States generally is treated with a single drug given on an outpatient basis. Aminopenicillins and tetracyclines are the most frequently prescribed drugs. The common use of cephalosporins in combination drug therapy raises concern over the adequacy of treating *Chlamydia trachomatis*, which is not sensitive to these antibiotics.

▶ This paper reviews the outpatient treatment of pelvic inflammatory disease in the United States between 1966 and 1983. Although therapy has probably changed somewhat in that time, it is clear that inadequate treatment as described above is still common. *Chlamydia trachomatis* and *Neisseria gonorrhoeae* are the most common causes of this disease. Treatment, therefore, should be effective against the organism. The Centers for Disease Control, recommend that outpatients receive doxycycline hydrochloride, 100 mg orally twice daily, and a single dose of ceftriaxone, 250 mg intramuscularly. Ampicillin, 3.5 gm, plus probenecid, 1.0 gm, may be substituted for the ceftriaxone. Hospitalized patients should receive cetoxitin and doxycycline or clindamycin and gentamicin.—S.S. Howards, M.D.

221

33 Infection and Urethritis

▶ ↓ The comments for this chapter were written by Dr. Jackson E. Fowler, Jr., Clarence C. Saelhof Professor of Urology, University of Illinois College of Medicine, Chief of the Division of Urology at University of Illinois Hospital.— J.Y. Gillenwater, M.D.

Necrotizing Soft-Tissue Infections of the Perineum and Genitalia: Etiology and Early Reconstruction
Peter R. Carroll, Eugene V. Cattolica, Charles W. Turzan and Jack W. Mc-Aninch (Univ. of California at San Francisco, Kaiser Permanente Med. Ctr., Oakland, and San Francisco Gen. Hosp.)
West. J. Med. 144:174–178, February 1986   33–1

In 1883 abrupt, rapidly progressive, gangrenous infection of the genitalia was described in five otherwise healthy young men. Since that time, approximately 400 similar patients have been reported. These infections probably represent a spectrum of disease best characterized as a fulminant soft tissue infection that may spread along subcutaneous planes and be followed by necrosis of the skin, fascia, or subcutaneous tissue. Despite the development of new antibiotics and improved methods of organ support, mortality and morbidity remain high. A review was made of experience with necrotizing soft tissue infections of the perineum and pelvis in 13 males and 1 female whose average age was 52 years (range, 18–81 years).

The patients had a wide range of symptoms; the delay between onset of local symptoms and presentation averaged 6 days. There were underlying or contributing conditions in several patients, including alcohol abuse in eight (57%), diabetes mellitus in three (21%), and genitourinary disease in three (21%). The source of the infection was traced to the rectum in seven patients, the skin in four, and the genitourinary tract in two. The source was not clear in one patient. Leukocytosis was almost uniformly present, and infection tended to be polymicrobial, with an average of 3.4 organisms identified in each specimen. The combination most frequently found was *Escherichia coli* with either *Bacteroides* sp or anaerobic cocci and *Bacteroides* sp with aerobic cocci. All patients underwent repeated surgical débridement and drainage, and local reconstruction was successfully carried out in 11 patients. Complications included renal failure in six, death (three), respiratory failure (four), cardiovascular collapse (four), coagulopathy (two), and in one patient each, urethral stricture, infertility, and fistula.

Early, aggressive surgical débridement and drainage are recommended to reduce morbidity and mortality. Other measures include prompt institution of antimicrobial therapy directed at both aerobic and anaerobic organisms, with subsequent tailoring to the specific bacteria cultures, and early surgical reconstruction to avoid extensive scarring and cosmetic deformity and allow earlier skin closure and a reduced hospital stay.

▶ Our experience with necrotizing soft tissue infections of the perineum and genitalia parallels the observations in this report. In one recent case at our institution, grossly apparent necrosis extending approximately 10 cm into the medial aspect of the thighs occurred during a three-hour period required for débridement of the lower abdominal wall, perineum, and genitalia. This experience, while anecdotal, underscores the potential fulminating behavior of this fortunately unusual infectious process.—J.E. Fowler, Jr., M.D.

Detection of *Chlamydia trachomatis* in Genital Specimens by the MicroTrak™ Direct Specimen Test
Philip E. Coudron, Daniel P. Fedorko, Marilyn S. Dawson, Lisa G. Kaplowitz, Richard R. Brookman, Harry P. Dalton, and Bettie A. Davis (Med. College of Virginia and Richmond Fan Free Clinic)
Am. J. Clin. Pathol. 85:89–92, January 1986   33–2

Chlamydia trachomatis, one of the most common sexually transmitted pathogens in the United States, affects both sexes. Although chlamydial infections may lead to serious complications, they are not always clinically apparent. Further, laboratory isolation of *C. trachomatis* in cell culture is expensive, technically difficult, and requires at least 2 days to complete. An immunofluorescent technique was developed to identify chlamydial inclusions that involves application of a fluorescein-labeled monoclonal antibody directly to smears containing genital scrapings; it requires less than 1 hour. Results obtained with this nonculture method (MicroTrak™) were compared with those of cell culture. The 251 cervical and 209 male urethral specimens were applied directly onto microscope slides (8-mm well) and stained with fluorescein-labeled monoclonal antibody. The slides were then examined for 10–15 minutes at 1,000 magnifications with an epifluorescent microscope. Results were considered positive if five or more typical elementary bodies were observed.

Sensitivity, specificity, and positive and negative predictive values for the direct smear were 89%, 97%, 85%, and 98% for males and 93%, 96%, 85%, and 98% for females.

This appears to be a satisfactory method for detecting *Chlamydia* in male and female genital specimens. Culture-positive, direct immunofluorescence-negative results could arise from artifacts and from mucus on the slides.

▶ The development of a monoclonal antibody that recognizes the intracellular elementary bodies of *C. trachomatis* constituted a quantum leap for the practical and clinically useful identification of *C. trachomatis* infections. This experience is consistent with past reports that immunofluorescent detection of the organism is sensitive and specific. The practicing physician should remember that the elementary bodies are intracellular, and that specimens suitable for analysis must include epithelial cells from the mucosal surface under investigation. This study also suggests that mucus in the specimen makes proper visualization of the cells more difficult, thus inclusion of this material should be avoided.—J.E. Fowler, Jr., M.D.

Treatment of Sexually Transmitted Chlamydial Infections

Lawrence L. Sanders, Jr., H. Robert Harrison, and A. Eugene Washington (Ctrs. for Disease Control, Atlanta)
JAMA 255:1750–1756, Apr. 4, 1986   33–3

Chlamydial infection is recognized as the most frequent bacterial sexually transmitted disease in this country. Both prevention and control require safe, effective antimicrobial therapy. The occurrence of urethral *C. trachomatis* infection in up to 30% of men with gonococcal urethritis requires the inclusion of appropriate antimicrobial agents in regimens used for gonorrhea. The current treatment of choice for nongonococcal urethritis is tetracycline, 500 mg four times daily for 1 week. Doxycycline and minocycline also are effective and may be given less frequently. Erythromycin may be given to patients who do not tolerate tetracyclines. Sulfonamides are effective in most cases of chlamydial urethritis, and amoxicillin in high dosage has been effective against *C. trachomatis* urethral infections in males.

Chlamydia trachomatis also is a frequent cause of mucopurulent cervicitis. Women have responded well to tetracycline therapy and to tetracycline analogues. Erythromycin base was poorly tolerated in clinical trials, but erythromycin stearate is effective. Sulfonamides may be used to treat chlamydial cervical infections in men. The optimal treatment of chlamydial infections in pregnant women remains uncertain.

Chlamydia trachomatis is an important cause of acute pelvic inflammatory disease, regardless of the findings at cervical culture. Broad-spectrum treatment effective against all potential pathogens, including *C. trachomatis*, is necessary in patients with acute pelvic inflammatory disease. Timely treatment of symptomatic and asymptomatic endocervical infections will reduce the occurrence of acute pelvic inflammatory disease and its long-term sequelae.

▶ This well-documented article from the Centers for Disease Control provides a review of treatments for sexually transmitted chlamydial infections and current treatment recommendations. By and large, treatment recommendations in the past decade have remained unchanged. For nongonococcal urethritis in the male and mucopurulent cervicitis in the female, tetracycline hydrochloride, 500 mg orally four times a day for 7 days, constitutes optimal treatment. Erythromycin, 500 mg orally four times a day for 7 days, is an equally effective alternative for patients who cannot tolerate tetracycline. The sexual partners of affected patients should be examined promptly and treated with the same regimen if a chlamydial infection is documented.—J.E. Fowler, Jr., M.D.

Treatment of Uncomplicated Infections Due to *Neisseria gonorrhoeae:* A Review of Clinical Efficacy and In Vitro Susceptibility Studies From 1982 Through 1985
Roselyn J. Rice and Sumner E. Thompson (Ctrs. for Disease Control, Atlanta)
JAMA 255:1739–1746, Apr. 4, 1986   33–4

Antimicrobial resistance in the gonococcus continues to evolve, and coinfection with *Chlamydia trachomatis* is a serious problem. More than half of the penicillinase-producing *Neisseria gonorrhoeae* infections in the United States have occurred in endemic foci in California, New York, and Florida. Aqueous penicillin G procaine is effective against uncomplicated anogenital tract infections in adults. Tetracycline minimal inhibitory concentrations appear to be increasing in the United States. Spectinomycin is effective against most strains of penicillin-resistant and tetracycline-resistant *N. gonorrhoeae*. The β-lactamase inhibitors clavulanic acid and sulbactam may be useful adjuncts. The quinolone derivative rosoxacin is relatively effective against penicillinase-producing and other isolates. Second-generation and third-generation cephalosporins are more active than earlier agents against *N. gonorrhoeae*. Patients with coexisting gonococcal and chlamydial infections have been treated with aqueous penicillin G procaine, probenecid, tetracycline, and trimethoprim-sulfamethoxazole (TMP-SMX). Penicillin G may also cure incubating syphilis coexisting with penicillin-sensitive gonorrhea. Sexual partners of gonorrhea patients ideally should be treated on the basis of the sensitivity of the strain isolated from the index case. Patients with pharyngeal infection by resistant gonococci are treated with TMP-SMX. Active surveillance detects treatment failures and helps to guide effective treatment. Resistance patterns must be monitored to avoid increased costs from blind application of newer agents.

▶ Recent experience in the treatment of gonococcal infections and current treatment recommendations from the Centers for Disease Control are summarized in this article. The good news is that chromosomally mediated and plasmid-mediated resistance has not increased substantially, and that most gonococcal infections in the United States are still susceptible to penicillin, ampicillin, or tetracycline. Spectinomycin remains the drug of choice for resistant infections. A course of tetracycline for 7–10 days in addition to the primary therapy for gonorrhea is advisable to eradicate chlamydial infections that may coexist with gonococcal infections. A wide variety of new agents have substantial activity against gonorrhea, but the precise role of these agents as primary treatment remains to be defined.—J.E. Fowler, Jr., M.D.

The following article is recommended to the reader:

Frangos, D.N., Nyberg, L.M., Jr.: Genitourinary fungal infections. *South. Med. J.* 79:455, 1986.

34 Scrotum and Testis

Scrotal Reconstruction After Fournier's Gangrene
Jørgen Hesselfeldt-Nielsen, Erik Bang-Jensen, and Per Riegels-Nielsen (Rigshospitalet, Copenhagen)
Ann. Plast. Surg. 17:310–316, October 1986   34–1

The primary treatment of Fournier's gangrene of the male genitalia requires removal of all necrotic and undermined tissue, leaving areas denuded of skin. Many workers suggest split-thickness skin transplantation for partial scrotal defects, whereas, with total loss of the scrotum, the testes usually are placed in subcutaneous pockets in the thighs. Primary scrotal reconstruction by flap methods has yielded suboptimal esthetic results. Complete scrotal reconstruction was achieved using split-thickness skin grafts alone in three men having extensive Fournier's gangrene.

Man, 67, with Parkinson's disease, had redness, edema, and warmth of the genital skin; incision of a perianal abscess revealed findings typical of Fournier's gangrene. Propagation had stopped anterior to the anus, at the glans, and in the groins. Treatment with broad-spectrum antibiotics and hyperbaric oxygen was given. After surgical revisions produced clean, granulating defects, split-skin grafts from the thighs were used to reconstruct the defect, starting at its posterior border in the perineum. Grafts were wrapped loosely around the testes and penis. All skin surfaces healed after three supplemental stamp graft transplants. The only complaint 2 years later was lack of scrotal contractility.

Minimal functional sequelae have occurred when using split-skin grafts to reconstruct skin defects primarily in the genital region resulting from débridement of Fournier's gangrene. Good cosmetic results have been obtained with this approach. Scrotal reconstruction with split skin is recommended only in patients with Fournier's gangrene.

▶ The authors recommend débridement and delayed split-graft coverage of the penis and scrotum for management of Fournier's gangrene. Their results are impressive.—J.Y. Gillenwater, M.D.

Sclerotherapy for Hydroceles and Epididymal Cysts With Ethanolamine Oleate
P. Hellström, L. Malinen, and M. Kontturi (Univ. Central Hosp., Oulu, Finland)
Ann. Chir. Gynaecol. 75:51–54, 1986   34–2

Ethanolamine oleate was used as a sclerosant for hydroceles (11 men) and epididymal cysts (6 men). The median age of the former group was 67 years (range, 53–84 years), and that of the latter, 64 years (range, 38–83 years). Treatment was by tapping and injection with ethanolamine oleate. The median length of follow-up was 8 months (range, 3–15 months). All 11 patients with hydroceles were cured. Six patients were treated once, four twice, and one patient three times.

In five patients small cysts ranging in size from 1 cm to 4 cm were detected with ultrasonography after treatment. Two of these were palpable. These cysts were regarded as epididymal cysts. In one patient a hydrocele and an epididymal cyst were treated at the same time, with cure of the hydrocele. One patient died of unrelated causes. Complications included severe pain (one patient), moderate pain (three), and mild pain (one) after treatment. Fever occurred in five patients.

Three of the six patients with epididymal cysts were cured; treatment failed in two who had multilocular cysts that precluded successful subsequent sclerotherapy. In one patient with a 44-mm cyst, a 32-mm multilocular cyst developed after two treatments. Yet, the patient was satisfied with the result. Two patients experienced severe pain, and one mild pain, after treatment. No complications were observed except for pain and mild fever.

Only 50% of patients with epididymal cysts were totally cured. It is probably not worth a trial to treat multilocular epididymal cysts by sclerotherapy. Recurrence is likely. Complications after sclerotherapy have been few, with pain being the basic problem. The pain lasted for only a few days, was easily controlled by analgesics orally, and required no hospitalization. Young men have not yet been treated with sclerotherapy, as more experience is needed with sclerosant agents regarding antifertility effects. Ethanolamine oleate should be used as primary treatment in men older than age 50 years with the conditions of hydroceles and epididymal cysts.

▶ The authors report good success with ethanolamine oleate sclerotherapy of hydroceles and epididymal cysts. We have not used sclerotherapy and still repair hydroceles surgically when therapy is needed.—J.Y. Gillenwater, M.D.

Primary or Secondary Extragonadal Germ Cell Tumors?
A. Böhle, U.E. Studer, R.W. Sonntag, and J.R. Scheidegger (Univ. of Berne, Switzerland)
J. Urol. 135:939–943, May 1986   34–3

It is controversial at present whether germ cell tumors can first appear at extragonadal sites, or whether the primary lesion is always testicular. The current treatment for extragonadal tumors is chemotherapy; however, this is inadequate for testicular tumors because of the presence of the blood-testis barrier. A retrospective study was conducted to determine the primary site of extragonadal germ cell tumors.

Sixteen patients with primary extragonadal tumors underwent scrotal palpation to exclude the presence of testicular tumors. Twelve patients had retroperitoneal tumors and four had mediastinal germ cell tumors. Eight patients received ultrasound scans of the testes after treatment for the extragonadal tumor. The other eight underwent palpation, biopsy, orchiectomy, or soft tissue radiography during treatment, which consisted of a combination of radiotherapy, chemotherapy, and/or surgery. During the average follow-up of 28 months, occult testicular primary tumors were found in 10 of 12 patients with retroperitoneal tumors; none was found in patients with mediastinal germ cell tumors. Of the eight who had ultrasound scans after therapy, three had pathologic ultrasound findings that were confirmed by histologic evaluation.

So-called primary extragonadal germ cell tumors in the retroperitoneum should be assumed to be testicular in origin and should be followed carefully with ultrasound scan during chemotherapy. Suspicious ultrasound findings should be followed by testicular biopsy and hemicastration if necessary.

Orchiectomy in Advanced Germ Cell Cancer Following Intensive Chemotherapy: A Comparison of Systemic to Testicular Response
Clayton Chong, Christopher J. Logothetis, Andrew von Eschenbach, Alberto Ayala, and Melvin Samuels (Univ. of Texas at Houston)
J. Urol. 136:1221–1223, December 1986   34–4

Patients with extensive, advanced germ cell cancer may require immediate chemotherapy, but testicular cancer may persist even if systemic disease is eradicated. Experience with postchemotherapy orchiectomy was reviewed in 16 patients seen at three centers in 1977–1985 who had advanced disease and underwent radical orchiectomy after initial chemotherapy. In three cases a primary testicular tumor was unrecognized at the outset. The median age was 30 years. Five patients had pure seminoma and 11 had nonseminomatous germ cell tumors. Fourteen patients received cyclic chemotherapy with two noncross-resistant drug combinations.

Viable residual tumor was found in four patients (25%). Three of 13 patients in complete systemic remission had residual viable tumor. All of them were well within 12–30 months after orchiectomy without further treatment. One patient without residual tumor relapsed 1 month after orchiectomy. The other patients have all remained in complete remission. One of three patients in partial remission had persistent testicular tumor and progressive disease developed later despite continued chemotherapy.

Viable testicular disease has been documented in the presence of durable complete remission after initial chemotherapy for advanced germ cell cancer. Eradication of primary disease in the presence of persistent or recurrent systemic disease also has been documented. The postchemotherapy orchiectomy findings are not predictive of patient outcome, and treatment decisions must be based on the status of systemic disease. Delayed postchemotherapy orchiectomy may be done, when necessary, without compromising survival.

► The preceding papers (Abstracts 34–3 and 34–4) make important observations that need to be verified in a larger series of patients. The paper by Chong et al. (Abstract 34–4) documents that chemotherapy does not cure tumor in the testis in 23% of patients, which failure may or may not be caused by the blood-testis barrier. That some primary testis tumors are cured by chemotherapy and others are not suggests that the blood-testis barrier may not be the only reason for the lack of tumor eradication. There may be differences in tumor sensitivities to the various chemotherapeutic agents used.

The paper by Böhle et al. (Abstract 34–3) shows that, in the presence of retroperitoneal germ cell tumors, 10 of 12 patients had evidence of occult testicular primary tumors. Böhle's admonition to follow patients who have "primary" retroperitoneal extragonadal germ cell tumors with scrotal ultrasound is appropriate. We need to separate in our thinking extragonadal tumors of the retroperitoneum and mediastinum as to possible testicular primaries.—J.Y. Gillenwater, M.D.

Carcinoma in Situ of Contralateral Testis in Patients With Testicular Germ Cell Cancer: Study of 27 Cases in 500 Patients

Hans von der Maase, Mikael Rørth, Sven Walbom-Jørgensen, Bent L. Sørensen, Ivan Strøyer Christophersen, Tage Hald, Grete Krag Jacobsen, Jørgen G. Berthelsen, and Niels E. Skakkebaek (Rigshospitalet, Copenhagen, Denmark)
Br. Med. J. 293:1398–1401, Nov. 29, 1986   34–5

Patients with germ cell cancer of the testis are at an increased risk for the development of a tumor in the other testis, but the course of contralateral carcinoma in situ is unknown. Carcinoma in situ of the contralateral testis was detected in 27 of 500 patients with unilateral testicular germ cell cancer screened in 1972–1985. Carcinoma in situ was defined as the intratubular presence of atypical germ cells. These cells are usually found in a single layer close to the basement membrane, but they may invade the interstitial tissue.

The incidence of contralateral carcinoma in situ in this series was 5%. In six patients contralateral testicular cancer developed 7–45 months after the diagnosis of carcinoma in situ. One patient had early invasive growth of undifferentiated germ cell cancer adjacent to the carcinoma in situ in the initial biopsy. All patients were classified as having stage I disease at the second orchidectomy and received no further treatment. One patient had seminomatous metastatic disease and was well after chemotherapy. Contralateral cancer developed only among patients not given systemic treatment. The estimated risk of invasive cancer developing in 21 patients not given systemic treatment was 40% at 3 years and 50% in 5 years. Eight patients received chemotherapy after contralateral carcinoma in situ was diagnosed. There was one death from spread of initial cancer. None of the 473 patients without contralateral carcinoma had contralateral testicular cancer during a median follow-up of 46 months.

Patients with testicular cancer should have the contralateral testis biopsied. If carcinoma in situ is found, invasive growth can be diagnosed at an early stage. Patients not given chemotherapy initially might usefully be given local radiotherapy to eradicate the carcinoma in situ. A dose of 2,000 rad will not appreciably alter Leydig cell function.

▶ This is an important observation that the incidence of carcinoma in situ was 5.4% in the contralateral testis in patients with testicular germ cell tumor. That 50% of these patients not receiving chemotherapy had testicular cancer, with one metastasizing, shows the malignant potential of these tumors. No contra- lateral testicular tumors developed in those patients with negative biopsies. The lesson is clear: We need to biopsy the opposite testis when removing a testicular cancer.—J.Y. Gillenwater, M.D.

Selection of Testicular Tumor Patients for Omission of Retroperitoneal Lymph Node Dissection
Harry W. Herr, Willet F. Whitmore, Jr., Pramod C. Sogani, Robin C. Watson, and William R. Fair (Mem. Sloan-Kettering Cancer Ctr., New York)
J. Urol. 135:500–503, March 1986   34–6

An attempt was made to determine which patients with testicular cancer would be optimal candidates for entry into a surveillance protocol as an alternative to retroperitoneal node dissection. Seventy-three patients with nonseminomatous germ cell tumors of the testis were evaluated in 1979– 1983. Disease was staged an average of 6 weeks after orchiectomy. Patients aged 15–40 years who had clinical stage I disease and were followed monthly for at least 2 years were eligible.

Ten (14%) of the 73 patients evaluated were entered into the surveillance study and followed for longer than 2 years. Three of them had relapses in the retroperitoneum after 4–7 months, but were salvaged by retro- peritoneal node dissection and, in 2, chemotherapy also; they were free from disease 24–29 months after treatment. All three patients had pure

---

Reasons for Exclusion of 63 Patients (86%) From Observation Alone
After Orchiectomy

	No.(%)	Surgical Stage Pos.	Neg.
Refused	2 (3)	0	2
Abnormal lymphangiogram	16 (25)	8	8
Pos. CT scan	22 (40)	12	10
Elevated tumor markers	6 (9)	4	2
Age <15 or >40 yrs.	3 (5)	0	3
Prior scrotal violation or orchio- pexy	8 (13)	1	7
Vascular involvement of sper- matic cord	4 (6)	2	2
Unavailable for monthly followup	2 (3)	0	2

(Courtesy of Herr, H.W., et al.: J. Urol. 135:500–503, March 1986, © Williams & Wilkins, 1986.)

embryonal cell carcinoma. One had vascular invasion within the tumor, and another had spermatic cord involvement. The most frequent reasons for excluding patients from surveillance were abnormal CT findings and an abnormal lymphangiogram (table). Forty-three percent of the patients who were operated on had pathologic stage II disease.

Patients with nonseminomatous germ cell tumors of the testis who are followed expectantly must be assessed carefully for extent of local tumor and potential sites of metastasis to minimize the risk of tumor recurrence. Expectant management of clinical stage I disease will probably increase, because three fourths of the patients followed for longer than 2 years are probably cured by orchiectomy alone.

▶ Twenty-five percent of clinical stage I nonseminomatous testicular tumors will metastasize. The clinical problem is how to predict which patients need retroperitoneal node dissection. The authors suggest that closer examination of the primary testicular tumor will help to determine prognosis. Invasion of the epididymis and spermatic cord, the primary cell type, and the presence of intratumoral vascular invasion were associated with increased metastasis. The practical problem is that most patients, and some urologists, do not realize how rapidly metastatic testicular tumor can grow and are not careful enough about follow-up when a surveillance protocol is instituted.—J.Y. Gillenwater, M.D.

Cyclic Chemotherapy With Cyclophosphamide, Doxorubicin, and Cisplatin Plus Vinblastine and Bleomycin in Advanced Germinal Tumors: Results With 100 Patients

Christopher J. Logothetis, Melvin L. Samuels, Debra E. Selig, Sheryl Ogden, Francisco Dexeus, David Swanson, Douglas Johnson, and Andrew von Eschenbach (Univ. of Texas at Houston)
Am. J. Med. 81:219–228, August 1986   34–7

Recent experience with cyclic chemotherapy was evaluated in 100 patients having metastatic germinal cell tumors who received a course of cyclophosphamide, cisplatin, and doxorubicin, alternating with vinblastine and bleomycin therapy (cyclic CISCA$_{II}$/VB$_{IV}$). The CISCA$_{II}$ regimen consists of 1 gm/sq m of cyclophosphamide and 80–90 mg/sq m of doxorubicin on days 1 and 2, and 100–120 mg/sq m of cisplatin on day 3. Vinblastine was given in a dose of 3 mg/sq m for 5 days, and bleomycin in a dose of 30 mg daily for the same period. Five patients with active infection first received a course of vincristine, bleomycin, and cisplatin. Total courses of therapy were individualized.

Ninety-one patients had tumors of primary testicular origin, whereas nine had extragonadal lesions. The disease-free survival rate was 89%. Four patients had resection of viable disease. Only five of nine patients with extragonadal tumors were alive without disease. None of 32 patients who were explored after the institution of chemotherapy had viable cancer. Considerable acute toxicity occurred, but only one patient had a fatal complication of treatment and long-term toxic effects were infrequent. One patient each had cardiac toxicity and bleomycin-induced lung toxicity.

Cyclic chemotherapy with $CISCA_{II}/VB_{IV}$ is an effective regimen that is indicated for patients at high risk of failure with cisplatin/vinblastine/ bleomycin chemotherapy, and also in those having extragonadal tumors. A higher complete disease-free response rate is obtained with cyclic therapy, with a lower rate of long-term toxicity.

▶ Cyclic chemotherapy with cyclophosphamide, doxorubicin, cisplatin, vinblastine, and bleomycin produced better results than conventional chemotherapy with vinblastine, bleomycin, and cisplatin (89% disease-free status and 2% relapse rate). This is in comparison to the 70% complete remission reported by Einhorn in disseminated disease plus the one third remission rate achieved by surgical excision in the remaining patients (*N. Engl. J. Med.* 305:927, 1981). Interestingly, the authors found exploratory surgery beneficial with persistently elevated α-fetoprotein levels after chemotherapy. Three of four patients were cured of a persistent focus of endodermal sinus tumor.— J.Y. Gillenwater, M.D.

Teratoma Following Cisplatin-Based Combination Chemotherapy for Nonseminomatous Germ Cell Tumors: A Clinicopathological Correlation
Patrick J. Loehrer, Sr., Siu Hui, Steven Clark, Mark Seal, Lawrence H. Einhorn, Stephen D. Williams, Thomas Ulbright, Isadore Mandelbaum, Randall Rowland, and John P. Donohue (Indiana Univ. at Indianapolis)
J. Urol. 135:1183–1189, June 1986   34–8

The clinical significance of pure teratoma, resected after chemotherapy for disseminated nonseminomatous germ cell tumor, is uncertain, although patients have been thought to have a good outlook after successful cisplatin-based combination chemotherapy. Fifty-one consecutive patients with primary testicular carcinoma or, in five, mediastinal germ cell tumors, underwent resection of teratoma from residual disease between 1975 and 1981. Thirty-five patients were first seen with stage C disease and 11 with advanced stage II disease. Most patients received vinblastine and bleomycin as well as cisplatin; nine were given cisplatin plus etoposide as salvage therapy. Maintenance chemotherapy was administered to 22 patients.

Teratomatous elements were found in nearly three fourths of 46 primary tumor specimens (table). Sixty-one percent of the patients were in complete remission for longer than 4 years after resection of teratoma. Ten patients each had recurrences of carcinoma and teratoma. Four patients relapsed initially more than 2 years after resection. Nine patients died, including one in whom angiosarcoma developed. Primary tumor in the mediastinum was the most significant adverse prognostic factor. Survival and relapse-free rates in patients with immature teratoma were similar to those in patients with mature teratoma.

Patients with resected teratoma and either nongerm cell elements or a large tumor burden should be followed closely beyond 2 years for recur-

Classification of Primary and Postchemotherapeutic Neoplasms

Primary Histology		Mature Teratoma (%)	Immature Teratoma (%)	Immature Teratoma With Nongerm Cell Elements (%)
		Post-Chemotherapy		
Embryonal Ca	9	6 (66)	3 (33)	
Seminoma	1			1 (100)
Embryonal Ca plus teratoma	21	12 (55)	5 (25)	4 (20)
Other Ca* plus teratoma	9	6 (66)	2 (22)	1 (11)
Other Ca* without teratoma	3	2 (66)	1 (33)	
Mature teratoma	1	1 (100)		
Immature teratoma	2		2 (100)	
Not available or unclassified	5	2 (40)	2 (40)	1 (20)
Totals	51	29 (58)	15 (29)	7 (13)

*Choriocarcinoma, embryonal carcinoma, endodermal sinus tumor, seminoma, or combination of these.
(Courtesy of Loehrer, P.J., Sr., et al.: J. Urol. 135:1183–1189, June 1986. © Williams & Wilkins, 1986.)

rence, especially patients with primary mediastinal disease. Operation alone may allow long-term, disease-free survival, even in patients with extensive teratoma.

▶ Residual disease after chemotherapy for nonseminomatous germ cell tumors has been found to consist of carcinoma (20%), necrotic fibrous tumor (40%), or teratoma (40%). This paper evaluated 51 patients whose surgically excised mass was teratoma. Most recurrences were local, so meticulous resection of the teratoma was stressed. The worst prognosis was observed in those patients who had nongerm cell elements and an increased tumor burden, and in those with primary mediastinal tumors. Nine of 51 patients died.— J.Y. Gillenwater, M.D.

Sequential Excision of Residual Thoracic and Retroperitoneal Masses After Chemotherapy for Stage III Germ Cell Tumors

Peter Tiffany, Michael J. Morse, George Bosl, E. Darracott Vaughan, Jr., Pramod C. Sogani, Harry W. Herr, and Willet F. Whitmore, Jr. (Mem. Sloan-Kettering Cancer Ctr., New York, and Cornell Univ.)
Cancer 57:978–983, March 1, 1986   34–9

Twenty-three patients with stage III mixed germ cell tumors received chemotherapy in 1968–1984 followed by excision of residual thoracic, cervical, and retroperitoneal masses. Various chemotherapeutic protocols were used. All tumors but one were testicular in origin. Twenty-one patients had measurable thoracic disease, and two had neck disease that had not responded fully to chemotherapy. Eighteen patients had retroperitoneal masses after chemotherapy. Eighteen had thoracotomy or sternotomy with resection of pulmonary deposits, with or without removal of mediastinal nodes or masses. Three patients had retroperitoneal node dissection, and two had radical neck dissection.

In one third of the patients the resected neck or chest disease differed pathologically from the retroperitoneal tissue. Usually, the latter specimen had less favorable histologic features. Four of 11 patients with fibrosis or necrosis in thoracic or neck specimens had malignancy in the retroperitoneum. Nine patients (39%) in all had residual malignancy after chemotherapy. Three of these patients remain alive, two without disease. One patient died postoperatively of aortic bleeding, and another of respiratory failure and sepsis.

All residual masses must be removed after chemotherapy for germ cell tumor, even if tumor marker levels return to normal. Some patients with residual malignancy may be salvaged by appropriate surgical treatment.

► This study correlated the histology of metastatic germ cell tumors in the head/neck with retroperitoneal metastasis. In 8 of 23 patients (35%) there were different pathologic findings, those with retroperitoneal metastasis usually having a worse prognosis. Four of 11 patients with fibrosis in the head/neck had malignancy in the retroperitoneum. Thus when the pathologic finding of the metastasis in the head/neck is benign, the retroperitoneal mass still has to be surgically excised.—J.Y. Gillenwater, M.D.

Sexual and Marital Relationships After Radiotherapy for Seminoma
Leslie R. Schover, Mario Gonzales, and Andrew C. von Eschenbach (Univ. of Texas at Houston and Rio Grande Cancer Treatment Ctr., Houston)
Urology 27:117–123, February 1986   34–10

A follow-up study of men treated for nonseminomatous tumors indicated a higher rate of erectile and orgasmic dysfunction in irradiated patients than in those treated by other means. This finding prompted a study of sexual function and fertility in 84 men surviving after radiotherapy for seminoma in 1963–1983. The mean age at diagnosis was 36 years, and at follow-up, 45 years. Two thirds of the patients had stage I tumors and 5% had stage III disease. In addition to orchiectomy and radiotherapy, seven men were treated for a second, asynchronous testicular primary tumor.

Significant sexual dysfunction was identified in up to 20% of the study group. One third of the men reported less intensity and pleasure at orgasm, and nearly half noted a reduced semen volume. The various sexual problems were highly interrelated. Men who were more anxious about cancer and sexuality had poorer sexual function than the others. Disease stage itself was not predictive of sexual function, but men given more extensive radiotherapy expressed less overall sexual satisfaction. The age at diagnosis was not significantly predictive of sexual function. Men having bilateral orchiectomy did not account for the sexual problems of the group as a whole. The ability to father children after treatment was not significantly related to cancer stage, radiation dosage, or extent of treatment.

Sexual function is an important concern for some men treated for seminoma. A high radiation dose to the para-aortic field may impair sexual function. The mechanisms by which irradiation affect sexual function remain to be determined. All men treated for testicular cancer should be counseled with regard to sexual function, marital communication, and infertility.

▶ Fifteen percent of the 84 men receiving radiation for seminoma had erectile dysfunction. The etiology of this dysfunction was not identified.—J.Y. Gillenwater, M.D.

The following review articles are recommended to the reader:

Cosentino, M.J., Cockett, A.T.K.: Structure and function of the epididymis. *Urol. Res.* 14:229, 1986.

Doll, D.C., Weiss, R.B.: Malignant lymphoma of the testis. *Am. J. Med.* 81:515, 1986.

Einhorn, L.H.: Cancer of the testis: A new paradigm. *Hosp. Pract.* (Off.)21:165, 1986.

Freeman, D.A.: Steroid hormone-producing tumors in man. *Endocr. Rev.* 7:204, 1986.

Friedrichs, R., Rubben, H., Lutzeyer, W.: Differential diagnosis and therapy of rare testicular tumors. *Eur. Urol.* 12:217, 1986.

35 Penis

Priapism: A Refined Approach to Diagnosis and Treatment
Tom F. Lue, Wayne J.G. Hellstrom, Jack W. McAninch, and Emil A. Tanagho
(Univ. of California at San Francisco and San Francisco Gen. Hosp.)
J. Urol. 136:104–108, July 1986   35–1

During a 2-year period, seven patients aged 21–57 years were treated for priapism. Because priapism can be ischemic or nonischemic, blood gas measurements were done to document the degree of ischemia. The degree of priapism was documented by intracorporeal pressure recording before and after correction.

Two patients had papaverine-induced priapism. One required two injections of diluted metaraminol bitartrate, which resulted in the penis becoming completely flaccid 3 hours later. In the second patient, aspiration of blood was necessary to achieve resolution. Four patients had ischemic spontaneous priapism. One with sickle cell trait required a small Winter shunt after saline irrigation and injection of norepinephrine. The second patient also responded to similar treatment. The third patient, an insulin-dependent diabetic, responded to aspiration and saline irrigation followed by shunting. Adequate erections were achieved 6 months postoperatively, although the penis was much shorter and thinner than before. The fourth patient, who had a long psychiatric history, had been taking lithium and thorazine, as well as disulfiram occasionally because of alcoholism. He required saline irrigation and aspiration followed by shunting. A patient with nonischemic priapism had a 1-month history of nephrolithotomy for which he took allopurinol to correct an elevated uric acid level. Aspiration and irrigation followed by bilateral shunting alleviated his condition.

In patients with early, mild ischemic priapism, aspiration alone or combined with instillation of α-adrenergic agents is recommended. This usually permits the cavernous and arteriolar smooth muscles to regain contractility. This treatment is also recommended for papaverine-induced priapism and early spontaneous priapism. To avoid systemic side effects, norepinephrine should not be given in doses larger than 15 μg and at intervals of more than 5 minutes. In late and severely ischemic stages, the shunt procedure usually is necessary, providing fresh blood for metabolic replenishment and tissue repair. To determine the effect of shunting, intracorporeal pressure should be monitored; a unilateral shunt should be effective for pressure less than 40 mm Hg, and a bilateral shunt for pressure of more than 50 mm Hg. The size and number of shunts should be minimized to avoid postoperative impotence.

▶ A corollary of the developing experience with papaverine and α blockade injections to create erection is that α-adrenergic agents are a logical choice to treat priapism. Certainly, as the authors recommend, this therapy plus irrigation is a first line of defense. If this fails, surgery is necessary. We start with a Winters shunt made with a true-cut biopsy needle. If this fails, we go to one or two corpus spongiosum-corpus cavernosum shunts. Houri and associates (1984 YEAR BOOK OF UROLOGY; *Urol. Int.* 38:138, 1983) suggested that there are two types of priapism: low flow with decreased Po₂ and high flow with normal Po₂. Correction of high-flow priapism requires a larger shunt but carries a better prognosis because the tissue remains well oxygenated and viable.—S.S. Howards, M.D.

Prevalence and Significance of Tobacco Smoking in Impotence
Michael Condra, David H. Surridge, Alvaro Morales, Janet Fenemore, and James A. Owen (Kingston Gen. Hosp. and Queen's Univ., Kingston, Ont.)
Urology 27:495–498, June 1986   35–2

Smoking is the major causative factor of peripheral vascular disease. However, the effect of smoking on male erectile dysfunction, which is often associated with vascular problems, is not well documented. A study was undertaken to determine the prevalence of smoking among impotent patients and the physiologic differences between smokers and nonsmokers that might play a part in impotence.

The 178 patients studied underwent urologic, psychiatric, vascular, hormonal, and metabolic examinations and two nights of monitoring nocturnal penile tumescence. Full histories of cigarette use were obtained. Among the impotent patients, the proportions of current smokers, 51.4%, and combined smokers and ex-smokers, 81.0%, were significantly higher than in the general population (38.6% and 58.3%, respectively). Smokers and nonsmokers had similar hormone levels; however, smokers had significantly lower mean penile blood pressure.

These findings indicate a significantly increased prevalence of cigarette smoking among impotent men compared with the general population. Although several indices of impotence were similar between smokers and nonsmokers, the measure of small penile vasculature function, penile blood pressure, was much lower in smokers. Smoking may be a risk factor for impotence.

▶ It is well established that smoking increases the risk of many forms of vascular disease. It is therefore not surprising that it would be a risk factor for impotence. Surprisingly, this has never been well documented. Condra and associates present evidence that supports, but does not prove, the hypothesis. No statistical analysis is presented, and the source of the population estimates is not given. An epidemiologically sound case-control study would seem appropriate. Dr. Tom Lue and associates at UCLA (*J. Urol.,* 1987; in press) have data on the monkey, demonstrating impotence in "smoking" monkeys, which also supports this concept.—S.S. Howards, M.D.

Reduction of Serum Testosterone Levels During Chronic Glucocorticoid Therapy

Michael R. MacAdams, Richard H. White, and Bradley E. Chipps (Univ. of California, Davis, at Sacramento)
Ann. Intern. Med. 104:648–651, May 1986   35–3

Glucocorticoids reduce testosterone concentrations in men and interfere with ovulation in women, partly because of direct suppression of gonadal steroid secretion. Pituitary gonadotropin secretion is inhibited in women, but the effects of long-term glucocorticoid therapy on the male hypothalamic-pituitary-gonadal axis are unknown. Sixteen men with a mean age of 67 years who had chronic obstructive lung disease were studied after at least 1 month of prednisone or methylprednisolone therapy. Eight patients were treated on a daily basis and eight on alternate days. Eleven age-matched and disease-matched patients not receiving glucocorticoids were also evaluated.

The mean serum testosterone concentration was 211 ng/dl in the glucocorticoid-treated patients and 449 ng/dl in the controls. Only two of the former had values of more than 300 ng/dl, whereas all but one of the controls had such values. The average daily steroid dose was inversely related to the serum testosterone concentration. The proportions of total testosterone not bound to protein were similar in the study and control groups. Basal gonadotropin concentrations were also similar, and peak gonadotropin responses to gonadotropin-releasing hormone were comparable in the glucocorticoid-treated and control men.

Long-term glucocorticoid administration often lowers the serum testosterone concentration in men with obstructive lung disease. Prednisone dosages as low as 15 mg daily may have this effect. Impotence and loss of libido in such patients may be the result of steroid-induced hypogonadism. Further, a low serum testosterone concentration may be responsible in part for glucocorticoid-induced osteopenia, because the bone mineral content is directly related to the circulating testosterone concentration, and testosterone may be useful in preventing or treating osteoporosis in men receiving glucocorticoid therapy.

▶ This finding is clinically significant and surprising. It is significant because the steroid-induced reduction in serum testosterone may cause or contribute to impotence, and surprising because men with untreated congenital adrenal hyperplasia have a normal serum level of testosterone. The mechanism of the reduced testosterone level has not been elucidated. Glucocorticoids are known to reduce sex binding globulin levels, and this may explain some but not all of the effect. Glucocorticoids can also directly reduce androgen synthesis. The basal and peak gonadotropin levels were similar to those in controls, but the authors argue that basal levels should have been elevated in the treatment group because the serum testosterone levels were reduced.—S.S. Howards, M.D.

Noninvasive Device to Produce and Maintain an Erection-Like State

Perry W. Nadig, J. Catesby Ware, and Ronald Blumoff (Humana Hosp., San Antonio, Tex.)

Urology 27:126–131, February 1986   35–4

A nonoperative mechanical method of producing a rigid penis is available allowing impotent men to engage in sexual intercourse. The device (Fig 35–1), which uses a vacuum to produce an erection-like state and rubber bands to maintain it, was evaluated in 35 men aged 45–83 years with organic impotence secondary to various causes who refused placement of a penile prosthesis. After placing the open end of the cylinder over the penis and pressing against the skin at the base, a vacuum is created by withdrawing air with the syringe; rubber bands are then applied to constrict the base of the penis.

An erection-like state was produced in all but three men, two of whom had too large a penis. Rigidity was considered adequate in 27 men. From 3 to 7 minutes were required to reach maximal rigidity. The penile skin temperature fell by nearly 1F in 30 minutes, but plethysmography showed continued blood flow into the penis in all instances. Twenty-four men use the device regularly, including several whose penile rigidity was less than satisfactory. Penile and brachial blood pressures were unchanged in nine men restudied after using the device for a mean of 10 months.

Eighty percent of men in this study with organic impotence who had refused a penile prosthesis have regularly used the vacuum device for sexual intercourse. Penile blood flow continues with the rubber bands in place, but men at risk of priapism should not use this device. The system has the advantage of being reversible, and impotent men may be able to use newer methods of correcting impotence as they become available.

▶ A device for a vacuum-induced erection was patented by Otto Lederer in 1917. There is no doubt that this method is effective in some patients. How-

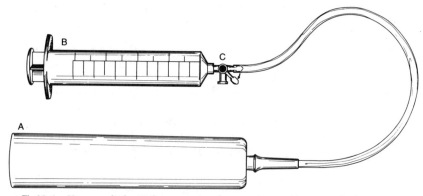

Fig 35–1.—Vacuum cylinder (A) fits over penis and vacuum is created by repeatedly drawing air from cylinder with piston syringe (B) and expelling it by means of a three-way stopcock (C). (Courtesy of Nadig, P.W., et al.: Urology 27:126–131, February 1986.)

ever, our experience with the device is much less favorable than that of Nadig and associates. The vast majority of our patients are not interested. Among those who try, a large percentage either find the procedure distasteful or unsuccessful. Nevertheless, we do have several very satisfied users and mention the device to all our impotent patients.—S.S. Howards, M.D.

Impotence: Evaluation With Cavernosography

Christian Delcour, Eric Wespes, Ghislain Vandenbosch, Claude C. Schulman, and Julien Struyven (Hôpital Erasme, Univ. Libre de Bruxelles, Brussels)
Radiology 161:803–806, December 1986   35–5

The mechanisms of erection have not been established. Nevertheless, the arterial anatomy of the penis is well known. Because arterial lesions are present in only 46% of patients with proved organic impotence, it was suggested that abnormal venous drainage from the corpora cavernosa may be a cause of impotence. During normal erection, occlusion of the venous drainage of the penis probably results in part from an active, neurologic mechanism and in part from a passive mechanism. The function of the venous system in erection was investigated.

The study population consisted of 187 impotent men in whom cavernosography was performed during artificial induction of erection with monitoring of intracavernous pressure and inflow. In addition to undergoing investigation of the mechanism of active erection, 69 patients received intracavernous injections of papaverine. Venous leakage was discovered in 88 patients. In these patients, a higher than normal rate of flow of diluted, heparinized contrast medium was required to initiate and maintain erection. Moreover, opacification of the prostatic plexus occurred during erection in these patients. In all patients who received papaverine, the flow rates necessary to initiate and maintain erection decreased. Cavernosography and cavernometry are essential in the workup of impotence, and studies with papaverine may be helpful in clarifying the active mechanism of erection.

Functional Evaluation of Penile Veins by Cavernosography in Papaverine-Induced Erection

Tom F. Lue, Hedvic Hricak, Richard A. Schmidt, and Emil A. Tanagho (Univ. of California at San Francisco)
J. Urol. 135:479–482, March 1986   35–6

The role of penile veins in erection, and whether their drainage increases or decreases during erection, is a matter of debate. Previous researchers have used erotic motion pictures to produce erections in their patients before making measurements of venous flow. A study was made of the use of papaverine, a smooth muscle relaxant, to induce erections for the performance of cavernosography. The study included 49 patients with impotence who had an excellent arterial response to papaverine as evaluated by pulsed Doppler analysis and sonography. Injections of 60 mg of papaverine in 20 ml of saline were made into the patient's penis and the pressure of the corpora cavernosa was measured with a butterfly needle connected to an arterial pressure monitor.

In the 11 patients who responded with full erections to the papaverine injections, normal veins were seen in their cavernosograms. Of the 33 patients who responded to papaverine with poor erections, 5 had severe venous leakage and 28 had arterial insufficiency and venous leakage, as demonstrated by cavernosography. The complications were severe dizziness in 4 patients and hematomas at the injection site in 22.

Papaverine injection is a useful tool in conjunction with cavernosography for detecting impotence caused by venous leakage. Once correctly located, the leak can be closed by venous ligation. Cavernosography is not recommended in patients with a poor arterial response to papaverine, because they are unlikely to be helped by venous ligation.

▶ Recently, considerable attention has been focused on "venous leak impotence" (please see the 1986 YEAR BOOK OF UROLOGY, pp. 283–286). Several groups have reported correction of impotence with surgical or balloon occlusion of "leaking" veins (please see 1986 YEAR BOOK and below). The two articles above (Abstracts 35–5 and 35–6) review experience with dynamic cavernosography. It is still not clear how common venous leak impotence is. We think that it is certainly less frequent than Delcour and associates suggest (Abstract 35–5). Lue's population (Abstract 35–6) was highly selected. We agree with Lue and associates that cavernosography should be reserved for men with organic impotence and good arterial inflow. Patients should be screened with the usual careful history, physical examination, and endocrine evaluation. Those with a suboptimal papaverine response should have Doppler evaluation of arterial blood flow if available. If not available, younger men (under age 55 years) without known vascular disease should be selected for cavernosography. Interpretation of these studies is subjective. However, if there is significant venous outflow during a papaverine infusion-induced erection, venous occlusion therapy should be offered. It is not certain how many men will benefit from this approach. We remain unconvinced that it will be more than a small percentage of all those who present with impotence.—S.S. Howards, M.D.

Erectile Dysfunction Caused by Venous Leakage: Treatment With Detachable Balloons and Coils
Patrick Courtheoux, Dominique Maiza, Jean-Paul Henriet, Claude D. Vaislic, Claude Evrard, and Jacques Theron (Centre Hosp. Régional et Univ. de Caen, Côte de Nacre, Caen, France)
Radiology 161:807–809, December 1986   35–7

Vascular impotence results from insufficient blood flow to the corpora cavernosa or from venous leaks and subsequent blood loss from the corpora cavernosa. The treatment for patients with venous leakage has not been well studied and is therefore not well established. A treatment for venous leakage consists of embolizing the deep dorsal vein of the penis by implanting detachable balloons and coils.

In a series of 135 patients with erectile dysfunction, 40 had venous leakage. These patients were classified into three groups according to findings on cavernosograms, and 31 were treated with implantation of balloons and coils. After treatment, 26 of these patients had normal sexual function. This technique is simple, safe, and effective for the treatment of impotence caused by venous leakage.

▶ These authors found a high incidence of venous leak impotence (40 of 135 patients, or 31%) and had a remarkable success rate. Their method of treatment is quite rational: a combined surgical/radiologic approach with radiologic confirmation. If results like this can be duplicated in other centers, the concept of venous leak impotence and its treatment will both become legitimized.— S.S. Howards, M.D.

Deep-Penile-Vein Arterialization for Arterial and Venous Impotence
Alexander Balko, Chander M. Malhotra, John P. Wincze, Jacques G. Susset, Sudhir Bansal, Wilfred I. Carney, and Robert W. Hopkins (Providence VA Med. Ctr., Rhode Island Hosp., and Miriam Hosp., Providence)
Arch. Surg. 121:774–777, July 1986   35–8

Penile prostheses, used to treat vasculogenic impotence, destroy the corpora cavernosa and do not restore normal physiology. Virag et al. reported encouraging short-term results with deep penile vein arterialization in patients with both arterial and venous impotence. A modified Virag procedure was evaluated in 11 important men after multidisciplinary evaluation that included Doppler penile pressure recording, testosterone estimation, and nocturnal penile tumescence testing. Arterial insufficiency was diagnosed in three patients and venous leakage in four; mixed factors were responsible in four others. The mean age was 53 years. A femoral artery to deep penile vein saphenous bypass was carried out, and the superficial veins at the base of the penis were ligated in cases of venous leakage.

Graft patency was confirmed by Doppler study in all patients but one after a mean follow-up of 13 months. One graft in the arterial group occluded 3 weeks postoperatively. Hypervascularization occurred in two patients in the mixed-factors group, in both of whom a side branch of the deep penile vein was joined directly to the neighboring corpus cavernosum. Edema resolved after the side branches were ligated, and the bypass was banded in one case. Postoperative nocturnal penile tumescence testing indicated excellent results in seven cases and a good result in another.

Deep penile vein arterialization is recommended for patients having vasculogenic impotence secondary to venous leakage. Intracavernosal papaverine injections may prove to be a better approach when arterial insufficiency is evident, or if mixed factors are responsible for impotence.

▶ This report is of anecdotal interest, but is uninterpretable for the following reasons: (1) The authors do not tell us how many patients they screened to find the 11 they treated. (2) The series is very small. (3) The etiologies are mixed and it is unclear whether the successes resulted from arterialization of the venous obstruction. (4) Amazingly, they do not tell us how many patients are functioning sexually. (5) The nocturnal penile tumescènce results are excellent in only three of nine patients with an arterial component.—S.S. Howards, M.D.

Intracavernous Drug-Induced Erections in the Management of Male Erectile Dysfunction: Experience With 100 Patients

Abraham Ami Sidi, Jeffrey S. Cameron, Linda M. Duffy, and Paul H. Lange (Univ. of Minnesota and VA Med. Ctr., Minneapolis)
J. Urol. 135:704–706, April 1986   35–9

Intracavernous vasoactive drug-induced erection is a promising approach to the management of impotence. One hundred men with organic impotence participated in a trial of intracavernous injections. A mixture of 25 mg of papaverine and 0.8 mg of phentolamine per ml was used. The initial doses were 0.25 ml in patients with a penile-brachial index of more than 0.85, 0.5 ml in those with a lower index, and 0.15 ml in those with neurogenic impotence. Injections were made with a 28-gauge or 30-gauge needle, unilaterally into the base of the cavernous body.

All patients with neurogenic impotence had functional erections, as did about two thirds of those with vasculogenic impotence and a similar proportion with neurogenic-vascular impotence. The response rate in those with idiopathic impotence was 90%. About half of the nonresponders had vascular arterial impotence. Patients with purely neurogenic impotence required much less medication than those in the other groups (table). Complications included sustained erection in 4 patients with pure neurogenic impotence, two of whom had cord injuries. Sixty-six responders elected to use this treatment, and none nad major complications during an average follow-up of 4 months. Most men who currently do not use self-injection have no available partner.

Intracavernous drug-induced erection has been well accepted by men with organic impotence. Those with pure neurogenic impotence have responded consistently. If complications prove to be relatively minor over the long term, intracavernous drug-induced erection undoubtedly will be an important treatment for impotence.

ETIOLOGIC GROUPS, DOSE RANGE, AND AVERAGE DOSE
± SD REQUIRED TO INDUCE FUNCTIONAL ERECTION

Etiology Group	Dose Range (ml.)	Av. Dose
Neurogenic	0.10–1.0	0.36 ± 0.22
Vascular	0.5–1.5	0.73 ± 0.30
Neurogenic/vascular	0.25–1.25	0.65 ± 0.33
Undetermined organic	0.25–1.5	0.75 ± 0.45

(Courtesy of Sidi, A.A., et al.: J. Urol. 135:704–706, April 1986. © Williams & Wilkins, 1986.)

▶ Intracavernous vasoactive drugs are now widely used in North America for impotence. Brindley's dramatic demonstration at the 1984 AUA meeting has even been discussed recently in the *Wall Street Journal.* We had been using papaverine, 30–60 mg in 10 of sterile saline, but have switched to 0.5–1.0 cc of the mixture used by Zorgniotti and Lefleur (*J. Urol.* 133:39, 1985) and the Minnesota group. The reasons for the change are that the latter approach avoids mixing and allows for the use of insulin syringes, which are convenient and almost painless. The great concerns with cavernous injections are priapism and the possibility of fibrosis with long-term use. There are several studies documenting Peyronie-like disease after injection in man, and Dr. Tom Lue has shown the same phenomenon in monkeys. Therefore, patients must be warned of this complication, and long-term use in patients with psychogenic impotence probably should be avoided.—S.S. Howards, M.D.

Effect of Chronic Oral Testosterone Undecanoate Administration on the Pituitary-Testicular Axes of Hemodialyzed Male Patients

A. van Coevorden, J.-C. Stolear, M. Dhaene, J.-L. van Herweghem, and J. Mockel (Univ. of Brussels)
Clin. Nephrol. 26:48–54, July 1986   35–10

Androgens are used to augment erythropoiesis in patients with end-stage renal disease, and oral testosterone therapy now is feasible in uremic males with hypogonadism. The effects of testosterone on the hypothalamus-pituitary-gonadal system were studied in a double-blind trial in 19 males

---

EFFECT OF TESTOSTERONE UNDECANOATE ON BASAL HORMONAL VALUES (MEAN + SD)

Parameters		Normal value	Group A = Treated Group		Group P = Placebo Group	
			Before treatment	After treatment	Before treatment	After treatment
Testosterone	ng/ml	(4–12)	5.6 ± 3	7.6 ± 4.3	4.9 ± 2.1	6 ± 1.74
Free testosterone	ng/dl	(8–32)	21.5 ± 11.9	45.9 ± 35.9	24.1 ± 15.4	24.3 ± 9.64
DHT	ng/ml	(0.3–1.0)	0.31 ± 0.14	1.13 ± 0.6	0.28 ± 0.13	0.25 ± 0.11
Androstenedione	ng/ml	(0.5–2.5)	0.85 ± 0.45	1.4 ± 0.7	0.83 ± 0.16	0.69 ± 0.2
11OH androstenedione	ng/ml	(0.5–3.6)	1.13 ± 0.7	1.44 ± 0.6	1.15 ± 0.6	1.25 ± 0.4
Dehydroepiandro-sterone sulfate	ng/ml	(1900–3300)	1269 ± 1135	1822 ± 990	1261 ± 394	1246 ± 518
FSH	ng/ml	(1.3–2.3)	5.51 ± 8.2	1.84 ± 1.9	8.33 ± 6	8.2 ± 6
LH	ng/ml	(1.2–2.2)	5.51 ± 4.3	2.13 ± 1.24	8 ± 4.8	8.7 ± 4.8
PRL	µU/ml	(110–250)	376 ± 271	306 ± 213	331 ± 120	359 ± 195
Estradiol	pg/ml	(<80)	33 ± 15	45 ± 16	52 ± 20	48 ± 23
Sex hormone binding globulin	nmoles/dl	(<9)	4.9 ± 4.3	3.8 ± 3.8	1.9 ± 0.7	3.2 ± 1.5

Student's *t* test paired variables: DHT $P < .01$

A
110A
DHEAS } $P < .05$
FSH
LH
PRL

(Courtesy of van Coevorden, A., et al.: Clin. Nephrol. 26:48–54, July 1986.)

undergoing chronic hemodialysis, using testosterone undecanoate and placebo in matched patient groups. Study patients received 80 mg of testosterone daily, orally, for 6 months.

Total and free testosterone levels were higher in treated patients at the end of the study, but the difference was not significant. The level of gonadotropins was significantly lower in the treatment group, however (table). A sustained rise in 5α-dihydrotestosterone was noted in the treatment group. Four of ten study patients reported increased libido and sexual activity, but no placebo patient noted such improvement. Renal and hepatic functions were unchanged. The number of transfusions decreased significantly in the testosterone-treated patients. In three patients prostatitis developed, in conjunction with septicemia in one. Hypertriglyceridemia was not observed.

Testosterone undecanoate is an effective, well-tolerated treatment for hypogonadal uremic men. Treatment restores the pituitary-testicular axis to normal in men receiving chronic hemodialysis, but further studies are needed to evaluate its effects on libido and sexual performance, alone and in conjunction with bromocriptine therapy.

Transdermal Testosterone Substitution Therapy for Male Hypogonadism
Monika Bals-Pratsch, Ulrich A. Knuth, Yong-Dal Yoon, and Eberhard Nieschlag (Univ. of Münster, West Germany)
Lancet 2:943–945, Oct. 25, 1986   35–11

Treatment of male hypogonadism requires replacement of testosterone, the most important androgen secreted physiologically by the testes. Testosterone cannot be administered orally because it undergoes hepatic metabolism and elimination. To avoid the first-pass effect of the liver, testosterone may be esterified with a long aliphatic side chain so that it can be absorbed via the lymph after ingestion, or testosterone esters can be injected intramuscularly. However, these preparations do not produce the constant serum testosterone levels observed physiologically. To achieve more constant serum testosterone levels, a transdermal therapeutic system for testosterone was devised that consists of testosterone-impregnated film. Results with this system in normal and hypogonadal men were reviewed.

The study population consisted of nine healthy normal men aged 23–37 years and seven hypogonadal patients aged 31–37 years. A testosterone-loaded film was applied to the scrotal skin. The transdermal therapeutic system was designed to last for 22 hours. In this time period, serum testosterone levels in normal men were moderately increased, with concentration curves almost parallel to basal levels. The seven hypogonadal patients also experienced an increase in serum testosterone levels during the 12-week treatment period. None of the patients experienced side effects. This approach appears to represent an alternative approach to androgen substitution therapy.

▶ Androgen replacement therapy in hypogonadal men has always been a problem. The available nonparenteral preparations are poorly absorbed and have significant hepatic toxicity. Testosterone undecanoate is reasonably well absorbed and appears to be free of hepatic complications. However, the drug is very short-acting and, as far as we can determine, it is not available in the United States. Transdermal preparations provide another alternative to injection therapy. We have participated in an experimental trial of a transdermal testosterone. It worked rather well and we expect it will be used in the future. It is not yet available and may be more expensive than parenteral forms of testosterone.—S.S. Howards, M.D.

Sexual Dysfunction in the Male Dialysis Patient: Pathogenesis, Evaluation, and Therapy
C.J. Foulks and H.M. Cushner (Brooke Army Med. Ctr., Fort Sam Houston, Tex.)
Am. J. Kidney Dis. 8:211–222, October 1986   35–12

At least half of the men undergoing dialysis become impotent. Uremic men usually have low testosterone levels, and evidence of primary hypogonadism has been reported in these patients. Testicular biopsies have shown markedly reduced production of spermatocytes and spermatocyte precursors; most patients have little maturational progression beyond the primary spermatocyte stage. A baseline level of testosterone seems necessary for maintenance of normal libido and potency. Hyperprolactinemia occurs in many men with end-stage renal disease and is a factor in male hypogonadism associated with impotence.

Studies of the causes of impotence in dialysis patients and of the outcome of treatment are lacking. Estimates of testosterone, prolactin, and gonadotropin levels might prove useful in planning treatment in individual cases. If impotence is secondary to medication, discontinuance of the responsible drug should help. However, antihypertensive medication must be withdrawn cautiously if a rebound rise in blood pressure is to be avoided. Neither stamp testing nor nocturnal penile tumescence testing is an infallible means of distinguishing between organic and psychological impotence. When conventional medical or psychological measures have failed, papaverine injection or use of an inflatable prosthesis might be worthwhile.

Improved libido and frequency of sexual intercourse have been described in males with functioning renal transplants. If a second transplant is necessary in a patient with reduced penile blood flow, an end-to-side anastomosis of the second graft into the common iliac artery might be helpful.

▶ Impotence is a major problem in patients with renal failure. As pointed out by the authors of this review, the etiology is multifactorial. In the last few years papers describing good therapeutic results with a variety of unrelated forms of treatment have been published. These include testosterone undecanoate (please see Abstract 35–10), zinc (1983 YEAR BOOK OF UROLOGY, p. 75), and bromocriptine (1984 YEAR BOOK OF UROLOGY, p. 151). These patients should be evaluated with a thorough history, physical examination, and laboratory studies, and then treated appropriately. Whether or not zinc and bromocriptine will prove useful is unclear.—S.S. Howards, M.D.

Intracavernous Injection of Noradrenaline to Interrupt Erections During Surgical Interventions
Jean M. de Meyer and Walter A. De Sy (Univ. Hosp., Ghent, Belgium)
Eur. Urol. 12:169–170, May–June 1986   35–13

Erections occurring during transurethral and urethral surgery cause excessive bleeding and make surgery difficult, and augmenting the depth of anesthesia is of little help. In an attempt to interrupt such erections during surgery, seven adults undergoing transurethral resection of the prostate and ten children having hypospadias repair or circumcision were given norepinephrine. Approximately 0.5–1.0 μg was injected into the dorsolateral side of the base of the penis. Two minutes after injection, tumescence subsided in all patients, although four adults required a second injection 30 minutes later. Injection was needed on only one side as the drug diffused easily to the other side. There were no complications. Epinephrine administration is recommended as the primary means of suppressing erection during surgery as it is safer and more successful than deepening the level of anesthesia.

▶ This paper presents a simple, logical solution based on recent knowledge to what has occasionally been a difficult problem.—S.S. Howards, M.D.

The following review articles are recommended to the reader:

Metz, P.: Arteriogenic erectile impotence. *Dan. Med. Bull.* 33:134, 1986.
Morley, J.E.: Impotence. *Am. J. Med.* 80:897, 1986.
Pohl, J., Pott, B., Kleinhans, G.: Priapism: A three-phase concept of management according to etiology and prognosis. *Br. J. Urol.* 58:113, 1986.

36 Cancer of the Penis

Penile Cancer: Aspiration Biopsy Cytology for Staging
Pierantonio Scappini, Francesco Piscioli, Teresa Pusiol, Albert Hofstetter,
Karlheinz Rothenberger, and Lucio Luciani (S. Chiara Hosp., Trento, Italy, and
Univ. of Lübeck, West Germany, and Ludwig-Maximilians Univ., Landshut,
West Germany)
Cancer 58:1526–1533, Oct. 1, 1986   36–1

At least half of the patients with penile cancer are likely to have regional
node metastases at the time of diagnosis, and survival falls sharply when
the inguinal or pelvic nodes are involved. The role of aspiration biopsy
cytology in staging penile carcinoma was examined in a series of 29 patients
aged 39–81 years, 28 with squamous cell carcinoma and 1 with malignant
melanoma. Aspiration was performed with fluoroscopic aid, usually with
a 22-gauge or 23-gauge Chiba needle. Computed tomography guidance
was used in one instance. Twenty-one patients were treated by local excision combined with laser irradiation. Two others had local excision
alone, and three patients each underwent total and partial penectomy.

Aspiration biopsy cytology correctly identified the true stage of disease
in all 20 patients having lymphadenectomy with histologic study of node
tissue. Two other patients with negative biopsy results but no histologic
control died of metastatic disease after 34 months and 53 months, respectively. One false negative cytologic result was found among 84 node
chains removed. Pedal lymphography resulted in false negative and false
positive rates of 12% and 4%, respectively.

Aspiration biopsy cytology is the procedure of choice for the preliminary
detection of metastatic node involvement by penile carcinoma. Some patients can thereby be spared the unnecessary removal of uninvolved ilioinguinal lymph nodes.

► We have had similar good results with cytologic studies from fine-needle
aspirations, and I believe that this is the method of choice for initial evaluation
of inguinal nodes.—J.Y. Gillenwater, M.D.

Value of the Neodymium-YAG Laser in the Therapy of Penile Carcinoma
K.H. Rothenberger (Municipal Hosp., Landshut, West Germany)
Eur. Urol. 12 (Suppl. 1) 12:34–36, September 1986   36–2

Mutilation associated with functional loss is characteristic of current
penile carcinoma therapy. Recurrence rates of 40% can be expected after
local tumor excision. Evaluation was made of treatment with the neodym-
ium-yttrium/aluminum/garnet (Nd:YAG) laser in management of T_1 and

T_2 tumors. Treatment includes radical circumcision followed by tourniquet application at the penis base. The macroscopically visible carcinoma is removed with a scalpel. Laser treatment of the base and margins of the excised area is carried out immediately. The aim is to achieve a reproducible, homogeneous, end deep necrosis to ensure complete devitalization of any remaining tumor cells with the Nd:YAG laser. The laser is used solely for coagulation.

Thirteen men aged 33–77 years with stage $T_1N_0M_0$ tumors and six aged 42–86 years with $T_2N_0M_0$ carcinomas were treated. In two patients with T_1 tumors, treatment of a carcinoma in situ with the laser was required within the first year. After 59 months, Bowen's disease of the glans developed in one patient, who then was treated successfully with the laser. No pathologic changes occurred in the other patients in the area of the glans during a period of 6.5 years. Of 17 patients followed for 43–77 months, one died of metastases from the penile carcinoma with no evidence of local tumor recurrence. Three died of other diseases. Two patients with T_1 and T_2 carcinomas underwent therapeutic lymphadenectomy for lymph node metastases. No metastases were found locally. One patient died of a bladder carcinoma after 59 months, and the second patient lived for 62 months after primary therapy with no complaints or evidence of disease.

No patient was lost to recurrent tumor; the disease in one patient was understaged. Neodynium-YAG laser therapy should be the method of choice for treatment and excision of penile carcinomas. Its advantages include maintenance of micturition and cohabitation functions, minimal cosmetic defects, no scarring with meatus constrictions, and a low local recurrence rate.

▶ The author uses a scalpel to excise the tumor with a 0.5-cm wide margin and then treats the base with the Nd:YAG laser. The report of no local recurrence is impressive.—J.Y. Gillenwater, M.D.

Treatment of Carcinoma of the Penis: The Case for Primary Lymphadenectomy

W. Scott McDougal, Fred K. Kirchner, Jr., Robert H. Edwards, and Linza T. Killion (Vanderbilt Univ.)
J. Urol. 136:38–41, July 1986   36–3

Only about half of the patients with node involvement by squamous cell cancer of the penis at presentation have been cured, making it necessary to determine preoperatively who is most likely to harbor metastases in the regional nodes. An attempt was made to determine who should have lymphadenectomy by reviewing the records of 65 patients followed for at least 5 years after presenting with squamous cell carcinoma of the penis. The average age was 59 years, and the average interval before treatment was 8 months.

One of two patients treated primarily by irradiation had local recurrence. Recurrence rates were 32% in 19 patients having circumcision or local

TREATMENT OF THE REGIONAL LYMPH NODES BY CLINICAL STAGE

	Stage I No./Total	Stage II No./Total	Stage III No./Total
Total No. pts.	19	23	23
Procedure.*			
Primary lymphadenectomy	--	8/9†	10/15
Delayed lymphadenectomy	--	0/1	--
No lymphadenectomy	19/19	5/13	0/3
Groin irradiation	--	--	0/5

*Number free of disease at 5 years/number of patients.
†Of nine patients with clinical stage II disease, six had microscopic nodal metastases.
(Courtesy of McDougal, W.S., et al.: J. Urol. 136:38–41, July 1986. © by Williams & Wilkins, 1986.)

excision, 6% in 35 undergoing partial penectomy, and 0% in 9 having total penectomy. All five patients undergoing irradiation of metastatic groin nodes died of disease. No patient with stage I disease underwent node dissection, and none died of disease. Patients with clinical stage II disease who underwent lymphadenectomy had a survival rate of 88% (table). When lymphadenectomy was not done in those with stage II tumors, only 38% lived without disease. Incapacitating lymphedema followed 4 of 25 groin dissections. Three patients required wound resurfacing. Two patients had groin wound abscesses.

Lymphadenectomy is not necessary in patients with stage I penile carcinoma if it is localized and well differentiated. Inguinal adenectomy seems wise in those with stage II disease. If the groin nodes are positive, iliac dissection should be carried out. Ilioinguinal lymphadenectomy is an established procedure in patients with stage III tumors.

▶ The problems of deciding whether or not to do an inguinal node dissection in patients with penile cancer are related to the high morbidity from the procedure and the fact that only 50% of palpable adenopathies have cancer in the nodes. We have favored excision of the "sentinel node" (Fowler, J.E.: *Urology* 23:352, 1984; 1985 YEAR BOOK OF UROLOGY, p. 247). We have also had excellent results with fine-needle aspiration and have had no false positive findings. This is a small series. Whether early node dissection is justified in those with stage II cancer of the penis with no preoperatively proven positive nodes remains to be clarified.—J.Y. Gillenwater, M.D.

The following review article is recommended to the reader:

Persky, L., deKernion, J.: Carcinoma of the penis. CA 33:258, 1986.

PEDIATRIC

37 Newborn and Neonatal Urology

Catheter Shunts for Fetal Hydronephrosis and Hydrocephalus: Report of the International Fetal Surgery Registry
Frank A. Manning, Michael R. Harrison, Charles Rodeck, and members of the International Fetal, Medicine and Surgery Society (Women's Hosp., Winnipeg)
N. Engl. J. Med. 315:336–340, July 31, 1986   37–1

High-resolution dynamic ultrasonography allows the detection and surgical treatment of fetal structural problems. Surgical interventions to treat obstructive uropathy and hydrocephalus have been attempted. A retrospective study of these procedures was made to analyze their efficacy. The records of fetuses undergoing invasive surgery to place catheters or shunts were obtained from an international registry of fetal surgery begun in 1982. Procedures included 73 vesicoamniotic shunt placements to treat obstructive uropathy and 44 ventriculoamniotic shunt placements or serial ventriculocentesis to treat obstructive hydrocephalus. Many of these procedures were repeated several times before the shunts were in place.

Decompression of the obstructed fetal urinary tracts had a 41% success rate and a procedure-related mortality of 4.6%. The major cause of death in treated and untreated fetuses was pulmonary hypoplasia. The survival rate of fetuses undergoing shunt placement for obstructive hydrocephalus was 83%; however, 52.9% are severely neurologically handicapped and 11.8% are less severely handicapped; 35.3% are developing normally. Procedure-related mortality was 10.25%.

Treatment of fetal hydronephrosis seems worthwhile for selected conditions, e.g., posterior urethral valve syndrome. The benefits of fetal surgery for obstructive hydrocephalus are not obvious because treatment does not appear to decrease morbidity among survivors. A prospective study is needed to assess the efficacy and safety of surgical intervention in the fetus.

▶ Intrauterine intervention for hydronephrosis is very exciting and tempting advanced technology. However, the evidence for its efficacy is totally circumstantial. The experimental data reported in the 1986 YEAR BOOK (p. 297) were overoptimistically interpreted, and the same can be said for this clinical survey. Clearly, much if not all of the damage of obstructive uropathy is done before the lesion can be detected and treated in utero. There is a developing consensus that this experimental form of therapy should be used only in selected centers under good controls. The best candidates are those with oligohydramnios obstruction of both kidneys or a solitary kidney and documentation of progression of the problem. We hope that the precise role of this technology will be defined in the near future. Anecdotal retrospective comparisons of small groups of patients will not define its role.—S.S. Howards, M.D.

Corroborative Evidence for the Decreased Incidence of Urinary Tract Infections in Circumcised Male Infants
Thomas E. Wiswell and John D. Roscelli (Brooke Army Med. Ctr., Ft. Sam Houston, Tex.)
Pediatrics 78:96–99, July 1986   37–2

A decreased incidence of urinary tract infection has been reported in circumcised compared with noncircumcised male infants. A two-part study was conducted to determine the incidence of urinary tract infection during the first year of life.

Of 3,924 infants born during a 4-year period, urinary tract infection developed in 16 (0.41%) during the first year of life. The incidence of urinary tract infection was significantly greater in noncircumcised male infants than in both female and circumcised male infants. Of the 422,328 infants born in army facilities worldwide during a 10-year period, 1,825 (0.43%) had a urinary tract infection during the first year of life. Overall, there was no male preponderance for infections in early infancy. An equivalent incidence of infection occurred in both sexes during the first month of life, with a female preponderance thereafter. However, noncircumcised male infants had a significantly increased incidence of urinary tract infection compared with female infants and a tenfold greater incidence compared with circumcised male infants. A significant decrease in circumcision frequency occurred during the 10-year study period, with a concomitant increase in the overall incidence of urinary tract infections in males.

The risk for urinary tract infection is increased in noncircumcised male infants. Additionally, as the circumcision rate decreases, the incidence of urinary tract infection in male infants increases. A reduced incidence of urinary tract infection may be at least one medical benefit of routine neonatal circumcision.

▶ The American Academy of Pediatrics has maintained since 1975 that there is no medical indication for circumcision. Nevertheless, large numbers of boys in the United States (unlike Europe) are circumcised. The argument over infant circumcision seems endless. This paper confirms the authors' original observation that uncircumcised boys had a higher incidence of urinary tract infections than did circumsised males. Additional reasons for infant circumcision are the problems associated with doing the procedure later in life and the risk of carcinoma of the penis developing. It is true that with good hygiene the chances of cancer of the penis developing are virtually eliminated, but if circumcision were denied in economic ghettos there is a definite possibility that 40 or 50 years later penile cancer could be a genuine problem in parts of the population. On the other hand, we see complications with circumcision, and it could be argued that circumcision does more harm than good. We have always thought that the medical issues are relatively balanced and that circumcision is a personal decision.—S.S. Howards, M.D.

38 Anomalies of the Kidney

Multicystic Dysplastic Kidney in Utero: Changing Appearance on US
Beverly E. Hashimoto, Roy A. Filly, and Peter W. Callen (Univ. of California at San Francisco)
Radiology 159:107–109, April 1986   38–1

Ultrasound is useful in the diagnosis of multicystic dysplastic kidney and can be used in utero. Six serial ultrasound examinations of fetal multicystic dysplastic kidneys revealed progressive enlargement of the affected kidney in four instances. In one case the kidney was reduced in size. In another the kidney first enlarged and then shrank.

Serial ultrasound examination of multicystic dysplastic kidneys in utero may show changes in size and appearance of the kidney. This should not cause a change in diagnosis.

Multicystic Dysplastic Kidneys: Spontaneous Regression Demonstrated With US
Gabriel Pedicelli, Sigrid Jequier, A'Delbert Bowen, and Jacques Boisvert (Montreal Children's Hosp., Children's Hosp. of Pittsburgh, and Hôpital St. Justine, Montreal)
Radiology 160:23–26, October 1986   38–2

In 1955, multicystic dysplastic kidney (MCDK) was first identified as an entity distinct from polycystic kidney. Multicystic dysplastic kidney, which is often found on the first day of life, is the second most frequent abdominal mass occurring in the neonate. Multicystic dysplastic kidney is usually diagnosed by ultrasonography, followed by nuclear renal scintigraphy and intravenous urography. Treatment is controversial with some investigators recommending nephrectomy. In nine children spontaneous regression of unilateral MCDK was demonstrated by repeated ultrasound examinations.

At the time of diagnosis the children ranged in age from 22 weeks' gestational age to 6 months. In three the diagnosis of MCDK was made in utero. Follow-up examinations at the ages of 3, 5, and 32 weeks postpartum revealed what would have been called unilateral agenesis of the affected side if no fetal ultrasound study had been carried out. In the remaining neonates, the diagnosis was made postnatally, and a substantial reduction in size or complete disappearance of the MCDK was observed on serial ultrasound examinations. Three neonates underwent surgical exploration, and there was no trace of a kidney, renal artery, or ureter found in two of these. In the third child a small MCDK was removed.

Ultrasonography reveals new features of the natural history of MCDK. Because malignant transformation of an MCDK is rare and because ultrasound provides a means of serial assessment, a more conservative, nonsurgical approach to management may be appropriate. An observation time of 1 year is recommended before the decision is made for surgical intervention unless other problems necessitate the surgical removal of the MCDK.

▶ These two papers (Abstracts 38–1 and 38–2) give us new insight into the natural history of MCDK. The observation that these kidneys sometimes enlarge in utero is not surprising because they must function at some point in utero to form their cysts and occasionally have limited function at birth. We have seen ten such patients recently, and others have also noted function at birth (Warshawsky, A. B., et al., *J. Urol.* 117:94, 1977). Pedicelli and associates' claim of spontaneous regression of MCDK is reasonably convincing. This observation would support the nonoperative approach to asymptomatic MCDK that most, but by no means all, pediatric urologists favor.—S.S. Howards, M.D.

Congenital Renal Arteriovenous Malformations
James B. Regan and Ralph C. Benson, Jr. (Mayo Clinic and Found.)
J. Urol. 136:1184–1186, December 1986   38–3

Fewer than 50 patients with congenital arteriovenous malformation of the kidney have been reported, but many undoubtedly are asymptomatic and are undetected. Fifteen patients in whom a congenital renal arteriovenous malformation was diagnosed in 1950–1984 were followed for an average of 13 years. The nine women and six men had a median age of 46 years when symptoms began and 48 years at diagnosis. Hematuria and hypertension were most frequent. One third of the patients had an abdominal bruit, and about one fourth had flank pain. One patient had bilateral lesions.

Ten patients had total nephrectomy, six because of actual hematuria or a presumed risk of bleeding and four to control hypertension. The latter patients remained hypertensive at last follow-up, but none required further surgery. Three patients were treated medically for hypertension and two were observed. All five of these patients had microhematuria. None required operative treatment.

Congenital renal arteriovenous malformations are most frequent in females and in the right kidney. Hypertension and hematuria are the most frequent presenting features. The presence of gross hematuria calls for intervention. Angiographically directed transcatheter embolization is an option in these patients. Microscopic hematuria itself may not warrant invasive measures. Hypertension has not been eliminated by nephrectomy, and medical management seems indicated unless lateralizing renin data are obtained.

▶ We suspect that small congenital renal arteriovenous malformations are much more common than indicated in this article or in the literature. The usual presentation is a young woman with intermittent gross hematuria and an unrevealing evaluation. The nephrectomy rate in the Mayo Clinic series seems high. One would hope with modern angiographic and surgical techniques that most kidneys with arteriovenous malformation could be salvaged.—S.S. Howards, M.D.

Use of a Monoclonal Antibody in Differential Diagnosis of Children With Haematuria and Hereditary Nephritis

Caroline O.S. Savage, A. Reed, M. Kershaw, J. Pincott, C.D. Pusey, M.J. Dillon, T.M. Barratt, and C.M. Lockwood (Hammersmith Hosp. and Hosp. for Sick Children, London, and Kingston Hosp., Surrey)
Lancet 1:1459–1461, June 28, 1986   38–4

Hereditary nephritis may be associated with abnormal antigenicity of the glomerular basement membrane; the glomerular and tubular basement membranes of some patients fail to bind a mouse monoclonal antibody, MCA-P1, which recognizes Goodpasture antigen, against which anti-GBM antibodies are directed in anti-GBM nephritis. A double-blind study was done on renal biopsy specimens obtained from 44 children with hematuria to determine whether MCA-P1 can identify patients with Alport's syndrome in whom Goodpasture antigen expression is abnormal. Thirteen children initially were thought to have definite and two possible hereditary nephritis. The most frequent diagnosis in the others was mesangial IgA disease.

All patients with diagnoses of nonhereditary glomerulonephritis had moderate or strong linear binding of MCA-P1 to the glomerular and distal tubular basement membranes. Nine of 13 patients with definite hereditary nephritis had no binding, and 3 others had only faint staining in some glomerular areas. Strong linear binding was found in the two patients in whom hereditary nephritis was considered a possibility. The degree of staining could not be related to the age at onset of illness, renal function, or degree of proteinuria.

Goodpasture antigen may be abnormal or absent from the glomerular basement membrane in hereditary nephritis. Use of MCA-P1 is helpful in diagnosing hereditary glomerulonephritis in many children presenting with hematuria, although not all will have abnormalities. The antibody binds to basement membranes in other organs involved in fluid filtration (e.g., the eye and cochlea), suggesting that abnormalities in Goodpasture antigen may underlie the pattern of organ involvement in Alport's syndrome.

▶ This paper documents the practical use of a monoclonal antibody. Urologists will not use this particular technique in their practice, but it is hoped that monoclonal antibodies will soon assist us both in diagnosis and therapy.—S.S. Howards, M.D.

39 Anomalies of the Ureter

Experience With Endoscopic Incision and Open Unroofing of Ureteroceles
Edward S. Tank (Oregon Health Sciences Univ., Portland)
J. Urol. 136:241–242, July 1986   39–1

Endoscopic incision of ureteroceles does not have a good reputation. Its efficacy, simply as a method to relieve obstruction, was examined in 40 children. Twenty improved to such an extent that nephroureterectomy was considered to be unnecessary; only two of these children later required reconstructive, nonextirpative operations for recurrent urinary tract infection. The other 20 underwent elective heminephroureterectomy with ureterocelectomy and lower ureteral reimplantation.

Endoscopic incision is easy and relieves obstruction, allowing the affected ureters to return to normal. Extirpation can be reserved for nonfunctioning segments when the children's age and size allow the procedure to be performed more easily.

▶ Tank's results clearly show that there is a place for endoscopic unroofing of ureteroceles in the treatment of children with this condition. Monfort has had excellent results with transurethral incision as the definitive treatment for ureteroceles to solitary ureters. A short incision should be made at the distal edge of the ureter to reduce the incidence of reflux. Gerridzen and Schillinger (1985 YEAR BOOK, p. 308; *Urology* 23:43, 1984) also reported excellent results with transureteral incision in three of four patients with ureteroceles to the upper pole ureter in duplicated ureters. These reports certainly suggest that careful transureteral resection of ureteroceles should be considered in selected patients.— S.S. Howards, M.D.

40 Vesicoureteral Reflux

Microproteinuria in Children With Vesicoureteric Reflux
F.G. Bell, T.J. Wilkin, and J.D. Atwell (Wessex Regional Ctr. for Paediatric Surgery and Gen. Hosp., Southampton, England)
Br. J. Urol. 58:605–609, December 1986   40–1

A relationship exists between renal parenchymal scarring and vesicoureteric reflux (VUR). However, the role of sterile reflux is less clear, although renal scars have been induced using high-pressure sterile reflux in animals. Increased excretion of protein in the urine is also a useful prognostic indicator of renal disease, and recent evidence suggests that "microproteinuria" may precede the development of overt renal disease. The incidence of microproteinuria was examined in patients with various grades of VUR in the absence of urinary infection.

Albumin, retinol binding protein, and creatinine concentrations were measured in random midstream urine samples collected from 36 children aged 1 week to 16 years who underwent VUR and in 36 controls aged 6 weeks to 17 years with no urologic complaints. Infection was excluded by culture and microscopy of urine specimens, and no patient was hypertensive. Albumin excretion increased in patients with increasing severity of VUR and renal scarring. Similar findings were noted with excretion of renal binding protein.

Glomerular and tubular handling of proteins is altered in VUR. The degree of microproteinuria correlates well with the severity of the VUR and is evidence of tubular dysfunction. The effects of medical management and antireflux surgery on microproteinuria require further evaluation.

▶ The data in this paper do not support the authors' conclusion that "the degree of microproteinuria correlates well with the severity of VUR." Only two patients had albuminuria out of the range of the control group and both of these had grade IV reflux and scarring. There was no statistical difference between the controls and those patients with grades I–III of VUR. The fact that some patients with scarred kidneys had microproteinuria is hardly surprising.— S.S. Howards, M.D.

Endoscopic Correction of Primary Vesicoureteric Reflux
Barry O'Donnell and Prem Puri (Children's Res. Ctr., Dublin)
Br. J. Urol. 58:601–604, December 1986   40–2

Management of vesicoureteric reflux (VUR) in children is controversial. Because reflux into a dilated system is unlikely to cease spontaneously in most patients, an operation may be needed. After a successful experimental study in piglets, attempts were made to correct VUR endoscopically in children starting in March 1984. Polytef paste was injected into the lamina propria of the bladder under the submucosal ureter. The series included 103 children followed for 3–23 months.

Overall, 75% of refluxing ureters showed absence of reflux after one injection of Polytef paste; 14% of ureters required 2–4 subureteric injections of Polytef paste for correction of VUR; 8% of ureters exhibited improvement in the grade of reflux after the initial injection of Polytef paste. Duplex systems were more difficult to correct and recurrence of reflux was much higher than in primary reflux. Follow-up intravenous urograms revealed no evidence of ureteric obstruction in the treated ureters.

The procedure is safe, simple, and effective in correcting all grades of VUR. To obtain the best results, attention should be paid to minute details of the technique and the injection should be made with pinpoint accuracy.

Endoscopic Correction of Vesicoureteric Reflux Secondary to Neuropathic Bladder
P. Puri and E.J. Guiney (Our Lady's Hosp. for Sick Children, Dublin)
Br. J. Urol. 58:504–506, October 1986   40–3

Vesicoureteric reflux (VUR) is a frequent problem in children with neuropathic bladder. When associated with urinary infection, progressive pyelonephritis scarring may result. Reimplantation of the ureters into a thick-walled trabeculated bladder has been unrewarding. Eleven children with neuropathic bladder and VUR were managed by endoscopic injection of Polytef paste. The patients, ten girls and one boy, had a mean age of 7 years. Seven had myelomeningocele, two had occult neuropathic bladder, and one each had sacral agenesis and spinal cord injury. Reflux was bilateral in four cases.

A 5F nylon catheter and 21-gauge needle were used cystoscopically to inject 0.2–0.9 ml Polytef paste at a site 0.5 cm into the space behind the intravesical ureter. Co-trimoxazole was administered for 2 weeks. Reflux disappeared in 13 of the 15 ureters evaluated, and it improved in one other. A second endoscopic injection was necessary in one instance. Postoperative urography showed no ureterovesical obstruction except in one ureter in which distention of the collecting system was slightly greater than in the preoperative study.

Limited experience with Polytef paste injection for reflux secondary to neuropathic bladder indicates good results, but longer-term follow-up is needed. The simplicity of the method makes it desirable for use in treating VUR. The procedure takes only about 15 minutes and may be done on an outpatient basis.

▶ Endoscopic correction of VUR is an exciting, if controversial, development. The technique was originally used by Politano, who reserves it for difficult situations, such as in patients in whom two or three previous operative repairs have failed. O'Donnell and Puri popularized the procedure and report excellent results with few complications (*Br. Med. J.* 289:7–9, 1984). They have even had success with neurogenic bladders, as documented in the second of the two papers abstracted above (Abstract 40–2). Others, including Dr. Claude Shulman of Brussels (*SPU Newsletter,* 5/2/86) and the pediatric urology group at Children's Memorial Hospital in Chicago are similarly enthusiastic. The advantages of the procedure are obvious: (1) It can be done on an outpatient basis. (2) It works. (3) It is cost effective. (4) Because of its simplicity it would seem reasonable to use it for many borderline cases (grade III/IV VUR) over which we have agonized in the past. There are disadvantages also: (1) Polytef paste is not FDA-approved for this purpose, although it is approved for injection into vocal cords. (2) There is some concern regarding migration and possible carcinogenesis. (3) There is the possibility of late destruction secondary to the inflammatory granulomatous reaction around the injection site. (4) There would be a very long-term liability problem if late serious complications occurred. Because of these concerns, certain groups, including Dr. Robert Jeffs' at Johns Hopkins, are experimenting with endoscopic injection of collagen-like compounds rather than Polytef.—S.S. Howards, M.D.

Follow-up of Renal Morphology and Growth of 141 Children Operated for Vesicoureteral Reflux: A Retrospective Computerized Study
J.-M. Ginalski, A. Michaud, and N. Genton (CMUV, Lausanne, Switzerland)
J. Pediatr. Surg. 21:697–701, August 1986   40–4

In the treatment of vesicoureteral reflux (VUR) in children, some authors favor ureterovesical reimplantation, whereas others recommend a conservative treatment, e.g., long-term prophylactic antibiotic therapy. A retrospective computerized study was made of the long-term morphological renal evolution in 141 children aged 10 years or younger operated on for VUR. All underwent ureterovesical reimplantation. Renal growth and morphology were evaluated 2 years and 5 years after surgery. Renal growth was estimated by measuring the ratio of the bipolar parenchymal thickness to the total length of the kidney.

Whatever the degree of reflux might have been, most of the kidneys partially or totally compensated for their growth failure, but growth resumption required many years for completion. Surgical correction of VUR had favorable consequences on the radiologic aspect of pyelonephritic scars only on some of the kidneys: in these cases, the child's age appeared to be the only factor that was of statistical importance affecting the postoperative evolution of the pyelonephritic scarring. The younger the children were at the time of surgery, the better the results. It is important that VUR be diagnosed early and that ureterovesical reimplantation be performed as soon as possible after diagnosis when surgical treatment is indicated.

► The data in this paper strongly suggest that correction of reflux has a beneficial effect on renal growth. Because the study was not controlled, it is unclear whether effective medical treatment would have produced a similar result. It is also interesting that younger children (less than 2 years of age) had a much higher incidence of increased parenchymal thickness at the site of scar than did older children.—S.S. Howards, M.D.

Renal Function Following Surgical Correction of Vesico-Ureteric Reflux in Childhood
D.J. Scott, H.N. Blackford, M.R.L. Joyce, A.R. Mundy, C.H. Kinder, G.B. Haycock, and C. Chantler (Guy's Hosp., London)
Br. J. Urol. 58:119–124, April 1986

40–5

The optimal therapy for children with severe vesicoureteric reflux (VUR) is undetermined. Surgery is beneficial in some instances, curing the reflux and allowing renal and physical growth to occur. A retrospective analysis was made of the changes in renal function after antireflux surgery in children aged 2–15 years who had no other urologic disease. All had glomerular filtration rates (GFRs) of less than 90 ml/minute/1.73 mm sq before or after surgery. Follow-up lasted for a mean of 2.7 years. Renal function was assessed by determination of serum creatinine levels and blood pressure, urine culture, and use of the Holtain Stadiometer. Renal scarring was visualized with ^{99m}Tc-dimercapto-succinic acid scanning.

Surgery cured reflux in 93% of the patients. Improvement in the GFR occurred in 75% of children undergoing bilateral reimplantation of ureters draining bilaterally scarred kidneys, the greatest improvement occurring when the GFR was less than 50 ml/minute/1.73 mm sq. Of 42 kidneys studied individually, 81% had an improved GFR. Hypertension occurred in 14.3% of the children. No new renal scars were detected after surgery.

Surgical correction of VUR improves renal function, especially in kidneys that are not severely damaged. Although reflux surgery inhibits further renal damage as a result of infection and continuing reflux, it is not certain whether nonsurgical management would have had similar results. Long-term follow-up is needed because children with scarred kidneys are at risk for the development of hypertension.

▶ This paper and several similar publications document that the scarred kidney continues to grow after ureteral neocystostomy. Unfortunately, none of these studies was controlled, so one cannot conclude from these data whether renal function is better after surgery than it would have been after continued medical treatment.—S.S. Howards, M.D.

41 Prune Belly

Total Abdominal Wall Reconstruction in the Prune Belly Syndrome
Richard M. Ehrlich, Malcolm A. Lesavoy, and Richard N. Fine (Univ. of California at Los Angeles)
J. Urol. 136:282–285, July 1986

41–1

The cause and pathophysiology of prune belly syndrome are uncertain, but insufficient attention has been given to the deficiency of abdominal musculature that accompanies urinary tract dilatation and intra-abdominal testes. The bizarre appearance of affected boys may have adverse psychological effects. Total abdominal wall reconstruction permits simultaneous access for bilateral orchiopexy and urinary tract reconstruction when necessary. After these procedures, the skin and subcutaneous tissue are sharply dissected from the muscle and fascia, laterally on either side to about the midaxillary line. After the umbilicus is removed, the fascial layers are advanced in a double-breasted, overlapping manner; both musculofascial layers are advanced laterally to the desired degree of tightness, and preplaced sutures are tied (Fig 41–1). The inferior fascial edges are then sewn to Cooper's ligament and the pubic tubercle, and excess medial skin is excised.

Six boys aged 1–12 years with severe abdominal wall laxity underwent total abdominal wall reconstruction. Five had simultaneous orchiopexy and one had partial cystectomy and urethrotomy. The average hospitalization was 6 days. There were no surgical complications and no vascular compromise. Cosmetic appearances were markedly improved and all chil-

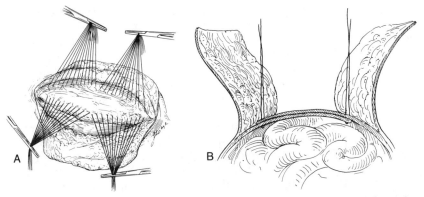

Fig 41–1.—**A,** musculofascial layers overlapped in double-breasted fashion. Preplaced sutures then are tied. **B,** sagittal section shows double-thickness overlap of musculofascial layers. Extent of overlap is determined by degree of tension and molding desired. (Courtesy of Ehrlich, R.M., et al.: J. Urol. 136:282–285, July 1986. © by Williams & Wilkins, 1986.)

dren and parents were pleased with the outcome. Laxity did not increase during follow-up for as long as 2 years. Binders were not used after the first 8–12 weeks. Testicular atrophy has not occurred.

Without reconstruction, the abdominal wall will not always improve, and the need to grow up wearing a corset or binder may be damaging emotionally. The operation should be performed soon after the first year to facilitate orchiopexy without the need to ligate the spermatic cord.

In an addendum, the authors report that two more recent patients have also done well after total abdominal wall reconstruction.

▶ There has been a long-standing controversy over whether or not abdominal wall pexy is beneficial in children with prune belly syndrome. Ehrlich and associates have documented that abdominal wall reconstruction can be successful and beneficial. In collaboration with Dr. Brad Rogers, a pediatric surgeon at the University of Virginia, we have taken a similar approach in the last several years with gratifying results. In boys whose testes are not in the scrotum, orchidectomy is combined with the abdominal wall surgery. It is interesting that some of those patients have transient, significant hypertension in the immediate postoperative period. The mechanism of this hypertension is unclear.— S.S. Howards, M.D.

A Broader Spectrum of Abnormalities in the Prune Belly Syndrome
Denis F. Geary, Ian B. MacLusky, Bernard M. Churchill, and Gordon McLorie (Hosp. for Sick Children, Toronto)
J. Urol. 135:324–326, February 1986   41–2

The medical literature has emphasized the genitourinary tract malformations associated with prune belly syndrome, but other organ systems may also be affected. A retrospective review of the clinical course of 25 children with prune belly syndrome was undertaken to assess the overall morbidity associated with this disorder, particularly that associated with nonurologic problems. The mean age at follow-up for the survivors was 8.5 years (range, 6 months to 19 years).

Three neonatal deaths occurred, mainly caused by renal or pulmonary diseases. Among the 22 survivors, 5 (23%) had chronic renal insufficiency or end-stage renal disease; all had impaired renal function in early infancy. The remaining 17 patients had mild renal insufficiency. Growth retardation was present in seven (32%) patients and correlated poorly with renal function. Clinically significant respiratory or orthopedic abnormalities occurred in 12 (55%) survivors. Chronic constipation was common. Developmental delay was documented in five children and suspected in one. Overall, nonurologic abnormalities occurred in 16 (73%) children.

Clinically significant extrarenal abnormalities are common in children with prune belly syndrome. Chronic renal disease remains a major cause of morbidity and mortality, but with appropriate care most patients, except those with renal impairment in infancy, retain adequate renal function.

▶ Nongenitourinary problems are frequent in children with prune belly syndrome. The pulmonary difficulties probably relate to the weak abdominal musculature and thoracic cage deformities (e.g., pectus excavation) that are common in these children.—S.S. Howards, M.D.

42 Urinary Tract Reconstruction

Urinary Tract Deterioration Associated With the Artificial Urinary Sphincter

David R. Roth, Parimal R. Vyas, R. Lawrence Kroovand, and Alan D. Perlmutter (Children's Hosp. of Michigan, Detroit, and Wayne State Univ.)

J. Urol. 135:528–530, March 1986   42–1

The artificial urinary sphincter provides long-term continence in most patients without pressure necrosis or periurethral fibrotic contraction, but many urologists report high rates of postimplantation complications. Upper tract deterioration is usually silent and therefore is potentially the most serious complication. Data were reviewed on 47 children in whom an artificial urinary sphincter was implanted between 1978 and 1985. All had detailed uroradiologic studies and most had urodynamic testing before operation.

Thirty-three of the 47 children are continent of urine and have stable upper urinary tracts and stable renal function. Two children required removal of the device because of erosion. Five continent patients had transient upper tract dilatation in association with unrecognized urine retention that resolved on intermittent catheterization and drug treatment. Seven children had late lower tract deterioration, and four had hydronephrosis. These patients were managed by bladder augmentation.

The reason underlying change in bladder function in these patients is unclear, but it may reflect the natural course of bladder function in myelodysplastic patients. Children with an artificial urinary sphincter should be closely followed for an indefinite time. Deterioration may take place without overflow incontinence. The upper tracts should be imaged semi-annually and renal function and bladder dynamics evaluated periodically.

▶ This is one of the largest series of pediatric patients to have received an artificial urinary sphincter. The surgical results are quite good, indeed, better than less experienced surgeons can expect. However, a significant minority of the patients had obstructive changes in their ureters, requiring intervention. This deterioration probably results from increased pressure in a noncompliant bladder. Some, but not all, of these complications might have been predicted by careful preoperative urodynamic studies. Good candidates for the sphincter should have a high-capacity, low-pressure bladder and low outlet resistance. Certainly, the authors' message that these children require careful follow-up is correct and very important. Because of the complications and the well-described surgical and mechanical problems with the artificial sphincter, we have been very selective in the use of this device. We prefer whenever possible to use pharmacologic management, intermittent catheterization, bladder augmentation, and/or continent diversion (please see Abstract 42–2).—S.S. Howards, M.D.

Continent Urinary Diversion: Variations on the Mitrofanoff Principle
John W. Duckett and Howard M. Snyder, III (Children's Hosp. of Philadelphia)
J. Urol. 136:58–62, July 19, 1986   42–2

In 1980, Mitrofanoff proposed implantation of the isolated appendix into the bladder as a catheter conduit for continent cystostomy. Use of the Mitrofanoff principle was applied in reconstructing a continent urinary diversion in ten patients.

TECHNIQUE.—The isolated appendix is implanted via an antirefluxing submucosal tunnel into the posterior bladder wall (Fig 42–1). The bladder neck is closed to prevent urethral incontinence, and the colonic end of the appendix is used as a catheter stoma. In patients with myelomeningocele and a neuropathic bladder, transureteroureterostomy may be performed. In this procedure the distal ureter is brought to the skin as a catheterizable continent ureterostomy (Fig 42–2). A sigmoid patch augmentation of the bladder is carried out to increase its capacity. The cecum also may be used for a reservoir if the segment is long enough for the pressure increase of a peristaltic wave to be dissipated in the reservoir.

The classical Mitrofanoff principle was used successfully in four patients. In two others with neurogenic bladder in whom the bladder was augmented, transureteroureterostomy allowed the distal ureter to be used as

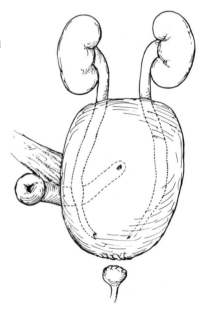

Fig 42–1.—Classic Mitrofanoff procedure. Isolated appendix is implanted with antirefluxing submucosal tunnel into posterior bladder wall. Bladder neck is closed to prevent urethral incontinence. Colonic end of appendix is used as stoma for catheterization. (Courtesy of Duckett, J.W., and Snyder, H.M., III: J. Urol. 136:58–62, July 19, 1986. © by Williams and Wilkins, 1986.)

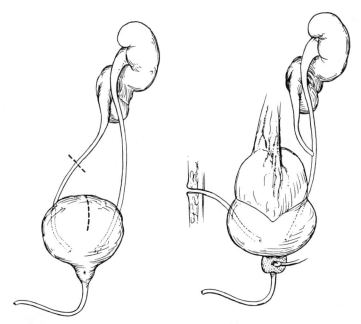

Fig 42–2.—Neuropathic bladder and myelomeningocele. Right-to-left transureteroureterostomy is done. Distal right ureter is brought to skin as catheterizable continent ureterostomy. Sigmoid patch augmentation of bladder is done to increase capacity. Artificial urinary sphincter was previously placed. (Courtesy of Duckett, J.W., and Snyder, H.M., III: J. Urol. 136:58–62, July 19, 1986. © by Williams & Wilkins, 1986.)

a conduit. In three patients a cecal segment was used. In one instance the ureteral orifice was transposed to the perineum as a neourethra, with the ureteral blood supply being based on detrusor remnants and the bladder mucosa excised. Another modification preserves the blood supply to part of the ureter derived from a previous skin ureterostomy stoma, which allows the ureter to be divided in the middle with maintenance of a blood supply to both parts. The Mitrofanoff principle is a valuable approach to continent reconstruction of the lower urinary tract.

▶ The Mitrofanoff principle was discussed in the 1986 YEAR BOOK, pp. 321–322. We have used the technique in six patients with five satisfactory results. It is definitely a useful method of continent diversion. In children with a neurogenic bladder who cannot be rendered continent by simple procedures (e.g., a Stamey operation or a sling as described by McGuire), either a Mitrofanoff procedure or a Kropp procedure should be considered. The choice depends on whether the patient would rather catheterize the urethra or an abdominal stoma, on the anatomy, and on the experience of the surgeon. Most children with neurogenic bladders who undergo these operations require bladder augmentation. We believe that these techniques are easier and more reliable than the Kock pouch and the artificial sphincter.—S.S. Howards, M.D.

Influence of Intestinal Segment and Configuration on the Outcome of Augmentation Enterocystoplasty

Abraham Ami Sidi, Yuri Reinberg, and Ricardo Gonzalez (Univ. of Minnesota)
J. Urol. 136:1201–1204, December 1986   42–3

Nearly all large and small bowel segments have been used for enterocystoplasty to augment the capacity of the contracted bladder. The clinical and urodynamic results of three different gut segments and configurations were compared in 34 patients examined after enterocystoplasty, 22 with neurovesical dysfunction and 12 with a normally innervated lower urinary tract. Fifteen patients had bladder outlet surgery in conjunction with enterocystoplasty. In 21 patients the ureters were implanted into the bowel. An intact ileocecal or cecal segment was used in 10 patients (group 1), a sigmoid tubular segment in 16 (group 2), and a sigmoid cup-patch segment in 8 (group 3).

The upper urinary tract and renal function remained stable or improved in all patients except for one with ureteral obstruction. Only one patient had postoperative urinary reflux. All patients had volume-dependent involuntary bladder contractions at the first follow-up visit; these were most marked in group 1 patients and least intense in group 3 patients. Functional bladder capacity and volume to the initial involuntary contraction increased in all groups at the last follow-up. Group 3 patients had lower peak pressures and larger volumes to initial contraction than the others had. Seven patients, four of them in group 2, required drugs to suppress intravesical contractions at last follow-up. All patients with a normally innervated urinary tract were continent. Continence was best in group 3 patients.

All of these techniques of enterocystoplasty resulted in increased functional bladder capacity and protected the upper urinary tract. The sigmoid cup-patch procedure provides a lower-pressure, higher-capacity reservoir than the tubular sigmoid segment and would appear indicated when simple augmentation enterocystoplasty without ureteral reimplantation is required. A tubular segment may be preferable in some patients with undiversion when there are short ureters and a small bladder.

▶ This paper provides interesting data relating to the controversy as to which type of bowel segment is best for bladder augmentation and continent diversion. Clearly, all of the segments become better reservoirs with time. The data are somewhat difficult to interpret because we do not know how large the various segments were when the reservoirs were originally constructed. It is clear that detubularization increases the capacity of a bowel segment by converting it from a cylinder to a sphere. Simple geometry validates that the sphere has a much larger capacity. What is not as certain is whether or not detubularization alters the neural and muscular physiology of the segment; i.e., given an equal resting volume, will a detubularized segment have a better filling capacity and lower pressure than a tubular segment? This study does not actually answer that question, although the last follow-up contraction incidence of only 10% in the detubularized sigmoid segments supports the concept that incising the bowel does have physiologic effects.—S.S. Howards, M.D.

43 Urethral Anomalies

Percutaneous Antegrade Ablation of Posterior Urethral Valves in Infants With Small Caliber Urethras: An Alternative to Urinary Diversion
Mark R. Zaontz and Casimir F. Firlit (Northwestern Univ.)
J. Urol. 136:247–248, July 1986   43–1

Antenatal ultrasonography has facilitated the early postnatal recognition of posterior urethral obstruction by valves; but in small infants, the urethra may not accept even the smallest resectoscope, precluding primary transurethral valve ablation. A percutaneous antegrade technique for valve ablation in such cases was developed and used successfully in six cases. A 12F suprapubic cystocatheter set is used. A 9.5F resectoscope may be

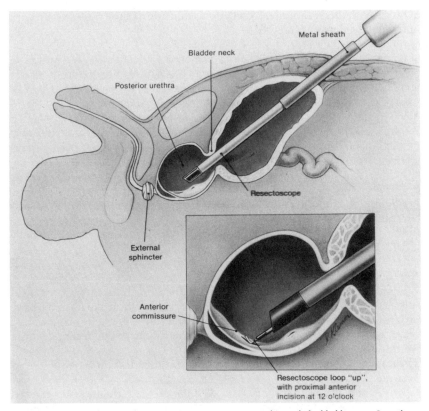

Fig 43–1.—Sagittal section demonstrates percutaneous suprapubic mode for bladder entry. Inset shows hooked electrode engaging valve leaflets at 12 o'clock position. (Courtesy of Zaontz, M.R., and Firlit, C.F.: J. Urol. 136:247–248, July 1986. © by Williams & Wilkins, 1986.)

placed through a precut trocar sheath so that the scope protrudes well beyond the sheath (Fig 43–1). After visualizing the valve leaflets, they are incised at the 12 o'clock or 5 o'clock and 7 o'clock positions, distally to proximally to avoid the external sphincter.

Six patients aged from 37 weeks' gestation to 8 weeks had posterior urethral valves amenable to percutaneous valve ablation. All had a poor urinary stream, and five had a distended bladder and/or palpable kidneys. Four patients had reduced renal function on scan study. The urethral caliber was 8F in four patients and less in the two premature neonates. Adequate valve ablation was evidenced by an excellent urethral stream immediately after incision of the leaflets. Voiding cystourethrography showed improvement in all cases. Renal scans at 6 months showed improvement in all patients with initially reduced renal function. All were thriving and gaining weight at follow-up.

Percutaneous antegrade ablation of posterior urethral valves is an alternative to primary transurethral valve ablation or urinary diversion in premature or underweight infants and those with a small-caliber urethra that will not accept the smallest resectoscope. Urethral instrumentation is avoided with this technique. Excellent visualization of the posterior urethra and valve leaflets is achieved.

▶ Percutaneous antegrade ablation of posterior urethral valves is a welcome addition to the urologist's armamentarium. The authors had excellent results and Dr. Richard Ehrlich added during the discussion at the pediatric meeting (J. Urol. 136:249–251, 1986) that he had successfully ablated valves in four children via a suprapubic approach. Dr. Terry Allen stated that he had attempted the procedure through a cutaneous vesicostomy and found it difficult. It should be remembered that even the authors do not advocate this approach in boys who are azotemic or septic.—S.S. Howards, M.D.

Predictors of Eventual End Stage Renal Disease in Children With Posterior Urethral Valves

Amir Tejani, Khalid Butt, Ken Glassberg, Anita Price, and K. Gurumurthy (SUNY, Downstate Med. Ctr.)
J. Urol. 136:857–860, October 1986   43–2

Despite corrective surgical relief of obstruction, children with renal insufficiency resulting from congenital posterior urethral valves may have progression to end-stage renal disease. To determine predictors of eventual end-stage renal disease with this obstructive uropathic condition, 25 boys were followed longitudinally for a mean of 9 years (range, 1–16 years). The patient age at diagnosis varied from 7 months intrauterine to 7 years post natal.

At the end of the follow-up period, 40% of the patients had retarded growth and 44% had end-stage renal disease. Only 5 of 18 children in whom the diagnosis of posterior urethral valves was made before age 2 years had end-stage renal disease, compared with 6 of 7 children whose diagnosis was delayed beyond age 2 years. Similarly, 7 of 9 children with persistent vesicoureteral reflux had end-stage disease compared with 4 of 16 who did not have reflux. End-stage disease was reached in varying intervals ranging from 6 months to 14 years after diagnosis.

Prolonged follow-up is necessary in children with congenital urethral valves, because end-stage renal disease can occur many years later despite adequate relief of obstruction. Delay in diagnosis and the presence of persistent vesicoureteral reflux are significant predictors of eventual end-stage renal status.

▶ The incidence (44%) of end-stage renal disease in this series is much higher than we currently see or have noted previously (Agusta, V.E., Howards, S.S.: *J. Urol.* 112:280, 1974). This is probably because the patients were selected from a nephrology transplant service. The poor prognosis with late diagnosis is not surprising and has been noted by others.—S.S. Howards, M.D.

Megalourethra
Robert A. Appel, George W. Kaplan, William A. Brock, and Decio Streit (Naval Hosp., Children's Hosp., and Univ. of California at San Diego)
J. Urol. 135:747–751, April 1986   43–3

Megalourethra is a rare congenital disease characterized by dilatation of the penile urethra and subdivided into two types, scaphoid and fusiform. A retrospective study was made of the authors' patients and of those reported in the literature who had megalourethra. The records of 41 patients were thus examined; 31 of these were classified as having the scaphoid type and 10, the fusiform type.

There was a wide range of corpora cavernosa defects, ranging from almost total absence to moderate amounts of erectile tissue. There was a significant association of this disease with upper urinary tract abnormalities. Of 34 patients for whom information was available, 32 had hydronephrosis, azotemia, cystic dysplasia, or pyelonephritis. Thirteen of 32 who were followed died.

The scaphoid and fusiform types of megalourethra represent varying degrees of the disease, because one patient had atresia of a single corpus cavernosum and four had a continuum in the degree of dysplasia of the corpus spongiosum. Investigation of the upper urinary tract in these patients is recommended, because the ultimate outcome of the disease depends on its functional status.

▶ This is a good review of a rare entity. The megalourethra results from a deficient corpus spongiosum. The authors' point that the syndrome represents a spectrum of the disease, rather than simply scaphoid or fusiform megalourethra, is well taken. The major lesson from this review is that there is a very high incidence of upper tract abnormalities in these patients.—S.S. Howards, M.D.

44 Myelomeningocele and Neuropathic Bladder

Urological Aspects of the Tethered Cord Syndrome
Wayne J.G. Hellstrom, Michael S.B. Edwards, and Barry A. Kogan (Univ. of California at San Francisco)
J. Urol. 135:317–320, February 1986   44–1

The tethered spinal cord syndrome is a developmental anomaly of the lumbosacral spinal cord common in children. Symptoms include bladder dysfunction, spastic gait, lower extremity weakness, muscle atrophy, foot deformities, progressive scoliosis, increasing pain, or abnormal reflexes and sensory patterns. Few studies document bladder changes in patients with the tethered cord syndrome. Eighteen patients, ranging in age from newborn to 29 years, with tethered spinal cord syndrome underwent complete urologic evaluation. The causes of tethering included a lipomeningocele in 14, postoperative adhesions in 3, and a thickened filum terminale in 1.

None of the patients had significant upper urinary tract abnormalities. Four had low-grade vesicoureteral reflux. Urodynamic studies showed a flaccid bladder in nine patients, including five with supersensitivity to bethanechol, an uninhibited bladder in five, mixed bladder dysfunction in two, and normal function in two. Repeat urodynamic studies were performed at least 6 months after release of the tethering in 15 patients. Six of eight patients who originally had flaccid bladders demonstrated significant changes: Two became normal, two had limited contractions, and two had evidence of upper motor neuron abnormalities. All four patients who had an uninhibited bladder improved postoperatively, and three became entirely normal.

Most patients with tethered spinal cord syndrome have significant bladder dysfunction. Early diagnosis and aggressive treatment of the tethering are warranted, because neurosurgical management unquestionably can improve bladder dysfunction.

▶ The tethered cord syndrome occurs when the spinal cord is fixed in a sacral position and fails to migrate upward during normal growth of the vertebral column. The importance of this syndrome to urologists is that children with this condition may present with voiding symptoms, as did ten of the patients in this series. Indeed, four of the children had voiding symptoms only. The authors nicely documented bladder dysfunction and the effects of surgical correc-

281

tion on that function. Fortunately, most of the patients had improved urody-namics after surgery. The critical point for the urologist is that, on rare occasions, he may be the first to see a child with the tethered cord syndrome. This condition should be suspected in children who have unexplained secondary voiding symptoms. The main dilemma for the urologist is knowing when to refer patients with secondary enuresis for neurosurgical evaluation, which is expensive and usually negative. There are two reasonable approaches: One is to refer all such patients; the other is to refer only those who have foot deformities and/or abnormal urodynamic studies.—S.S. Howards, M.D.

Urethral Lengthening and Reimplantation for Neurogenic Incontinence in Children
Kenneth A. Kropp and Fru F. Angwafo (Med. College of Ohio, Toledo)
J. Urol. 135:533–536, March 1986   44–2

The mechanical devices used in incontinent children with myelomeningocele have too short a life expectancy, and urethral lengthening alone has not helped. A procedure using the child's own tissues was evaluated in 13 children with myelomeningocele. Eleven had been undergoing intermittent clean catheterization and medication; the other two had had urinary diversion and underwent diversion.

TECHNIQUE.—An attempt is made to create a bladder tube acting as a one-way valve to allow a catheter to be passed into the bladder, without urine leakage. A rectangular pedicle flap of anterior bladder wall is based on the bladder neck. It is rolled into a tube over a catheter, sutured, passed through a broad submucosal tunnel, and sutured to the bladder neck. In three patients the tubularized flap was fashioned from posterior bladder wall.

All children operated on are out of diapers day and night. Three have occasional dribbling, but only one wears a minipad. One child later became incontinent but responded to removal of a bladder stone and treatment of infection. Four of six boys have had late problems with catheterization. Vesicoureteral reflux has occurred, but was not associated with progressive hydronephrosis or deteriorating renal function. One child with progressive hydroureteronephrosis successfully underwent bilateral ureterolysis.

The bladder tubularization procedure combines the advantages of using bladder musculature with a one-way valve. Patients must exhibit compliance with an intermittent clean catheterization program and must be able to catheterize themselves before being selected for this operation. The authors presently offer the procedure as a last resort before an artificial sphincter is considered.

▶ Dr. S. Kropp and Angwafo have designed an extremely clever and potentially very useful procedure. The success rate in their hands has been high. It should be stressed that this is a major operation and children with neurogenic bladders almost always require augmentation cystoplasty. One must also be absolutely certain that the child is willing to catheterize the urethra. In this type of patient we have been performing a Mitrofanoff procedure (please see 1986 YEAR BOOK

OF UROLOGY, p. 322; also, Abstract 42–2). After talking with Dr. Kropp about this operation, we now offer these children a choice between the two procedures. The decision is based on whether they would rather catheterize a perineal or an abdominal stoma. Of course, the condition of the urethra and appendix or ureters must also be considered.—S.S. Howards, M.D.

Modified Pubovaginal Sling in Girls With Myelodysplasia
Edward J. McGuire, Chi-Chung Wang, Howard Usitalo, and Joan Savastano (Univ. of Michigan)
J. Urol. 135:94–96, January 1986   44–3

Myelodysplasia is often associated with intractable incontinence in girls. Although most girls notice improved continence at the time of puberty, some do not, and even those who improve may still need to wear protective clothing. Because daily urinary incontinence has a deleterious effect on personality development in adolescents, urinary control is usually achieved using the artificial sphincter. However, this procedure often requires bladder flap urethroplasty in patients with myelodysplasia and is more difficult to perform than a pubovaginal sling. A review was made of experience using a modified pubovaginal sling in eight girls with total urinary incontinence and bladder pressures of 8–15 cm of water at the time of urethral leakage.

TECHNIQUE.—A vertical midline vaginal incision is made and the vaginal mucosa is lifted off the urethra and urethrovesical junction. The dissecting scissors are advanced through the pelvic floor adjacent to the symphysis on either side of the urethra. A 4-cm suprapubic incision is made, the rectus sheath is identified, and a strip of rectus fascia 1×3 cm in size is removed (Fig 44–1). Next, 2–0 polypropylene sutures are placed in each end of the fascia and anchored by a polytetrafluoroethylene pledget. Both ends of the polypropylene suture are placed through the Stamey needle, which is advanced into the retropubic space from below upward. The sutures are grasped and removed from the needle on both sides. This maneuver pulls the ends of the sling on either side of the urethra into the retropubic space. To ensure that the path is extraurethral and extravesical, endoscopic inspection of the urethra and bladder is performed with the needles in place. With the proximal urethra visualized, the sutures are drawn up until the bladder neck closes; they are then tied over the pledgets above the rectus fascia. The wounds are closed without drainage and an 18F catheter is left in place for 24 hours and then removed, after which self-catheterization is reinstituted.

All eight patients were dry on 4-hour to 6-hour intermittent catheterization schedules without stress incontinence. The bladder pressure responses to filling with the child at rest increased by 12–15 cm of water over the preoperative value at the time of urethral urinary leakage. The sling provided some compression of the urethra at rest, but this increased with an increase in intra-abdominal pressure when the urethra was driven into the rigid sling.

A pubovaginal sling provides excellent compression in girls with intractable incontinence owing to proximal urethral nonfunction. As long

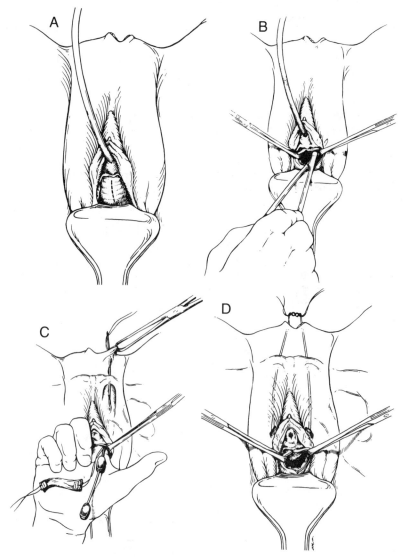

Fig 44–1.—A, vaginal incision *(dotted line).* **B,** dissection of vaginal mucosa off underlying bladder and urethra outlined by Foley catheter. **C,** technique of initial sling placement using Stamey needle. Note two pledgets to reinforce sutures at either end of sling. **D,** sling in place and sutures ready to be tied over polytetrafluoroethylene patches that are not shown. (Courtesy of McGuire, E.J., et al.: J. Urol. 135:94–96, January 1986. © by Williams & Wilkins, 1986.)

as patients are selected by simple urodynamic criteria, improvement in continence can be achieved by an operation.

▶ McGuire et al. describe a much simpler procedure than a Mitrofanoff or Kropp operation for girls with incontinence. It has worked well in their hands in properly selected patients. The child must have low leak pressure, good bladder capacity, and be willing to catheterize the urethra. A simple Stamey urethropexy or injection of polytetrafluoroethylene (1986 YEAR BOOK OF UROLOGY, p. 331) may also be effective in these children. In children who do not meet the criteria outlined above we have favored a Mitrofanoff procedure and would also consider Kropp's operation. One could certainly combine bladder augmentation with a pubovaginal sling, but we do not know of any series evaluating such an approach. We certainly would prefer the options listed above to placing an artificial sphincter in most of these patients (please see Chapter 42).—S.S. Howards, M.D.

Internal Urethrotomy in Girls and Its Impact on the Urethral Intrinsic and Extrinsic Continence Mechanisms
R. Kessler and C.E. Constantinou (Stanford Univ.)
J. Urol. 136:1248–1253, December 1986   44–4

The mechanisms of continence remain incompletely understood, but internal urethrotomy may have an effect on urinary incontinence in girls. Eleven girls (mean age, 18 years) who underwent internal urethrotomy in childhood were studied. All of them noted incontinence after the procedure, but leakage with stress was demonstrated in only one case. Leakage consistently was worsened by stress. The physical findings were normal in all patients. Urodynamic studies were done to characterize the detrusor, and urethral profiles were recorded to determine the effects of urethrotomy on the intrinsic and extrinsic mechanisms of urethral closure.

Four patients exhibited detrusor instability on cystometrography. Voiding was associated with high flow rates at low detrusor pressures in these patients. Low urethral resistance was apparent. The average maximum resting urethral closure pressure was significantly reduced at 62 cm of water, compared with findings in age-matched normal persons. Transmission pressures on coughing indicated substantial transmission to the distal and mid urethra. Vascular pulsations at amplitudes of 15–25 cm water were observed in 8 of the 11 patients.

Patients who complain of incontinence after internal urethrotomy may not exhibit signs of stress incontinence on physical examination because the extrinsic urethral mechanism is intact. Later urethral incontinence is, however, more likely if the intrinsic sphincteric mechanism is compromised by urethrotomy when transmission is lost through childbirth or aging.

▶ Kessler and Constantinou make a valuable contribution to the literature by documenting that internal urethrotomy can weaken the urethral continence mechanism in girls. We also have seen several patients with incontinence after internal urethrotomy. It is remarkable how widely practiced that procedure is in view of the lack of objective evidence for its efficacy in girls with urinary tract infections. We have even seen girls with enuresis treated by internal urethrotomy. Of course, they got worse. We hope that this paper will help to eliminate the practice.—S.S. Howards, M.D.

Detrusor Instability in Children With Recurrent Urinary Tract Infection and/or Enuresis: I. Clinical Conditions and Symptomatology

N. Qvist, E.S. Kristensen, K.K. Nielsen, D. Ehlers, K.M.E. Jensen, T. Krarup, and J. Christoffersen (Aalborg County Hosp., Denmark)
Urol. Int. 41:196–198, May–June 1986   44–5

Most urinary tract symptoms in children are caused by recurrent urinary tract infections (UTIs) and/or enuresis. To determine the incidence of detrusor instability in these children, 41 children aged 5–15 years referred for recurrent UTIs and/or enuresis were evaluated prospectively by CO_2 cystometry. Detrusor instability was defined as uninhibited bladder contractions with rises in pressure of more than 15 cm of water.

Detrusor instability was found in 18 children (44%). However, only 7 children (17%) would have presented with detrusor instability if complete reproducibility were to be requested in repeated tests. Detrusor instability did not correlate significantly with definite pathologic changes in the urinary tract or with irritative bladder symptoms, e.g., crossing legs, squatting, and urge incontinence.

Uncertainty remains regarding the importance of detrusor instability in children with urinary tract symptoms. It may be a secondary phenomenon to frequent UTIs, causing reactive changes in the bladder.

▶ This simple paper makes two very important points: First, it is not at all clear how to define detrusor instability. The contrast between an initial instability incidence of 44% and a reproducible rate of 17% is striking. What does a bladder contraction mean in a youngster who has had a recent UTI, is frightened, has a foreign body in her bladder, and is surrounded by strangers? Second, because we have no unequivocal definition of detrusor instability and no totally objective test to determine how common the finding is in normal persons and those with various pathologic conditions, we cannot be dogmatic regarding the role of detrusor instability in the disease process. Many of the studies on the subject are flawed and deal in phenomenology.—S.S. Howards, M.D.

Comparison of Desmopressin and Enuresis Alarm for Nocturnal Enuresis

Sören Wille (Open Pediatric Clinic, Falkenberg, Sweden)
Arch. Dis. Child. 61:30–33, January 1986   44–6

Bedwetting, a common problem in children, is usually treated by one of two methods: enuresis alarm or drugs. The enuresis alarm was invented in 1904 by Pfaundler and, even with the variety of devices available today, the principle is therapeutically effective and free of side effects. Treatment usually results in an initial cure rate of 65% to 100% with a 9% to 47% relapse rate. Drug therapy has centered on the use of tricyclic antidepressants, particularly imipramine, for which the total remission is 10% to 50% during treatment with a long-term cure of 5% to 40%. Reports of side effects with imipramine, some of which were lethal, have led to a reduction in its use. In 1977 Dimson reported the effects of an antidiuretic agent, desmopressin. Several double-blind, placebo-controlled studies have shown the drug to have a rapid effect but often with immediate posttherapy relapse. Desmopressin appears to be safe with few side effects.

The efficacy and safety of desmopressin were compared with an enuresis alarm in a controlled, randomized study of 3 months' duration. Forty-six patients older than age 6 years completed the study. Twenty-four received desmopressin, 20 μg intranasally, and 22 were given the alarm. Patients who relapsed were given the same treatment for 3 more months. The number of dry nights was evaluated weekly. An immediate and significant ($P < .001$) improvement was seen in the desmopressin-treated group during the first 3 weeks. In the last 9 weeks, the alarm-treated group was drier, a significant difference ($P < .002$) occurring in week 11. After treatment, both groups were significantly drier than before, with more favorable results occurring in the enuresis alarm group.

Even though desmopressin produced better results initially with its rapid onset of action, and although it is safe and produces lasting posttreatment improvement in about 30% of the patients, the enuresis alarm remains the treatment of choice for children with nocturnal enuresis. If the alarm proves impracticable or fails, desmopressin therapy is a safe and practical alternative.

▶ Desmopressin can eliminate nocturnal enuresis in some children. However, it is a rather awkward therapy, given intranasally. It is considered experimental when used in children for enuresis and is also rather expensive. We offer parents of enuretic children three choices: (1) no therapy, (2) an alarm system, or (3) tofranil and/or anticholinergic treatment. The alarm system should be given a trial period of 2–3 weeks before being judged a failure. Many parents use drugs only when the child is away from home to avoid embarrassment. Children's Memorial Hospital in Chicago has a clinic that uses psychological and dietary therapy in addition to conventional methods and has a very high cure rate. Although we do not believe that most enuresis is a psychological problem, we do think that, if available, a behavioral approach may be useful in some children.—S.S. Howards, M.D.

45 Genital Anomalies

Imperforate Anus in Females: Frequency of Genital Tract Involvement, Incidence of Associated Anomalies, and Functional Outcome
Susan E. Fleming, Robert Hall, Mathias Gysler, and Gordon A. McLorie (The Hosp. for Sick Children, Toronto)
J. Pediatr. Surg. 21:146–150, February 1986   45–1

Considerable progress has been made in understanding the anatomical and embryologic basis of imperforate anus. Surgical techniques have been refined and the outcome for these children, as far as fecal continence is concerned, is generally good. Unfortunately, little is known about the genital tract in these children, nor is much known about the ultimate reproductive function of women with imperforate anus. A determination was made of the frequency of genital tract involvement in imperforate anus, the incidence of associated anomalies, and functional outcome for the bowel, urinary tract, and vagina.

Data on 162 female children with imperforate anus treated since 1959 were reviewed. Of these, 21% had a noncommunicating and 79% had a communicating anomaly of the rectum or anus. The associated anatomical abnormalities were found in the lower urinary tract (15%), upper urinary tract (25%), lower genital tract (27%), upper genital tract (35%), and additional organ systems (51%). Death occurred in 26 patients and in 19 it resulted from the associated abnormalities. In those patients who were aged 13 years or older, functional outcome was assessed. Bowel function was normal or near normal in 85%, as was urinary and renal function. However, in 44% of the patients evaluated, there was persistent vaginal abnormality or scarring; in 25% this was severe enough to necessitate further surgery.

With modern approaches to the management of imperforate anus, most children will survive with good bladder and bowel function. On reaching adolescence, the major medical and psychosexual concerns of these girls will probably relate to their capacity for normal sexual function, their fertility potential, and their ability to sustain an ongoing pregnancy. The patient's capacity to achieve these aims depends on a detailed evaluation of the genital tract at an early stage in management, careful evaluation of the lower genital tract postsurgically, and optimal timing of vaginoplasty if indicated.

▶ This article provides a comprehensive review of data in a large series of girls with imperforate anus. The authors document that the results of reconstruction of the lower genital tract are not good. This is an important observation. The above data suggest that the mechanical problems secondary to inadequate reconstruction are significant. It is time for pediatric urologists and surgeons to review the subject and develop better strategies for correcting the anomalies and also surgical failures before they become psychologically permanent.—S.S. Howards, M.D.

Bilateral Rhomboid Flaps for Reconstruction of the External Genitalia in Epispadias-Exstrophy
Stephen A. Kramer, and Ian T. Jackson (Mayo Clinic and Found.)
Plast. Reconstr. Surg. 77:621–631, April 1986   45–2

Excision of superficial scar tissue or dartos fascia or skin procedures alone do not provide adequate cosmetic and functional results in epispadias. Hinman first described lengthening of the penis, and Johnston described a means of elongation involving dissection through a V-Y incision and partial detachment of the penile crura from the ischiopubic rami; the mobilized crura are advanced and approximated in the midline (Fig 45–1). Attempted coverage of the dorsal penile shaft with ventral penile skin may lead to recurrent dorsal chordee. A new penile elongation method makes use of an inverted-V incision on the lower abdominal wall to expose the crura, and of laterally based rhomboid flaps for dorsal skin coverage. This approach clearly defines the penopubic angle and lowers the risk of injuring the verumontanum and ejaculatory ducts. Ten males 4–23 years of age with epispadias-exstrophy complex had penile elongation and genital reconstruction with bilateral rhomboid flaps.

TECHNIQUE.—Exposure is via an inverted-V incision on the lower abdominal wall and penile base (Fig 45–2). Bilateral rhomboid flaps are outlined from the

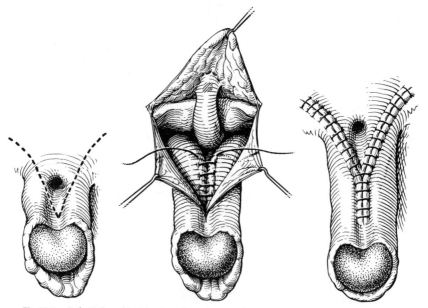

Fig 45–1.—**Left,** V-shaped incision is made on dorsum of penis. **Center,** mobilized crura are advanced and approximated in midline to lengthen penile shaft. **Right,** V-shaped incision is closed as Y. (Courtesy of Kramer, S.A., and Jackson, I.T.: Plast. Reconstr. Surg. 77:621–631, April 1986.)

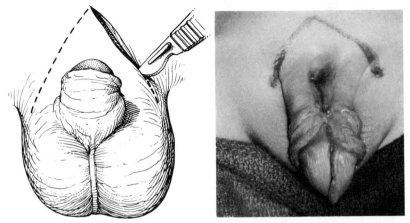

Fig 45–2.—Left and right, inverted V-incision incorporating all nonhair-bearing skin is made at base of penis. (Courtesy of Kramer, S.A., and Jackson, I.T.: Plast. Reconstr. Surg 77:621–631, April 1986.)

lateral pubic area.The corpora are widely mobilized and dissected proximally, partly detached from the ischiopubic bones, and then reapproximated in the midline dorsally or rotated ventrally. Residual dorsal chordee is eliminated by ventral dissection, with excision of transverse ellipses of tunica albuginea to produce a straight penis. Penile lengthening and urethroplasty may be done separately, or combined as a single-stage procedure using either full-thickness grafts or preputial flaps. The defect on the dorsal aspect of the penis is filled with two lateral rhomboid flaps elevated from the lateral pubic region.

This approach allows for considerable penile lengthening, and the bilateral rhomboid flaps provide ideal skin coverage. Satisfactory cosmetic rsults were obtained in all cases, and normal intercourse was made possible. All flaps have remained viable, and no patient has had recurrent penile contracture. This method also may be used in patients with a congenital or acquired short penis.

▶ There is a developing consensus that division of the urethral plate and partial mobilization of the crura with preservation of the nerve supply (Johnston, J.H.: J. Urol. 113:701, 1975) are important in reconstruction of the exstrophied or epispadiac penis. Modern principles of urethroplasty should also be employed. We favor vascularized preputial island flap grafts as advocated by Duckett and Mitchell (1985 YEAR BOOK, p. 315). Particularly in second operations, there may be a paucity of good dorsal skin to fill the defect created by mobilization. In these instances myocutaneous flaps are useful. The preceding article describes hairless rhomboidal flaps. Horton favors hairbearing inguinal groin flaps (Horton, C.E., et al.: *Clin. Plast. Surg.* 8:399, 1981).—S.S. Howards, M.D.

The following review article is recommended to the reader:

Barakat, A.V., Seikaly, M.G., Der Kaloustian, V.M.: Urogenital abnormalities in genetic disease. *J. Urol.* 136:778, 1986.
Josso, N.: Anti-Müllerian hormone. *Clin. Endocrinol.* 25:331, 1986.

46 Hypospadias

Hypospadias Repair Without a Bladder Drainage Catheter
Michael E. Mitchell and Thomas B. Kulb (Indiana Univ. at Indianapolis)
J. Urol. 135:321–323, February 1986   46–1

A catheter for bladder drainage is used in hypospadias repair to provide temporary urinary diversion, immobilize the suture line, and minimize reaction of tissue. However, the hospital stay is increased, patient mobility is limited, and there are risks of infection and problems with the mechanical catheter. A silicone pleated urethral stent, or splent, was used with short-term or no bladder drainage in 44 consecutive patients who had hypospadias repair and were followed for an average of 9.5 months.

After a strip is removed from the silicone splent, the split tube is passed through the neourethra (Fig 46–1). For a longer urethroplasty the neourethra is tubularized over the splent and secured to the glans with 2 mm of exposed tubing (Fig 46–2). Six types of single-stage hypospadias repair

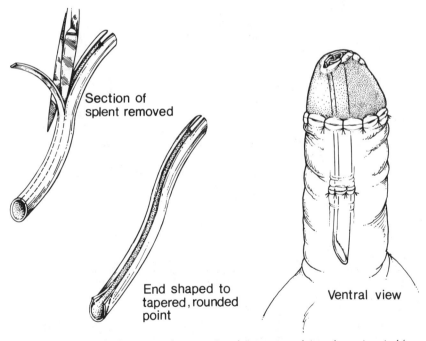

Section of
splent removed

End shaped to
tapered, rounded
point

Ventral view

Fig 46–1.—Longitudinal section equal to approximately one quarter of circumference is excised from section of silicone tubing. Length of tubing is situated so that proximal *(tapered)* end is about 1.5 cm proximal to beginning of neourethra. (Courtesy of Mitchell, M.E., and Kulb, T.B.: J. Urol. 135:321–323, February 1986. © by Williams & Wilkins, 1986.)

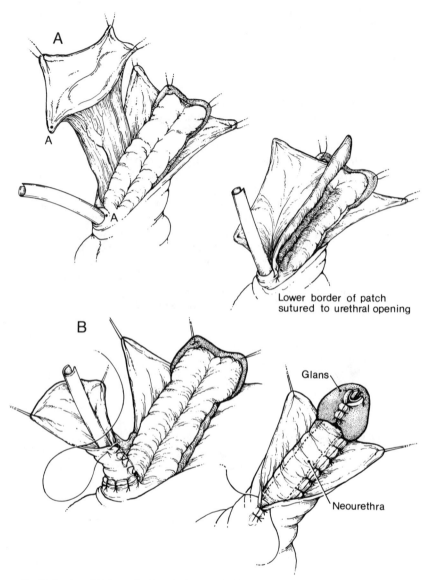

Fig 46–2.—A, and **B**, in application of splent to island preputial technique authors find it preferable to make proximal suture line first. Subsequently, patch is formed into tube over splent that is already in place. (Courtesy of Mitchell, M.E., and Kulb, T.B.: J. Urol. 135:321–323, February 1986. © by Williams & Wilkins, 1986.)

were carried out, usually the modified meatoplasty and glanuloplasty and the Duckett preputial graft procedures.

The first 15 patients had inpatient procedures with a suprapubic catheter placed to act as a "safety valve." All of the patients voided within 36 hours of surgery when the tube was removed. No infections occurred, but one patient had a fistula. The subsequent 29 patients had repair with the splent but without a bladder catheter. All 14 patients operated on in the hospital voided within 18 hours, and none required later catheterization. The 15 patients who had ambulatory surgery voided within 24 hours. One fistula developed, but there were no infections and no patient later had to be catheterized.

The splent was used more recently in 40 patients and was found to be applicable to vascularized grafts as well as to free graft urethroplasty and repair of fistulas. Hypospadias repair without drainage from a bladder catheter allows prompt ambulation and a brief hospital stay or even ambulatory surgery. The risks of infection and bladder spasm are reduced.

▶ We have found the stent designed by Mitchell and Kulb to be very useful. For boys in diapers we use a neurosurgical silicone stent as described by Duckett (Duckett, J.W.: Hypospadias, in *Adult and Pediatric Urology*. Chicago, Year Book Medical Publishers, 1987), which extends to the bladder neck and provides continuous drainage. For children out of diapers, however, we use the Mitchell stent. Both systems work well. Initially, the patients do have some discomfort when voiding with the Mitchell stent in place. The Mitchell stent can also be difficult to pass after the anastomosis is completed; therefore, the method of performing the proximal anastomosis first and then constructing the tube over the stent is advisable. The Duckett stent may cause bothersome bladder spasms.—S.S. Howards, M.D.

47 Testis and Scrotum

Elevation of Serum Gonadotropins Establishes the Diagnosis of Anorchism in Prepubertal Boys With Bilateral Cryptorchidism
Jonathan P. Jarow, Gary D. Berkovitz, Claude J. Migeon, John P. Gearhart, and Patrick C. Walsh (Johns Hopkins Univ.)
J. Urol. 136:277–281, July 1986   47–1

A nonoperative means to diagnose anorchism would be most useful. The reliability of determining the basal serum gonadotropin level alone in predicting anorchism was examined in more than 500 boys aged 1–15 years seen in 1972–1982 with bilateral cryptorchidism. Retractile testes were ruled out by repeated examination. Twenty-eight prepubertal boys failed to respond to a trial of human chorionic gonadotropin (hCG). All 21 boys with an adequate testosterone response to hCG and six of the other seven were explored.

Patients with normal testosterone responses to hCG had mean serum LH and FSH levels of 3.7 mIU/ml. In each case the testes were found at exploration and brought down to the scrotum. Six of the seven patients with no response to hCG had abnormally elevated serum gonadotropin levels. Six of these patients were explored, and no testes were discovered. One of two pubertal patients with impalpable testes was found to have testes at exploration despite a lack of testosterone response to elevated gonadotropins. Among three patients who were castrated postnatally, the two who were prepubertal had normal levels of serum gonadotropins, and the pubertal patient had markedly high levels.

The neonate with bilaterally impalpable testes should be karyotyped and undergo appropriate blood studies to rule out congenital virilizing adrenal hyperplasia. Retractile testes must be ruled out up to age 1 year. Serum gonadotropin levels should be estimated in all cases. Abnormal elevations in boys younger than 11 years indicate anorchism and thus preclude the need for exploration. However, normal gonadotropin levels do not exclude anorchism. All children with impalpable testes and normal basal gonadotropin levels should receive a trial of hCG or undergo exploration.

▶ The principles outlined in this paper are important and frequently misunderstood. It has been asserted that in boys with no palpable testes the absence of a response of serum testosterone activity to hCG stimulation rules out a testis. This is not correct. There are several case reports of testes present under these circumstances (Bartone, F.F. et al.: *J. Urol.* 132:563, 1984; 1985 YEAR BOOK OF UROLOGY, p. 333). However, there are no reports of prepubertal boys with no response to hCG and significantly elevated levels of gonadotropins who have testes. Thus if a boy is prepubertal, has no response to hCG, and has elevated levels of gonadotropins, exploration is not necessary. Jarow and associates point out that the opposite is not necessarily true, i.e., although most boys who do not respond to hCG but have normal gonadotropins do not have testes, some do.—S.S. Howards, M.D.

Boys With Late Descending Testes: The Source of Patients With "Retractile" Testes Undergoing Orchidopexy?

M.C. Pike and other members of the John Radcliffe Hosp. Cryptorchidism Study Group, Radcliffe Infirmary, Oxford, England
Br. Med. J. 293:789–790, Sept. 27, 1986   47–2

As part of a long-term study, all boys born at the John Radcliffe Hospital in Oxford were examined at birth. Those who were cryptorchid were reexamined 3 months later. A cryptorchid testis was defined as one in which the testicle center was less than 4 cm below the pubic tubercle (2.5 cm for infants weighing less than 2,500 gm) when measured at its lowest point after manipulation without applying tension. A nonscrotal cryptorchid testis was defined as one found outside the scrotum that can be manipulated inside it only with tension; a scrotal cryptorchid testis can be manipulated into the scrotum without tension.

At about 1 year of age, findings in 45 boys with late descending testes, i.e., descent by 3 months but not at birth, were compared with those in 20 infants whose testes were descended at birth. All of the latter still had descended testes. Of the former, 18 (40%) had a cryptorchid testis; the least descended testis was nonscrotal in 14 (78%) of the 18 boys. Of 29 (64%) boys with bilateral undescended testes at birth, a slightly decreased risk of being cryptorchid at 1 year was observed. A hydrocele was found either at birth or at 3 months in 7 (39%) of the 18 with late descending testes who had a cryptorchid testis at 1 year, compared with 5 (19%) of the 27 without a cryptorchid testis.

These patients with late descending testes probably account for the discrepancy between 0.8% of boys identified with true cryptorchidism in 1960 and 1.9% who underwent orchidopexy. Whereas resorption of an occult hernia was reported previously to lead to cryptorchidism, in the present study no hernias were observed, but a hydrocele was more common in the late descending testis group cryptorchid at 1 year. Any infant with undescended testes at birth should be reexamined at 3 months and then at 1 year. It is not known whether a late descending testis that becomes cryptorchid will again require treatment.

▶ This paper is interesting and provocative. It has been widely accepted from the data of Scorer and Farrington (*Congenital Deformities of the Testis and Epididymis,* London, Butterworths, 1971, pp. 15–27) that approximately 3.0% of term boys are born with undescended testes (UDT) and by 1 year of age two thirds of these testes have descended, so that the final incidence of UDT is 0.8%. However, later studies of the same population revealed a 1.9% orchidopexy rate (Chilvers, C., et al.: *Lancet* 2:330, 1984). This paper points out that in the original Scorer and Farrington study, boys whose testes descended between birth and 3 months of age were not reexamined at 1 year of age. To test the hypothesis that UDT redeveloped in some of these boys between 3 months and 12 months of age, the authors reexamined at 1 year boys whose testes had descended between birth and 3 months; they indeed found that 18 of 45 (40%) had cryptorchidism. This puts the true rate of UDT at approximately 2% at age 1 year and fits with the orchidopexy data.—S.S. Howards, M.D.

Effect of Age at Orchidopexy on Risk of Testicular Cancer
M.C. Pike, Clair Chilvers, and M.J. Peckham (Radcliffe Infirmary, Oxford, and Inst. of Cancer Res., Sutton, Surrey, England)
Lancet 1:1246–1248, May 31, 1986   47–3

The patient's age at time of surgery to correct undescended testis has steadily decreased in the past two decades. Many patients undergo orchidopexy before age 1 year in the belief that future risk of infertility and testicular cancer may be reduced if the problem is corrected early. A retrospective study sought to determine whether early orchidopexy does indeed reduce the risk of testicular cancer.

The 724 patients examined all had primary testicular cancer. Tumor histology, a history of undescended testis (UDT) and its treatment, and other testicular problems were noted. Of these patients, 69 had a history of cryptorchidism. The type of tumor, seminoma or teratoma, did not differ between those with and without UDT. Of the 69 patients with testicular cancer, 58 underwent either orchidopexy or orchidectomy. The age at surgery was almost identical to that expected for surgery of the whole population with UDT in whom testicular cancer did not necessarily develop.

The risk of testicular cancer developing does not appear to be dependent on the age at treatment of UDT. Other reasons for early orchidopexy (e.g., a decrease in risk of infertility) were not studied. As no decrease in the rate of testicular cancer with early orchidopexy was noted, physicians must carefully consider whether early surgery is warranted, because the risk of damage to the testis is increased in infancy.

▶ This is an important article. We have long been skeptical of the claims that early orchidopexy prevents cancer. Many of these assertions were made before significant numbers of boys who had earlier orchidopexy were old enough to be at risk for testis cancer. This paper does not resolve the issue, because there are very few patients who had orchidopexies at age 1–2 years in the series. However, the data suggest that early operation will not prevent cancer. This is not surprising, because the propensity to malignancy in these testes is probably genetic.—S.S. Howards, M.D.

Double-Blind, Placebo-Controlled Study of Luteinising-Hormone-Releasing Hormone Nasal Spray in Treatment of Undescended Testes

S.M.P.F. de Muinck Keizer-Schrama, F.W.J. Hazebroek, A.W. Matroos, S.L.S. Drop, J.C. Molenaar, and H.K.A. Visser (Erasmus Univ. and Univ. Hosp./Sophia Children's Hosp., Rotterdam, and Med. Dept., Hoechst Holland, Amsterdam)
Lancet 1:876–879, Apr. 19, 1986   47–4

The goals of treatment for undescended testes (UDT) are to improve potential fertility and improve the boy's psychosexual development. Early treatment for UDT is advocated because the chance of spontaneous descent is low after the first year of life, the number of spermatogonia in the undescended testis falls after the second year of life, and the prospect of fertility improves and the risk of malignant degeneration decreases with early treatment. Management options include hormonal or surgical treatment. Hormonal treatment formerly consisted of the administration of human chorionic gonadotropin (hCG). However, since 1976, luteinizing hormone-releasing hormone (LHRH) has been given in a nasal spray with success rates varying from 13% to 78%. This approach was used in 252 prepubertal boys with 301 undescended testes who were given LHRH, 1.2 mg/day intranasally.

After the 8-week double-blind trial, 10 placebo-treated (8%) and 14 LHRH-treated (9%) testes had descended completely. After a second LHRH course involving all of the patients in an open study, 48 testes (18%) had descended completely. The lowest success rate (7%) occurred in the youngest age group (1–2 years). Of the successfully treated testes, 75% could be manipulated at least to the scrotal entrance prior to treatment. When these findings were compared with those in age-matched controls, the cryptorchid boys' responses to LHRH and hCG before treatment did not suggest deficiencies in the hypothalamo-pituitary-gonadal axis or in Leydig cell function. Subsequent to treatment, there was no evidence of stimulation of the hypothalamo-pituitary-gonadal axis, and the serum testosterone level did not increase. Surgery, which was necessary in 170 patients (196 testes), revealed various anatomical anomalies.

Luteinizing hormone-releasing hormone nasal spray is useless for testes that are not palpable. These data do not support the presence of hormonal abnormalities in cryptorchid boys, but they may indicate damage of the germinal epithelium in some boys with bilateal cryptorchidism. Further, the hormonal data do not support the theory that the mode of action involves activation of the pituitary-gonadal axis. Hormonal evaluation is of no prognostic value for the success of hormonal therapy. Failure to respond to hormonal therapy was often accounted for by anatomical anomalies revealed at surgery.

Hormonal Therapy of Cryptorchidism: A Randomized, Double-blind Study Comparing Human Chorionic Gonadotropin and Gonadotropin-Releasing Hormone

Jacob Rajfer, David J. Handelsman, Ronald S. Swerdloff, Richard Hurwitz, Harold Kaplan, Thomas Vandergast, and Richard M. Ehrlich (Univ. of California at Los Angeles)
N. Engl. J. Med. 314:466–470, Feb. 20, 1986   47–5

Marked discrepancies exist in reports of the efficacy of hormonal treatment of cryptorchidism. Parenteral human chorionic gonadotropin (hCG) administration was compared with intranasal administration of gonadotropin-releasing hormone (GnRH) in 33 boys with unilateral or bilateral cryptorchidism. Five boys with retractile testes also were treated.

Only 1 of 17 boys treated with hCG had a testis descend into the scrotum during the study. Three of 16 boys treated intranasally with GnRH had descent of a testis. All five patients with retractile testes had descent after treatment with hCG. Pituitary-testicular axis stimulation was verified by increased circulating testosterone concentrations.

Hormonal therapy is generally ineffective for true cryptorchid patients, but it is highly effective in boys with retractile testes. The wide range of previously reported findings may be the result of the presence of a certain percentage of patients with retractile testes in samples of supposed cryptorchid patients. Use of these hormones may provide a diagnostic test to differentiate those with true cryptorchidism from those with retractile testes.

▶ These studies (Abstracts 47–4 and 47–5) document very poor results of hormonal therapy for undescended testes (UDT). We do not find these results surprising. The results of hCG therapy for unilateral UDT have always been modest. They are even worse in younger patients. With the current trend to treat patients earlier in life, hCG therapy becomes only marginally useful. Because luteinizing hormone-releasing hormone (LHRH) therapy presumably works by stimulting LH secretion, it would be expected that the results for LHRH and hCG would be similar. Of course, it is always possible that with a different LHRH analogue and different dosage schedules better results might be obtained. There are other studies that show better results. Hadžiselimović has data showing that LHRH treatment has beneficial effects on spermatogonia (*Horm. Res.* 13:358, 1980). If this effect proves to be permanent, LHRH therapy could be advisable to promote fertility even if it does not cause testicular descent.—S.S. Howards, M.D.

Undescended Testes: Is Surgery Necessary?
Arnold H. Colodny (Children's Hosp., Boston)
N. Engl. J. Med. 314:510–511, Feb. 20, 1986   47–6

An undescended testicle (UDT) is rare, occurring in about 2% to 3% of full-term male infants. At age 1 year, only 0.7% still have UDTs, and the chance of descent after this point is negligible. The reasons to intervene are numerous. For example, the UDT will not produce sperm needed to supplement the sperm from the contralateral testicle, which often has a deficiency of germ cells. The UDT has an increased incidence of cancer, which is easier to detect in scrotal testicles. Also, the UDT cannot substitute for the other testicle if the latter becomes diseased. The UDT is more subject to trauma if not residing in the free-swinging scrotum, and it is more likely to undergo torsion. The boy's self-image may also be harmed by not having both testicles in the scrotum.

Between ages 1 and 2 years, orchidopexy may decrease testicular degeneration and may also reduce the chance of cancer. However, the cancer rate in the contralateral testicle is higher than when both testicles are normal. The efficacy of gonadotropin-releasing hormone and human chorionic gonadotropin therapy to cause testicular descent is controversial and appears to depend highly on whether the study group included boys with retractile, rather than true, UDTs.

Two-stage therapy may become the treatment of choice. The child would first be given hormone therapy, which may partially or even fully cause the testicle to descend. If shown to transform gonadocytes to spermatocytes, this hormone therapy would be especially important. In those boys who do not have complete descent or experience a relapse after hormone therapy, orchidopexy should be done.

▶ Although one can make an argument for orchidectomy in patients with unilateral UDT, the consensus, for the reasons cited by Colodny and with which we concur, is that orchidopexy is the procedure of choice. We perform the operation at approximately 1 year of age even though the evidence that this is crucial is not convincing. As stated above, we do not believe that patients with unilateral UDTs should be treated routinely with hormones for the purpose of initiating descent. The issue of whether or not luteinizing hormone-releasing hormone (LHRH) therapy will improve future fertility remains open and, if the case is proven, routine LHRH therapy will be advisable. Thus we are in agreement with Colodny's position.—S.S. Howards, M.D.

The Fate of the Human Testes Following Unilateral Torsion of the Spermatic Cord

J.B. Anderson and G.C.N. Williamson (Royal Infirmary, Bristol, England)
Br. J. Urol. 58:698–704, December 1986   47–7

The long-term effects of torsion of the spermatic cord on the testis saved from infarction and its fellow are of considerable importance. It is possible that patients with torsion have preexisting abnormalities in spermatogenesis that can explain subsequent subfertility. Fifty-six patients seen from 1984 to 1986 with acute testicular torsion were studied prospectively. The median age was 17 years. Symptoms had been present for a median of 8 hours when the patient was first seen in the hospital. More than 25% had experienced similar episodes in the past. Orchiectomy was done in 13 patients, for an immediate testicular salvage rate of 77%.

Ten of 44 patients reviewed had previous orchiectomy. Of the others,

41% had more than 20% atrophy on the affected side, always after torsion of longer than 8 hours. Twenty of 35 patients having contralateral testicular biopsy exhibited partial maturation arrest in spermatogenesis, chiefly at the late spermatid stage. Fifteen of 32 patients studied after 3–6 months, including 4 of 6 having orchiectomy, had low sperm concentrations; moreover, 5 had reduced motility. Most patients with evidence of partial maturation arrest were oligozoospermic. A minority of oligozoospermic patients had elevated serum FSH levels. Sperm-agglutinating and sperm-immobilizing antibodies were infrequent. No specific antitestis antibodies were detected in the serum after torsion. These findings suggest that spermatogenesis is already impaired in the testes prone to torsion, and tend to reduce the relevance of autoimmunization in the occurrence of posttorsional oligospermia.

Testicular Histology in Children With Unilateral Testicular Torsion
F. Hadžiselimović, H. Snyder, J. Duckett, and S. Howards (Children's Hosp., Basel, Switzerland, and Children's Hosp. of Philadelphia)
J. Urol. 136:208–210, July 1986   47–8

A histopathologic review of testicular biopsy specimens from 30 adolescents and 8 prepuberal boys with unilateral testicular torsion was performed to examine the effect on the contralateral testis and to determine the preexisting histopathologic status of the testes. In 18 cases a specimen of the affected testis only was obtained, in 18 a specimen of both testes was obtained, and in 2 only the contralateral testis could be biopsied, as the affected testis was completely infarcted.

Significant preexisting testicular abnormalities were found in 53% of the patients. The Sertoli cell only syndrome was found in seven patients, the partial syndrome in four, defective spermatogenesis in eight and mucus plugs caused by cystic fibrosis inducing tubular changes in one. In 70% of the specimens from the prepuberal boys the number of spermatogonia was reduced. In adolescent boys the number of late spermatids was severely reduced in both testes. Atrophy of Leydig cells was common. The state of the blood-testis barrier did not affect the pathologic changes in the contralateral testis. These observations suggest that the infertility associated with unilateral testicular torsion may result from preexisting testicular abnormalities.

▶ The preceding two papers (Abstracts 47–7 and 47–8) both present similar evidence that patients who undergo torsion of the spermatic cord have a high incidence of preexisting abnormalities of spermatogenesis. Combined they are very convincing. This would explain the clinical observation (please see Abstract 47–9) that, as a group, patients who have had torsion have suboptimal semen quality without invoking an immunologic mechanism. This makes sense to us. We were not able to document contralateral effects of torsion of the testis in rats. We also believe that, although there is some evidence for a contralateral effect in animals with long-term torsion, the evidence for an immunologic mechanism is poor. Thus these findings in our view are consistent with the animal data.—S.S. Howards, M.D.

Seminal Fluid Changes After Testicular Torsion
O.A. Awojobi and E.O. Nkposong (Univ. of Ibadan, Nigeria)
Urology 27:109–111, February 1986   47–9

Changes in seminal fluid after unilateral testicular torsion were studied in adults undergoing orchiectomy for gangrenous testis and contralateral orchiopexy when seen within 12 hours of onset of symptoms and also in patients seen several days after onset of symptoms who merely had the contralateral testis fixed. Seminal fluid analysis was performed within 2 weeks of surgery and after 12–18 months.

Seven patients with a mean age of 21 years were evaluated, three after orchiectomy with contralateral orchiopexy and four after fixation of the contralateral testis. Sperm counts tended to increase in both groups, most markedly in the orchiectomy patients. Sperm concentrations remained relatively higher in this group; most patients had counts exceeding 20 million per ml 2 months postoperatively. Improvement in sperm quality was most apparent in patients having the infarcted testis excised. Changes in sperm motility paralleled those in sperm concentration. The only married patient had not had another child at follow-up, but his wife was using contraception.

Fertility is grossly impaired after unilateral testicular torsion. Sperm morphology and motility are more affected than sperm concentration. It appears best to excise the infarcted torsive testis. Autopsy studies of testes anatomically disposed to torsion in men of proved fertility and infertile men may show whether patients with testicular torsion have bilateral testicular abnormality resulting in reduced spermatogenesis.

▶ Krarup (*Br. J. Urol.* 50:43, 1978) and Bartsch et al. (*J. Urol.* 124:375, 1980) have presented data suggesting, but not proving, that patients who have had torsion of the testis have reduced fertility potential. The data in this report are difficult to interpret. Certainly, the two groups are too small to compare. Overall semen quality seems to improve with time after the acute insult. This is hardly surprising, because anesthesia alone can interfere with testis function. There is no normal control group, but one gets a hint that, over the long term, most of these patients have semen quality in the fertile range, although perhaps less good than a normal control group would demonstrate, particularly vis-a-vis morphology.—S.S. Howards, M.D.

The following review article is recommended to the reader:

Hutson, J.M., Donahoe, P.K.: The hormonal control of testicular descent. *Endocr. Rev.* 7:270, 1986.

48 Pediatric Oncology

The Current Management of Bilateral Wilms' Tumor
Robert Kay and Edward Tank (Cleveland Clinic Found. and Univ. of Oregon, Portland)
J. Urol. 135:983–985, May 1986   48–1

Chemotherapy has markedly improved the outlook for children with Wilms' tumor; progressively less extensive operative measures have been used, those most recently being limited to biopsy as the initial surgical approach. Eleven patients aged 6 months to 5 years were treated for bilateral Wilms' tumor in 1972–1984; four were younger than 1 year of age. Ten patients underwent surgery before chemotherapy, usually unilateral nephrectomy with contralateral tumor biopsy or bilateral biopsies of the renal masses. All patients received actinomycin D and vincristine therapy. Seven patients had further surgery 3–15 months after chemotherapy.

Eight patients (73%) were free of disease 18 months to 12 years postoperatively and three died of metastatic disease. Two patients who were seen initially with pulmonary metastasis are free of disease. Five patients with known residual tumor before chemotherapy have done well. All patients who died received radiotherapy as well as chemotherapy. No complications of radiotherapy were observed.

A conservative surgical approach to bilateral Wilms' tumor appears appropriate. Initial biopsy of both kidneys is followed by chemotherapy, with partial nephrectomy subsequently if necessary. Exploratory laparotomy at 3 months may be appropriate. Radiotherapy is given if unresectable disease is present. This approach is effective in a high proportion of patients.

▶ The treatment of unilateral Wilms' tumor is standardized and very successful. All patients should be entered into the National Wilms' Tumor protocol and treated in collaboration with a pediatric oncologist. Bilateral tumors require an individualized approach. Two others series of Wilms' tumors were discussed in the 1986 YEAR BOOK (pp. 349 and 350). Recommendations for children with synchronous bilateral tumors vary from biopsy and chemotherapy to unilateral nephrectomy and contralateral partial nephrectomy. We believe that one cannot generalize. It is important to determine whether the patient has nephroblastomatosis, in which case chemotherapy is appropriate, or only two tumors, in which case several options, including initial surgery, seem reasonable. Many of these children do very well. We have a long-term survivor treated with unilateral nephrectomy and chemotherapy without radiation. We prefer to avoid radiation whenever possible (please see Abstract 48–2).—S.S. Howards, M.D.

Outcome of Pregnancy in Survivors of Wilms' Tumor

Frederick P. Li, Kathreen Gimbrere, Richard D. Gelber, Stephen E. Sallan, Francoise Flamant, Daniel M. Green, Ruth M. Heyn, and Anna T. Meadows (Natl. Cancer Inst., Bethesda, and other medical institutions in the United States and France)

JAMA 257:216–219, Jan. 9, 1987   48–2

A pilot study indicated low birth weight in several infants whose mothers had received abdominal radiotherapy in childhood for Wilms' tumor. A larger study, undertaken at seven pediatric oncology centers, included 99 patients cured of childhood Wilms' tumor in 1931–1979 who subsequently carried or sired 191 singleton pregnancies of at least 20 weeks' gestation. The median age at diagnosis of Wilms' tumor was 4 years, and the median follow-up was 25 years. Nominal radiotherapy doses to the renal fossa or hemiabdomen were usually 2,000–3,500 rad. Twenty-six patients also received chest irradiation, and 44 patients were given dactinomycin.

An adverse outcome occurred in 30% of the pregnant women irradiated in childhood, compared with 3% in a comparison series of 77 nonirradiated women, a significant difference. Both fetal deaths and low-birth-weight infants were more frequent in the irradiated group. Increased perinatal mortality in the irradiated group resulted from both high fetal mortality and high neonatal mortality. Adverse outcomes usually preceded 37 weeks' gestation. Chest irradiation was not a significant independent factor in adverse pregnancy outcomes.

Adverse pregnancy outcomes among females irradiated for Wilms' tumor in childhood may reflect radiation-induced somatic damage to abdominopelvic structures. Nearly one in three pregnancies among irradiated females in the present series resulted in a low-weight infant or a late fetal death. These observations are relevant to the counseling and prenatal care of women given abdominal radiotherapy for Wilms' tumor. It is possible that the findings also apply to women given abdominal irradiation for childhood cancers other than Wilms' tumor.

▶ This study presents strong evidence that radiation therapy in girls results in fetal deaths and low birth rates in the patients' offspring. The study is uncontrolled but well done. It is unlikely, but possible, that the adverse pregnancy outcomes resulted from an independent variable, e.g., a genetic predisposition. These women are known to have a high incidence of shortened trunk, scoliosis, fibrosis of the abdominal muscles, and injury to visceral organs. The authors argue that the pregnancy outcomes can most likely be attributed to somatic injuries rather than to genetic damage, because males do not have a similar incidence of poor outcomes, nor do Japanese atomic bomb survivors, and animal studies do not produce the results seen in these women.—S.S. Howards, M.D.

Renal Parenchymal Carcinoma in Children

C.M. Booth (Dedham, Colchester, Essex, England)

Br. J. Surg. 73:313–317, April 1986   48–3

Data on renal parenchymal carcinoma in 14 patients younger than age 20 years, seen in British hospitals in 1957–1983, were reviewed. Hematuria, loin pain, and a mass were the most frequent presenting features, but no patient had all of these features. Urography showed a definite mass or major pelvicaliceal displacement in most instances. Eight patients underwent elective nephrectomy with removal of the perirenal fat and hilar lymph nodes, but no attempt was made to remove all para-aortic nodes. Two patients had nephroureterectomy and two had emergency nephrectomy. A child who had previous nephrectomy for Wilms' tumor underwent local enucleation of renal cell carcinoma. A patient with multiple metastases died preoperatively. Three patients were irradiated, but none received chemotherapy. None of six patients with stage I disease died of tumor, but four of eight patients with extrarenal spread died within 17 months of operation.

One hundred documented reports of renal parenchymal carcinoma in the pediatric age group were reviewed. Hematuria and loin pain each were present in about half of the patients, and nearly half of the children had a mass. Several children presented after minor trauma. Renal calcification was evident in 16% of the patients. All but five patients underwent nephrectomy, but only 16 had a true radical nephrectomy with excision of the para-aortic nodes. Adjunctive measures were most useful in those with stage II tumors. The corrected 5-year survival for 71 evaluable patients was 52%. The 10-year rate for 50 patients was 32%, but follow-up has been brief in many cases.

Renal parenchymal carcinoma should be considered in a child with a renal mass. The presentation may be precipitated by mild trauma. Nephrectomy is indicated in these cases. Radiotherapy and chemotherapy may have a role in patients with local extrarenal spread. Overall survival is about the same as in adults.

▶ This is a concise review of the world literature on renal cell carcinoma in children. One hundred of the 160 patients reported since 1934 were surveyed. The major points are that the disease is rare, occurring in less than 8% of children with renal tumors, and that its characteristics are not different from renal cell carcinoma in adults. The one exception is that, in younger patients, the sex distribution is equal, whereas in adults men predominate 2:1.—S.S. Howards, M.D.

Optimal Treatment of Clinical Stage I Yolk Sac Tumor of the Testis in Children
Francoise Flamant, Claire Nihoul-Fekete, Catherine Patte, and Jean Lemerle (Institut Gustave-Roussy, Villejuif, and Hôpital des Enfants Malades, Paris)
J. Pediatr. Surg. 21:108–111, February 1986 48–4

Malignant germ cell tumors of the testis comprise about 76% of childhood malignant testicular tumors. The remainder arise from interstitial tissues; rhabdomyosarcoma, occurring in paratesticular tumors, is not included. Clinicians disagree on the best treatment for yolk sac tumors, one category of malignant germ cell tumors, especially when the tumor is clinically localized.

Conservative treatment for early stage yolk sac tumor was attempted in 24 patients with clinical stage I tumor. All had undergone orchiectomy 10–25 days before referral. α-Fetoprotein was found in the serum or microscopic slides of 23 patients. None had detectable chorionic gonadotropin secretion or had undergone lymphadenectomy. Twelve received systemic chemotherapy every 3 months for 1 year or until relapse. Methotrexate, 7 mg/sq m; actinomycin D, 300 μg/sq m; and cyclophosphamide, 200 mg/sq m, were used. These patients also received physical examinations and had chest and abdominal x-ray studies, as well as α-fetoprotein level checks every 3 months for the first 2 years, every 6 months in the third year, then annually. The other 12 patients did not receive systemic chemotherapy but were examined similarly more often.

No significant difference was found between the groups in survival or relapse-free survival rate. The 3-year survival rate was 96%, with a plateau in 18 months; the 3-year relapse-free survival rate was 84%. Of the 12 receiving chemotherapy, 10 were "cured" (defined as remaining in first remission with a normal α-fetoprotein level 2 years after orchiectomy). One had recurrence in the para-aortic nodes in the seventh month and died after 15 months without node control, despite lymphadenectomy, radiation therapy, and chemotherapy every month. The second patient had pulmonary metastases within 12 months. The α-fetoprotein levels diminished too slowly in this patient after orchiectomy, only reaching a normal level 3.5 months after surgery and the first course of chemotherapy. This patient is alive and well 8 years after treatment with excision of metastases, radiation therapy, and chemotherapy every month. Of the 12 who did not receive chemotherapy, 10 are alive and well and 9 are considered cured. Two experienced relapse in the fourth and fifth months, respectively, with increased α-fetoprotein levels. After surgery and the chemotherapeutic regimen used to manage stage III tumors, both are considered cured.

Orchiectomy and noninvasive clinical evaluation are recommended for children with clinical stage I yolk sac tumors of the testis, omitting lymphangiography but using α-fetoprotein analyses. Scrupulous monthly follow-ups must show a steady decrease in the α-fetoprotein levels, with normal levels of less than 20 ng/ml reached within 3 months after orchiectomy. Increasing α-fetoprotein levels seen at two successive evaluations within 8 days is considered a sign of relapse. Immediate treatment is begun, using regimens for stage III or IV tumors, which offer a high possibility for cure. With this approach, which requires strict adherence to the follow-up program, 80% of patients with clinical stage I yolk sac tumor can be treated by orchiectomy alone.

▶ A paper with similar recommendations for the treatment of yolk sac or endodermal sinus tumors appeared in the 1986 YEAR BOOK (p. 354). Although the treatment of these tumors has been controversial, a consensus seems to be developing for careful observation of boys with stage I disease. Most of the literature reports less than 10% positive nodes in stage I patients. This, combined with the fact that Flamant and associates found that 23 of 24 patients had an elevated serum level of α-fetoprotein (making it a good marker), would support the argument for observation. However, it needs to be emphasized that observation for stage I testis tumors of all types is treacherous. The follow-up must be frequent and careful, because metastases can be asymptomatic and progress rapidly to a point where salvage is not good (please see Abstract 48–5).—S.S. Howards, M.D.

Testicular Tumours in Children
R.R. Livingstone and L.A. Sarembock (Univ. of Cape Town and Red Cross War Mem. Children's Hosp., Cape Town)
S. Afr. Med. J. 70:168–169, August 1986   48–5

Tumors of the testes, the seventh most common neoplasm, represent 1% of all malignant tumors in children. Although the numbers are small, 60% occur in children younger than age 3 years, and 80% are malignant. Thus all scrotal masses must be considered malignant until proved otherwise. Cancer of the testis usually presents as a slow-growing scrotal mass; the patient rarely has associated pain. Hydrocele may accompany the tumor. In the common fluid hernia of infancy, it is necessary to eliminate the possibility of a tumor by careful transillumination and ultrasonography.

All 23 children with testicular tumors seen between 1969 and 1984 were younger than age 12 years. There were ten germ cell tumors; six patients had non-Hodgkin's lymphoma and 7 had acute lymphoblastic leukemia. Of the ten germ cell tumors, nine were classified histologically as yolk sac tumors and one as a well-differentiated teratoma. All of the yolk sac tumors occurred in children younger than age 3 years. Eight of these had asymptomatic growing scrotal masses, and three of the eight had associated hydroceles. The remaining patient was initially thought to have chronic torsion of the testis. Eight of these nine patients underwent radical orchidectomy. Postorchidectomy treatment included prophylactic irradiation in four patients, chemotherapy in only one, prophylactic lymph node dissection in two, and no further treatment in two. Despite the varied management, eight of the nine patients with yolk sac tumor were well with no evidence of disease 6 months to 14 years after diagnosis. Of the six patients with non-Hodgkin's lymphoma, four had testicular tumors on initial presentation. There was only one short-term survivor in this group. None of the seven patients with acute lymphoblastic leukemia survived.

Yolk sac tumor differs from adult testicular cancer. It is less aggressive and usually affects very young children. Radical orchidectomy is adequate surgery for this tumor. Neither retroperitoneal node dissection, radiotherapy, nor prophylactic chemotherapy is recommended. Careful follow-up is necessary to detect metastatic disease or recurrence.

▶ There were only nine yolk sac tumors in this series, but the authors' results and recommendations are similar to those reported above. There is confusion regarding this malignancy because it is rare and is called by a number of names, including yolk sac tumor, endodermal sinus tumor, orchioblastoma, embryonal carcinoma of infancy, and Teilum's tumor, the latter after the man who first called it an endodermal sinus tumor (Teilum, C.: *Cancer* 12:1092, 1959). One small important point is made in this paper: Three of the patients with yolk sac tumors presented with hydroceles. We recently saw a 16-month-old boy with the recent onset of a hydrocele who had a testis tumor. It is important that boys with secondary hydroceles be evaluated immediately rather than merely observed.—S.S. Howards, M.D.

Nongerminomatous Malignant Germ Cell Tumors in Children: A Review of 89 Cases From the Pediatric Oncology Group, 1971–1984
Edith P. Hawkins, Milton J. Finegold, Hal K. Hawkins, Jeffrey P. Krischer, Kenneth A. Starling, and Arthur Weinberg (Baylor College of Medicine, Houston, Univ. of Florida, West Virginia Univ., and Southwestern Med. School)
Cancer 58:2579–2584, Dec. 15, 1986   48–6

Yolk sac tumors and embryonal carcinomas rarely occur in children; they affect the gonads and the sacrococcygeal region. The prognosis for gonadal tumors appears to be improved since the advent of chemotherapy. From 1971 to 1984, 89 patients with yolk sac tumors, embryonal carcinomas, and teratomas with foci of yolk sac or embryonal carcinoma were enrolled in the Rare Tumor Registry of the Southwest Oncology Group (1971–1979) and the Pediatric Oncology Group (1980–1984). A review was made of 9 clinical and 13 pathologic variables to determine the outcome of this cohort and to identify any prognostic correlates. Specific therapies could not be evaluated because there was too much variation.

There was an improved survival for each 5-year period regardless of tumor site. There was no statistically significant difference between "pure" tumors and those mixed with other teratomatous components. Further, no statistically significant difference was found between yolk sac tumors and embryonal carcinomas in children; a better than reported prognosis was noted for sacrococcygeal tumors occurring after the neonatal period. However, a particularly poor prognosis was found for neonatal "benign" sacrococcygeal teratomas resected without coccygectomy when they recurred as yolk sac tumors. Excellent survival was associated with all testicular tumors regardless of age or the presence of embryonal carcinoma, and the occurrence of mediastinal tumors in females was noted. The polyvesicular vitelline pattern of yolk sac tumor confers a better prognosis than other histologic forms of sacrococcygeal tumors.

Primary Site as a Prognostic Variable for Children With Pelvic Soft Tissue Sarcomas
Beverly Raney, Jr., Andrew Carey, Howard McC. Snyder, John W. Duckett, Louise Schnaufer, Henrietta K. Rosenberg, Soroosh Mahboubi, Jane Chatten, and Philip Littman (Children's Hosp. of Philadelphia and Univ. of Pennsylvania)
J. Urol 136:874–878, October 1986   48–7

The site of origin of soft tissue sarcomas in the pelvic region may have important implications with regard to disease control and survival. A review was made of the characteristics and clinical course of 16 consecutive children, aged 1–16 years, with pelvic soft tissue sarcomas. An incisional biopsy was obtained from each patient. Treatment consisted of the intravenous administration of vincristine, actinomycin D, and cyclophosphamide with or without doxorubicin, cis-platinum, and etoposide. Thirteen patients (81%) also received radiation therapy.

Eight children (median age, 3 years) had sarcomas arising in the bladder or the bladder-prostate region: seven had local tumor and one had lung metastasis. Presenting symptoms were urinary obstruction or gross hematuria. The median tumor diameter was 5 cm. All eight children had a complete response to treatment, which eventually included complete cystectomy and prostatectomy in three boys with persistent tumor. Six were alive and remained free of disease 1–9 years after initiation of therapy. The other eight children (median age, 7 years) had a pelvic mass at diagnosis that arose adjacent to but outside of the bladder or prostate; two had lung metastases at diagnosis. The median tumor diameter was 15 cm. Only five children had a complete response to treatment and only three survived and remained free of tumor for 1–8 years after therapy.

The primary site of sarcoma arising in the pelvic region has major implications for management and prognosis. Sarcoma arising in the bladder-prostate region are relatively small when discovered and present with early overt signs and symptoms demanding medical attention; they thus have better prognosis than tumors arising in the retroperitoneum-pelvis outside the bladder. Surgical removal of residual tumor and preservation of the bladder, when possible, should be attempted in all patients whose tumor does not respond completely to primary chemotherapy, with or without adjunctive radiation therapy.

▶ This is an encouraging report with much better results than reported by Ghavimi and associates (*J. Urol.* 132:313, 1984; 1985 YEAR BOOK, p. 339), who found that only 2 of 16 patients with bladder neck or prostate primaries survived with their bladder intact. We have used combination chemotherapy to treat these patients for the past 12 years with good results. The 100% complete response rate and 63% bladder retention rate reported above for patients with bladder and prostate involvement are most gratifying. Also encouraging is the report from Amsterdam that eight of nine patients treated with a very aggressive chemotherapeutic approach survived (Voûte, P.A., et al.: Natl. Cancer Inst. *Monogr.* 56:121, 1981). However, in spite of the success of chemotherapy, in some patients extirpative surgery is still required for nonresponders and partial responders and post complete response recurrences. The surgeon cannot be lulled into a false sense of security, but should be ready to intervene when indicated. The authors and the literature document that nonbladder-prostate pelvic sarcomas have a worse prognosis. In 101 such patients, a 42% 3-year relapse-free survival was reported (Crist, W.M., et al.: *Cancer* 56:2125, 1985).—S.S. Howards, M.D.

Pelvic Rhabdomyosarcoma: A Review of the RPMI Experience

Unyime O. Nseyo, Pinchas M. Livne, Richard M. Wolf, J. Edson Pontes, and Robert P. Huben (Roswell Park Mem. Inst., Buffalo)
Urology 28:456–461, December 1986   48–8

Management of rhabdomyosarcoma (RMS) has changed because of the use of multidisciplinary protocols that include surgery, radiotherapy, and multidrug chemotherapy. Although this approach has prolonged survival, it has resulted in significant functional and cosmetic morbidities in long-term survivors. To preserve function and minimize damage to regional organs, modifications were suggested in the extent of surgery and the dosage of radiation, and the sequence of administering these treatments was clarified. A review was made of experience with RMS at the Roswell Park Memorial Institute (RPMI).

Sixteen patients were treated for pelvic RMS at RPMI between 1959 and 1983; the nine males and seven females ranged in age from 1 year to 71 years (median, 12.5 years). The primary sites were the prostate in seven, vagina in six, bladder in two, and urovaginal in one. Five patients treated during the first decade of the study with limited surgery, various doses of radiation, and single-agent chemotherapy survived for 3–13 months (median, 10 months). During the second decade of the study, the multidisciplinary protocol of surgery, irradiation, and combined chemotherapy led to no evidence of disease in two patients, one prolonged survival, and one failure. One patient treated with bladder-sparing surgery and combination chemotherapy is alive with disease at 36 months. Limited surgery, irradiation, and combined chemotherapy were used in one patient who later underwent urinary undiversion; two others so treated survived for an average of 13.2 months. There were two other patients who had biopsy of their primary lesion prior to receiving radiation and multidrug chemotherapy, who survived for 20 months and 13 months, respectively. In one patient a transperineal needle biopsy specimen obtained from prostate and prostate ultrasound indicated complete local response 7 months after introduction of therapy; however, he died 6 months later of disseminated disease in the spine, brain, and long bones. The overall median survival in adults was 13 months; since 1972 this has been 24.5 months. Children had an overall median survival of 14 months, and 76 months since 1972.

Multidisciplinary protocols including surgery, irradiation, and combined chemotherapy resulted in prolonged survival despite the fact that 63% of the patients had advanced disease at diagnosis. Patients, including children, with symptoms of bladder outlet obstruction should be thoroughly investigated. Rectal examination should be routine along with the remainder of the physical examination in these patients.

Infants Younger Than 1 Year of Age With Rhabdomyosarcoma

Abdelsalam H. Ragab, Ruth Heyn, Melvin Tefft, Daniel N. Hays, William A. Newton, Jr., and Mohan Beltangady (Rhabdomyosarcoma Study Committee

of the Pediatric Oncology Group, The Children's Cancer Study Group, and the Pediatric Intergroup Statistical Ctr., Emory Univ. and other participating institutions)
Cancer 58:2606–2610, Dec. 15, 1986   48–9

Rhabdomyosarcoma, which occurs in almost all areas of the body, accounts for approximately 8% of all solid tumors found in children. The peak incidence is between ages 2 years and 6 years. A previously published study of death certificates of 1,170 children who died of rhabdomyosarcoma revealed two age peaks, the first at ages 1–4 years and the second at ages 15–19 years. Rhabdomyosarcoma may be present at birth, and the diagnosis has been made in infants younger than age 1 month; a comparison was made of the characteristics in infants younger than age 1 year and those in older children enrolled in the Intergroup Rhabdomyosarcoma Study.

Of the 1,561 patients registered in the Intergroup Rhabdomyosarcoma Study as of May 1983, 78 (5%) were younger than age 1 year. These infants did not differ from children aged 1–20 years with regard to male/female ratio, clinical grouping, or survival. However, the infants had a significantly greater frequency of undifferentiated sarcoma (18% vs. 7% in older children), as well as a markedly greater proportion of cancer with botryoid pathology (10% vs. 4% in older children). When reviewed by the newly proposed cytopathologic classification, there was no difference in pathologic type between the two age groups. The infants had a higher rate of bladder-prostate-vagina primary tumor involvement than found in older children (24% vs. 10%). Also, they tended to receive less of the prescribed doses of chemotherapy and radiation therapy than older children, and to experience more toxicity to treatment.

The overall survival curve for the two age groups appears to be similar. This is in contrast to that for Wilms' tumor and neuroblastoma, in which age (less than 1 year) is a favorable prognostic factor.

▶ This review makes two clinically relevant points: Rhabdomyosarcomas, although uncommon before the age of 1 year, do occur from birth to 12 months of age; further, the prognosis in these young patients is the same as that in older children, as distinguished from the prognosis for Wilms' tumor and neuroblastomas.—S.S. Howards, M.D.

Prognostic Value of Different Staging Systems in Neuroblastomas and Completeness of Tumour Excision
N.L.T. Carlsen, I.J. Christensen, H. Schroeder, P.V. Bro, U. Hesselbjerg, K.B. Jensen, and O.H. Nielsen (State Univ. Hosp., Rigshospitalet, and Finsen Lab., Copenhagen, Univ. Hosp., Aarhus and Odense, and Aalborg Hosp., Denmark)
Arch. Dis. Child. 61:832–842, September 1986   48–10

In all, 253 children with neuroblastoma seen in Denmark in 1943–1980 were retrospectively restaged according to eight different systems to assess individually the prognostic value of each staging system. The tumor in all but 18 was proved histologically. Patients lacking evidence of disease 2 years after diagnosis were considered cured.

The system proposed by Evans et al. was the most predictive and superior to the tumor-node-metastases (TNM) staging system. Age had independent prognostic significance regardless of the staging system used. The findings confirmed the existence of Evans stage IV-S, according a favorable prognosis to infants having metastatic disease in the liver and skin. All staging systems examined had some prognostic significance for survival.

The staging system for neuroblastoma proposed by Evans et al. was the best system in this analysis, apparently because factors other than resectability are important in survival. Tumor size in the Evans system is related to patient size, whereas this is not true in the TNM clinical stage grouping system. Prospective observations are needed to determine definitively the best staging system for neuroblastoma.

▶ This paper presents strong evidence that the staging system devised by Evans (*Cancer* 27:374, 1971) is the best method to predict prognosis in children with neuroblastoma. Age is an important independent variable, as it is with Wilms' tumors but not with rhabdomyosarcomas (please see Abstract 48–9). The study is of both academic and practical interest. It is interesting that the TNM system widely touted by oncologists was inferior to the Evans method. This seems to be because the relative size of the tumor (whether it crosses the midline) and factors other than resectability (stage IV-S) are important in this tumor. It is hard to understand why the authors did not omit the 18 patients without proven histology when elimination of these would have left 235 patients and a scientifically better investigation.—S.S. Howards, M.D.

Efficacy of Magnetic Resonance Imaging in 139 Children With Tumors
Mervyn D. Cohen, Robert M. Weetman, Arthur J. Provisor, Jay L. Gorsfeld, Karen W. West, David A. Cory, John A. Smith, and Warren McGuire (Indiana Univ. at Indianapolis and James Whitcomb Riley Hosp. for Children, Indianapolis)
Arch. Surg. 121:522–529, May 1986   48–11

Magnetic resonance imaging (MRI) was performed in 139 children with neoplasms and the findings were compared with those of CT. Sedation was most often required for children aged 6 months to 3 years. A wide range of pulse sequences was used, but all studies included at least two spin-echo pulse sequences. An inversion-recovery sequence also was obtained in the early part of the series. The most frequent malignant neoplasms were neuroblastoma, non-Hodgkin's lymphoma, Wilms' tumor, and Hodgkin's disease. Twenty patients had benign tumors.

All tumors were detected by MRI. Thoracic neuroblastomas appeared as posterior mediastinal masses. The origin of adrenal neuroblastomas from the adrenal could be inferred only from their suprarenal site. In most children with Hodgkin's disease and non-Hodgkin's lymphoma, the origin of tumor masses from nodes could be inferred. Ewing's tumor and osteogenic sarcoma sometimes could be identified through their location. Wilms' tumor was accurately distinguished from neuroblastoma by the varying internal appearances of hemorrhage and necrosis. Calcification usually was not detected by MRI. Extension of neuroblastoma across the midline, and marrow metastases on occasion, were apparent. Lung metastases of Wilms' tumor were identified in a few cases. Local spread of malignant bone tumors was well visualized on MRI. Resectability of both soft tissue and bone tumors could be appreciated. Follow-up studies were useful in many patients having only radiotherapy and/or chemotherapy.

Imaging with MR is a useful means of evaluating neoplasms in pediatric patients. No ionizing radiation is involved. Imaging is performed in multiple planes, high soft-tissue contrast is obtained, and there is excellent visualization of bone marrow and blood vessels. The study can be repeated at frequent intervals.

▶ In this series, MRI was often superior to CT scanning for determining the extent of disease in neuroblastoma (T2-weighted images) and thoracic lymphoma because the blood vessel could be better seen, but it was inferior to CT in detecting non-Hodgkin's lymphoma, cortical bone tumors, and tumor calcifications, according to the authors. We have been attempting to stage bladder and prostate tumors with MRI and have been disappointed. Although MRI gives some information that is not available from CT, for practical purposes it is not very useful except in the CNS. It is difficult at this time to justify the cost of these procedures except for very special situations.—S.S. Howards, M.D.

The following review articles are recommended to the reader:

Beckwith, J.B.: Wilms tumor and other renal tumors of childhood: Update. *J. Urol.* 136:320, 1986.

Senga, Y., Taguchi, H., Asao, T., et al.: Undifferentiated renal cell carcinoma in infancy: Report of a case and review of literature. *Pediatr. Pathol.* 5:157, 1986.

49 Pediatric Transplant

The Outcome of 304 Primary Renal Transplants in Children (1968–1985)
John S. Najarian, Samuel K.S. So, Richard L. Simmons, David S. Fryd,
Thomas E. Nevins, Nancy L. Ascher, David E.R. Sutherland, William D.
Payne, Blanche M. Chavers, and S. Michael Mauer (Univ. of Minnesota)
Ann. Surg. 204:246–258, September 1986   49–1

Data concerning 304 children who received primary renal transplants
between 1968 and 1985 were examined with regard to long-term outcome
and causes of primary graft failures and deaths. Of these children, 48
(16%) were younger than 24 months, 60 (20%) were aged 2–5 years, and
196 (64%) were aged 6–17 years. Sixteen received kidneys from human
leukocyte antigen (HLA)-identical siblings, 210 received kidneys from
HLA mismatched relatives, and 78 received kidneys from cadaver donors.
The primary cause of renal failure in the children aged 6–17 years was
glomerulonephritis; in children younger than 2 years of age the primary
cause was congenital hypoplasia-dysplasia; and for the group aged 2–5
years it was congenital nephrotic syndrome.

Currently, 254 patients are alive 2 months to 18 years after renal transplant; 77% have working grafts (188 first and 45 retransplants) and 7%
are undergoing dialysis. There were 116 (38.2%) primary renal allograft
failures, because of rejection in 73 (24%), recurrent disease in 16 (5.3%),
death caused by sepsis in 7 (2.3%), nonseptic deaths in 10 (3.3%), technical
failure in 8 (2.6%), and primary nonfunction in 2 (0.7%). Primary graft
function rates at 5, 10, and 15 years were 100%, 100%, and 90% in
HLA-identical sibling kidneys; 84%, 64%, and 52% in mismatched related
kidneys; and 72%, 54%, and 47% in cadaver kidneys. Patient survival
rates at 1, 5, and 10 years for mismatched related and cadaver kidneys
were not significantly different. Primary graft function at 1 and 5 years
for 0–1 HLA-AB antigen matched cadaver kidneys was similar to that of
2–4 HLA-AB antigen cadaver kidneys, with patient survival rates also
basically identical in these groups. The success rate in young children was
confirmed by the 1-year survival and primary graft function rates in 44
mismatched related recipients younger than 2 years of 92% and 88%. A
decreased rejection rate was associated with the use of pretransplant random blood transfusions. In children who were given standard immunosuppression for mismatched related kidneys, primary graft function improved from 78% at 1 year in the pretransfusion era to 92% in the
transfusion era. Recurrence of the original disease in the transplanted
kidney was the leading cause of graft failure in this group in the transfusion
era. The overall cadaver graft outcome in children given standard immunosuppression did not improve in the transfusion era.

Renal transplantation can be performed safely in children. No significant difference exists in overall patient and graft survival, compared with the primary graft outcome in nondiabetic adults.

▶ The authors report a very large series of pediatric transplants with excellent results. This certainly reflects their excellent surgical and medical management. It is especially impressive that the pediatric patients do as well as nondiabetic adults, because the former more frequently have recurrence of the original disease. Of interest to the nontransplanting urologist is that the second, third, and sixth leading causes of renal failure in this series were, respectively, congenital hypoplasia/dysplasia, obstructive uropathy, and pyelonephritis-reflux. The treatment protocol has changed over the years. Pretransplant random blood transfusion was introduced in 1979. Antilymphoid globulin was given from the beginning. Splenectomy was abandoned in 1984. More recently, cyclosporine and donor-specific transfusions have been given to some patients. A standard Politano-Leadbetter reimplant is reported, although recently, I believe, an extravesical approach has been adopted.—S.S. Howards, M.D.

Experience With Renal Transplantation in Children Undergoing Peritoneal Dialysis (CAPD/CCPD)

Heinz E. Leichter, Isidro B. Salusky, Robert B. Ettenger, Stanley C. Jordan, Teresa L. Hall, Jennifer Marik, and Richard N. Fine (UCLA Ctr. for the Health Sciences, Los Angeles)
Am. J. Kidney Dis. 8:181–185, September 1986   49–2

Renal transplantation remains the optimal therapeutic modality for children with end-stage renal disease, because it offers the potential of maximum rehabilitation. The clinical course and complications of 44 patients aged 3–21.5 years (mean, 12.0 years), previously maintained on continuous ambulatory peritoneal dialysis (CAPD) and/or continuous cycling peritoneal dialysis (CCPD) were reviewed retrospectively to determine the infectious risk of renal transplantation. These patients received 32 cadaver and 16 living-related donor renal grafts after being maintained on peritoneal dialysis for 756 patient-months (mean, 17.1 months). Dialysis catheters were left in situ at the time of transplantation and were removed electively when stable graft function was evident.

Twenty-five patients (57%) required posttransplant dialysis because of acute tubular necrosis or acute rejection. In five patients (11%), including two undergoing dialysis, peritonitis developed. Exit site and tunnel infections occurred in nine patients (20%). Antibiotic treatment and/or catheter removal were curative in all instances. Posttransplant ascites developed in 12 patients (27%) and responded to catheter drainage. The overall 1-year and 2-year actuarial graft survival rates were 65% and 55%, respectively. No graft was lost because of infectious complications, and only one death occurred, which was unrelated to peritoneal dialysis.

Pediatric patients maintained on CAPD and/or CCPD can safely receive transplants. The potential infectious risks related to peritoneal dialysis can be managed with appropriate management of the catheter and prompt antibiotic therapy. Patient and graft survival rates are comparable to those in patients receiving hemodialysis prior to transplantation.

▶ This is a smaller series with a higher percentage of cadaver transplants than the one reported from Minnesota. The authors document that children on continuous peritoneal dialysis can safely be given transplants with good results, although in 38% either peritonitis or ascites developed. The incidence of peritonitis is lower and the cadaver graft 1-year survival of 63% is higher than that previously reported. It is impressive that no graft was lost to infection.—S.S. Howards, M.D.

Subject Index

A

Abdomen
  wall reconstruction in prune belly
    syndrome, 269
Adenosine-deaminase-binding protein
  tubular injury in kidney transplant and,
    125
Adrenal
  cortex tumors, comparison of, 73
  diseases, functional, difficulties with CT,
    69
  mass, incidentally discovered, 72
  pseudocysts, vascular origin of, 74
Age
  at orchidopexy and testicular cancer
    risk, 299
Aged
  bacteriuria and mortality in, 32
  bacteriuria with no association with
    symptoms, 33
  males, uroflowmetry in, 145
Allopurinol
  to prevent calcium oxalate calculi,
    53
Alpha-mercaptopropionylglycine
  in nephrolithiasis, cystine, 55
Aluminum
  kidney disease and, 79
Amino
  -terminal sequence of fibroblast growth
    factor, 179
Anderson-Carr progression
  ultrasound demonstration of, 47
Anesthesia
  local
    in ESWL, 110
    for transurethral resection of prostate,
      184
Angiotensin
  II with chemotherapy in bladder cancer,
    168
Anogenital region
  cancer, after kidney transplant, 134
Anomalies
  arteriovenous, congenital renal, 260
  associated with imperforate anus in
    females, 289
  in prune belly syndrome, broader
    spectrum of, 270
Anorchism
  gonadotropin elevation in diagnosis of,
    297
Antibiotics
  in pelvic inflammatory disease, 221

Antibody(ies)
  monoclonal, in diagnosis of hematuria
    and hereditary nephritis, in
    children, 261
Antigen(s)
  tubular, in tubular injury in kidney
    transplant, 125
Arterialization
  of deep penile vein, for arterial and
    venous impotence, 243
Arteriovenous malformation
  kidney, congenital, 260
Aspiration
  fine needle, of abnormal prostate, 193
Atherogenesis
  diet and vasectomy (in monkey), 215
Atrial
  natriuretic factor, renal and systemic
    effects, 75
Autotransfusion
  intraoperative, in urologic oncology, 43

B

Bacillus Calmette-Guerin
  in bladder carcinoma
    monitoring by serial flow cytometry,
      163
    skin test and granuloma formation in,
      161
    transitional cell, two courses of, 162
  effect on bladder carcinoma, 160
  immunotherapy in bladder cancer,
    complications of, 165
Bacteria
  adherence to bladder uroepithelial cells
    in urinary tract infection, 25
  pathogens and urinary tract infection, 26
Bacteriuria
  mortality and, in aged, 32
  no association with symptoms, in aged,
    33
  screening, evaluation of rapid methods
    to detect, 27
Balloons
  for erectile dysfunction due to venous
    leakage, 242
Biopsy
  cytology in penile cancer, 249
  prostatic needle, ultrasound vs. digitally
    directed, 194
  after radiotherapy in prostate cancer,
    195
  transrectal aspiration, in prostate
    cancer, 193

Author Index